Comparative Veterinary Pharmacology, Toxicology and Therapy

Comparative Veterinary Pharmacology, Toxicology and Therapy

Proceedings of the 3rd Congress of the European Association for Veterinary Pharmacology and Toxicology, August 25-29 1985, Ghent, Belgium
Part II, Invited Lectures

Edited by
A.S.J.P.A.M. Van Miert
M.G. Bogaert and M. Debackere

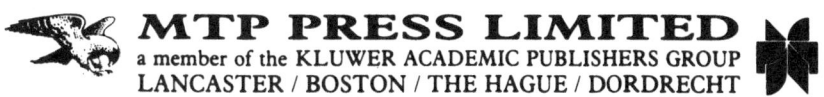
MTP PRESS LIMITED
a member of the KLUWER ACADEMIC PUBLISHERS GROUP
LANCASTER / BOSTON / THE HAGUE / DORDRECHT

Published in the UK and Europe by
MTP Press Limited
Falcon House
Lancaster, England

British Library Cataloguing in Publication Data
European Association for Veterinary Pharmacology and
   Toxicology. *Congress (3rd : 1985 : Ghent)*
   Comparative veterinary pharmacology, toxicology and
   therapy: proceedings of the Third EAVPT Congress,
   Ghent, Belgium, August 25-29, 1985.
   Part 2: Invited lectures
   1. Veterinary pharmacology—Europe 2. Veterinary
   toxicology—Europe
   I. Title   II. Miert, A.S.J.P.A.M. van
   III. Bogaert, M.G.   IV. Debackere. M.
   636.089'5'094   SF915

ISBN-13: 978-94-010-8343-0   e-ISBN-13: 978-94-009-4153-3
DOI: 10.1007/978-94-009-4153-3

Published in the USA by
MTP Press
A division of Kluwer Academic Publishers
101 Philip Drive
Norwell, M.A. 02061, USA

Library of Congress Cataloging-in-Publication Data
European Association Veterinary Pharmacology and
   Toxicology. Congress (3rd: 1985: Ghent, Belgium)
   Comparative veterinary pharmacology, toxicology, and
   therapy.

Includes bibliographies.
   Contents: —pt. 2. Invited lectures.
   1.Veterinary pharmacology—Congresses. 2. Veterinary
   toxicology—Congresses. 3. Animals—Diseases—
   Chemotherapy—Congresses. I. Van Miert,
   A. S. J. P. A. M.   II. Bogaert, M. G., 1937-
   III. Debackere, M., 1930-   IV. Title.
   SF915.E87   1985   636.089'51   86-19134

   ISBN-13: 978-94-010-8343-0

Contents

DRUG RESIDUE TOXICOLOGY

INFLAMMATION AND ANTI-INFLAMMATORY DRUGS
IMMUNOMODULATION

DRUG BIOTRANSFORMATION

OPIATES, OPIOIDS AND NEUROPEPTIDES

DRUG USE AND REGULATION

Preface

The third congress of the European Association for Veterinary Pharmacology and Toxicology (EAVPT) was held in Ghent, Belgium, from 25 to 29 August 1985. Part I of the Proceedings of this congress contains the abstracts of all invited lectures, oral communications and poster communications, presented at the congress. The invited lectures are now published (this volume) in extenso as Part II of the Proceedings.

The editors wish to thank all invited speakers for their active contribution to the success of the third congress of EAVPT. They are very grateful to Dr. P. De Backer for compiling all manuscripts, Dr. P. Lees for scientific amendments, Miss B. Vermeesch and Dr. R. Lefebvre for preparing the camera ready copy and MTP Press for literary advice and publishing.

A. S. J. P. A. M. van Miert
M. G. Bogaert
M. Debackere

Contributors

AMEND J.F.
Department of Anatomy and Physiology, Atlantic Veterinary
College, University of Prince Edward Island, Charlotte-
town, P.E.I. C1A 4P3, Canada.

ANIKA S.M.
Department of Veterinary Physiology and Pharmacology,
University of Nigeria, Nsukka, Nigeria.

ARGENZIO R.A.
Department of Anatomy, Physiological Sciences, and Radio-
logy, School of Veterinary Medicine, North Carolina State
University, Raleigh, NC 27606, USA.

ARONSON A.L.
Clinical Pharmacology Unit, School of Veterinary Medicine,
North Carolina State University, Raleigh, North Carolina
27606, USA.

AUCOIN D.P.
The Animal Medical Center, 510 E 62nd Street, New York,
New York 10021, USA.

BAARS A.J.
Central Veterinary Institute, P.O. Box 65, 8200 AB Lely-
stad, The Netherlands.

BAGGOT J.D.
Department of Veterinary Pharmacology and Toxicology, University of California, Davis, California 95616, USA.

BAI S.A.
Clinical Pharmacology Unit, School of Veterinary Medicine,
North Carolina State University, Raleigh, North Carolina
27606, USA.

BARDON T.
Department of Physiology, Ecole Nationale Vétérinaire, 23,
chemin des Capelles, 31076 Toulouse Cedex, France.

BELPAIRE F.
J.F. and C. Heymans Institute of Pharmacology, University
of Ghent, Medical School, De Pintelaan 185, B-9000 Gent,
Belgium.

BENARD P.
Ecole Nationale Vétérinaire, Laboratoire de radioéléments
et d'études métaboliques (I.N.R.A.), 23, chemin des Capelles, F-31076 Toulouse Cedex, France.

BINGEFORS K.
Department of Social Pharmacy, Uppsala University Biomedical Center, PO Box 586, S-751 23 Uppsala, Sweden.

BOGAERT M.G.
J.F. and C. Heymans Institute of Pharmacology, University
of Ghent, Medical School, De Pintelaan 185, B-9000 Ghent,
Belgium.

BREIMER D.D.
Center for Bio-Pharmaceutical Sciences, Division of Phar-
macology, University of Leiden, P.O. Box 9503, 2300 RA
Leiden, The Netherlands.

BREUKINK H.J.
Large Animal Clinic of Internal Diseases, Faculty of
Veterinary Medicine, University of Utrecht, The Nether-
lands.

BUENO L.
Station de Pharmacologie-Toxicologie, INRA, 180, chemin de
Tournefeuille, 31300 Toulouse, France.

BURGAT-SACAZE V.
Ecole Nationale Vétérinaire, Laboratoire de radioéléments
et d'études métaboliques (I.N.R.A.), 23, chemin des Capelles, F-31076 Toulouse Cedex, France.

CALDWELL J.
Department of Pharmacology, St. Mary's Hospital Medical
School, London W2 1PG, England.

CHERBUT C.
Department of Physiology, Ecole Nationale Vétérinaire, 23,
chemin des Capelles, 31076 Toulouse Cedex, France.

CONLON P.D.
Department of Biomedical Sciences, Ontario Veterinary
College, University of Guelph, Guelph, Ontario N1G 2W1,
Canada.

CRAIGMILL A.L.
Veterinary Extension, University of California, Davis, CA
95616, USA.

DE BACKER P.
Department of Veterinary Pharmacology and Toxicology,
Faculty of Veterinary Medicine, University of Ghent,
Casinoplein 24, B-9000 Ghent, Belgium.

DEBACKERE M.
Department of Veterinary Pharmacology and Toxicology,
Faculty of Veterinary Medicine, University of Ghent,
Casinoplein 24, B-9000 Ghent, Belgium.

DE GRAAF G.J.
Central Veterinary Institute, P.O. Box 65, 8200 AB Lely-
stad, The Netherlands.

DEGRYSE A.-D.
Department of Veterinary Research, Janssen Pharmaceutica,
B-2340 Beerse, Belgium.

DE JONG W.H.
National Institute of Public Health and Environmental
Hygiene (RIVM), Laboratory for Pathology, P.O. Box 1, 3720
BA Bilthoven, The Netherlands.

DE JONGE H.R.
Department of Biochemistry I, Medical Faculty, Erasmus
University, P.O. Box 1738, 3000 DR Rotterdam, The Nether-
lands.

DE MOOR A.
Large Animal Surgical Clinic, Faculty of Veterinary Medi-
cine, University of Ghent, Casinoplein 24, B-9000 Ghent,
Belgium.

DE RICK A.
Department of Small Animal Medicine, Faculty of Veterinary
Medicine, University of Ghent, Casinoplein 24, B-9000
Ghent, Belgium.

DE ROIJ T.A.J.M.
Animal Health Division, Duphar B.V., C.J. van Houtenlaan 36, 1381 CP Weesp, The Netherlands.

DROUMEV D.
Department of Pharmacology, Faculty of Veterinary Medicine, Higher Institute of Zootechnics and Veterinary Medicine, D. Blagoev str. 62, 6000 Stara Zagora, Bulgaria.

DURANTON A.
Station de Pharmacologie-Toxicologie, INRA, 180, chemin de Tournefeuille, 31300 Toulouse, France.

ELEZOGLOU V.
Department of Pharmacology, Veterinary Faculty, Aristotelian University of Thessaloniki, 54006 Thessaloniki, Greece.

ENGELS F.
Institute of Veterinary Pharmacology, Pharmacy and Toxicology, Faculty of Veterinary Sciences, University of Utrecht, P.O. Box 80.176, 3508 TD Utrecht, The Netherlands.

EYRE P.
Department of Biomedical Sciences, Ontario Veterinary College, University of Guelph, Guelph, Ontario N1G 2W1, Canada.

FARGEAS M.J.
Station de Pharmacologie-Toxicologie, INRA, 180, chemin de Tournefeuille, 31300 Toulouse, France.

FERRE J.P.
Department of Physiology, Ecole Nationale Vétérinaire, 23, chemin des Capelles, 31076 Toulouse Cedex, France.

FINK J.
Institute for Pharmacology, Toxicology and Pharmacy, Tier-
ärztliche Hochschule Hannover, FRG.

FIORAMONTI J.
Station de Pharmacologie-Toxicologie, INRA, 180, chemin de
Tournefeuille, 31300 Toulouse, France.

FOLKERTS G.
Institute of Veterinary Pharmacology, Pharmacy and Toxicology, Faculty of Veterinary Sciences, University of
Utrecht, P.O. Box 80.176, 3508 TD Utrecht, The Netherlands.

FREELAND L.R.
Department of Anatomy and Physiology, Atlantic Veterinary
College, University of Prince Edward Island, Charlotte-
town, P.E.I. C1A 4P3, Canada.

FUCHS V.
Department of Veterinary Pharmacology, Pharmacy and
Toxicology, Karl-Marx-University of Leipzig, Zwickauer
Strasse 55, 7010 Leipzig, GDR.

GASTHUYS F.
Large Animal Surgical Clinic, Faculty of Veterinary Medi-
cine, University of Ghent, Casinoplein 24, B-9000 Ghent,
Belgium.

GINGERICH D.A.
Veterinary Research Department, Bristol-Myers Company,
Syracuse, New York, USA.

GOLBS S.
Department of Veterinary Pharmacology, Pharmacy and
Toxicology, Karl-Marx-University of Leipzig, Zwickauer
Strasse 55, 7010 Leipzig, GDR.

GORDON L.L.
Veterinary Research Department, Bristol-Myers Company, Syracuse, New York, USA.

GRONDEL J.L.
Section Cell Biology, Department of Experimental Animal Morphology and Cell Biology, Agricultural University, P.O. Box 338, 6700 AH Wageningen, The Netherlands.

HALL L.W.
Department of Clinical Veterinary Medicine, University of Cambridge, Madingley Road, Cambridge CB3 OES, England.

HARTMAN E.G.
Department of Veterinary Bacteriology, Utrecht University, P.O. Box 80 171, 3508 TD Utrecht, The Netherlands.

HEKSTER Y.A.
Department of Clinical Pharmacy, Sint Radboud Hospital, University of Nijmegen, Nijmegen, The Netherlands.

HEYKANTS J.
Department of Drug Metabolism and Pharmacokinetics, Janssen Pharmaceutica, B-2340 Beerse, Belgium.

HONDE C.
Station de Pharmacologie-Toxicologie, INRA, 180, chemin de Tournefeuille, 31300 Toulouse, France.

JAGER L.P.
Central Veterinary Institute, P.O. Box 65, 8200 AB Lelystad, The Netherlands.

JANSSEN P.A.J.
Janssen Pharmaceutica, B-2340 Beerse, Belgium.

KALPRAVIDH M.
Veterinary Research Department, Bristol-Myers Company, Syracuse, New York, USA.

KIDD A.R.M.
Ministry of Agriculture Fisheries and Food, Central Veterinary Laboratory, New Haw, Weybridge, Surrey KT15 3NB, United Kingdom.

KING R.S.
Department of Anatomy and Physiology, Atlantic Veterinary College, University of Prince Edward Island, Charlottetown, P.E.I. C1A 4P3, Canada.

KLEIN W.R.
Institute for Veterinary Surgery, Faculty of Veterinary Medicine, State University Utrecht, The Netherlands.

KOUNENIS G.
Department of Pharmacology, Veterinary Faculty, Aristotelian University of Thessaloniki, 54006 Thessaloniki, Greece.

KOUTSOVITI-PAPADOPOULOU M.
Department of Pharmacology, Veterinary Faculty, Aristotelian University of Thessaloniki, 54006 Thessaloniki, Greece.

KUEHNERT M.
Department of Veterinary Pharmacology, Pharmacy and Toxicology, Karl-Marx-University of Leipzig, Zwickauer Strasse 55, 7010 Leipzig, GDR.

LEFEBVRE R.A.
J.F. and C. Heymans Institute of Pharmacology, University of Ghent, Medical School, De Pintelaan 185, B-9000 Ghent, Belgium.

LEIBETSEDER J.
Institute of Nutrition, University of Veterinary Medicine,
Linke Bahngasse 11, A-1030 Vienna, Austria.

MALLON F.M.
Department of Anatomy and Physiology, Atlantic Veterinary
College, University of Prince Edward Island, Charlotte-
town, P.E.I. C1A 4P3, Canada.

MASSAT F.
Ecole Nationale Vétérinaire, Laboratoire de radioéléments
et d'études métaboliques (I.N.R.A.), 23, chemin des Capelles, F-31076 Toulouse Cedex, France.

NABUURS M.J.A.
Central Veterinary Institute, P.O. Box 65, 8200 AB Lely-
stad, The Netherlands.

NICHELSON R.L.
Department of Anatomy and Physiology, Atlantic Veterinary
College, University of Prince Edward Island, Charlotte-
town, P.E.I. C1A 4P3, Canada.

NIEUWENHUIJS J.
Institute of Veterinary Pharmacology, Pharmacy and Toxicology, Faculty of Veterinary Medicine, University of
Utrecht, P.O. Box 80.176, 3508 TD Utrecht, The Netherlands.

NIJKAMP F.P.
Institute of Veterinary Pharmacology, Pharmacy and Toxicology, Faculty of Veterinary Sciences, University of
Utrecht, P.O. Box 80.176, 3508 TD Utrecht, The Netherlands.

NOUWS J.F.M.
Meat Inspection Service, R.V.V.-District 6, P.O. Box
40010, Nijmegen, The Netherlands.

OGUNBIYI P.O.
Department of Biomedical Sciences, Ontario Veterinary College, University of Guelph, Guelph, Ontario N1G 2W1, Canada.

OOMS L.A.A.
Department of Veterinary Research, Janssen Pharmaceutica, B-2340 Beerse, Belgium.

PAIRET M.
Department of Physiology, Ecole Nationale Vétérinaire, 23, chemin des Capelles, 31076 Toulouse Cedex, France.

POWERS J.D.
Department of Veterinary Physiology and Pharmacology, College of Veterinary Medicine, The Ohio State University, 1900 Coffey Road, Columbus, OH 43210, USA.

POWERS T.E.
Department of Veterinary Physiology and Pharmacology, College of Veterinary Medicine, The Ohio State University, 1900 Coffey Road, Columbus, OH 43210, USA.

REHM W.F.
F. Hoffmann-La Roche & Co. Ltd., 4002 Basle/Switzerland.

REITZ R.H.
Mammalian and Environmental Toxicology Research Laboratory, Dow Chemical, Midland, Michigan, USA.

RICO A.G.
Ecole Nationale Vétérinaire, Laboratoire de radioéléments et d'études métaboliques (I.N.R.A.), 23, chemin des Capelles, F-31076 Toulouse Cedex, France.

RIVIERE J.E.
College of Veterinary Medicine, North Carolina State University, Raleigh, NC 27650, USA.

ROURKE J.E.
Veterinary Research Department, Bristol-Myers Company,
Syracuse, New York, USA.

RUCKEBUSCH Y.
Department of Physiology, Ecole Nationale Vétérinaire, 23,
chemin des Capelles, 31076 Toulouse Cedex, France.

RUITENBERG E.J.
National Institute of Public Health and Environmental
Hygiene (RIVM). Laboratory for Pathology, P.O. Box 1,3720
BA Bilthoven, The Netherlands.

RUTTEN V.P.M.G.
Department of Immunology, Faculty of Veterinary Medicine,
State University Utrecht, The Netherlands.

SCHATZMANN U.
Klinik für Nutztiere und Pferde der Universität Bern, 3012
Bern, Switzerland.

SOLDANI G.
Farmacologia e Farmacodinamia Veterinaria, Università de-
gli Studi di Pisa, Via delle Piagge 2, 56100 Pisa, Italy.

SPIERENBURG T.H.J.
Central Veterinary Institute, P.O. Box 65, 8200 AB Lely-
stad, The Netherlands.

STEERENBERG P.A.
National Institute of Public Health and Environmental
Hygiene (RIVM), Laboratory for Pathology, P.O. Box 1, 3720
BA Bilthoven, The Netherlands.

STROM P.W.
Veterinary Research Department, Bristol-Myers Company,
Syracuse, New York, USA.

STROUP W.W.
Department of Anatomy and Physiology, Atlantic Veterinary College, University of Prince Edward Island, Charlotte-town, P.E.I. C1A 4P3, Canada.

SUNDLOF S.F.
College of Veterinary Medicine, University of Florida, Gainesville, FL 32611, USA.

VAANDRAGER A.B.
Department of Biochemistry I, Medical Faculty, Erasmus University, P.O. Box 1738, 3000 DR Rotterdam, The Nether-lands.

VAN DEN HENDE C.
Large Animal Surgical Clinic, Faculty of Veterinary Medicine, University of Ghent, Casinoplein 24, B-9000 Ghent, Belgium.

VAN DER MOLEN E.J.
Central Veterinary Institute, P.O. Box 65, AB Lely-stad, The Netherlands.

VAN DUIN C.T.M.
Institute of Veterinary Pharmacology, Pharmacy and Toxico-logy, Faculty of Veterinary Medicine, University of Utrecht, P.O. Box 80.176, 3508 TD Utrecht, The Nether-lands.

VAN KLINGEREN B.
National Institute of Public Health and Environmental Hy-giene, P.O. Box 1, 3720 BA Bilthoven, The Netherlands.

VAN MIERT A.S.J.P.A.M.
Institute of Veterinary Pharmacology, Pharmacy and Toxico-logy, Faculty of Veterinary Medicine, University of Utrecht, P.O. Box 80.176, 3508 TD Utrecht, The Nether-lands.

VAN MUISWINKEL W.B.
Section Cell Biology, Department of Experimental Animal
Morphology and Cell Biology, Agricultural University, P.O.
Box 338, 6700 AH Wageningen, The Netherlands.

VAN PEER A.
Department of Drug Metabolism and Pharmacokinetics, Janssen Pharmaceutica, B-2340 Beerse, Belgium.

VAN REE J.M.
Rudolf Magnus Institute for Pharmacology, Medical Faculty,
University of Utrecht, Vondellaan 6, 3521 GD Utrecht, The
Netherlands.

VARMA K.J.
Department of Veterinary Physiology and Pharmacology,
College of Veterinary Medicine, The Ohio State University,
1900 Coffey Road, Columbus, OH 43210, USA.

VERSCHUUREN H.G.
Department of Toxicology, Dow Chemical Europe, Horgen,
Switzerland.

VREE T.B.
Department of Clinical Pharmacy, Sint Radboud Hospital,
University of Nijmegen, Nijmegen, The Netherlands.

WALKER C.H.
Department of Physiology and Biochemistry, University of
Reading, P.O. Box 228, Whiteknights, Reading RG6 2AJ, U.K.

WATSON A.D.J.
Department of Veterinary Clinical Studies, The University
of Sydney, New South Wales, 2006, Australia.

WEYNS A.
Department of Veterinary Anatomy and Embryology, Faculty
of Veterinary Medicine, RUCA Antwerpen, Belgium.

Welcome address

M. DEBACKERE
Chairman Organizing Committee

Mr. Rector and members of the Honorary Committee, dear
ladies, dear colleagues, dear friends,

It is a privilege and a pleasure for me, as Chairman, to
welcome you, on behalf of the organizing committee, to
this 3rd Congress of our European Association for
Veterinary Pharmacology and Toxicology. Although this
Association is relatively young, being founded only seven
years ago, this third congress demonstrates that the EAVPT
has taken an honoured place as an international scientific
association specifically devoted to pharmacology and
toxicology. As in other branches of veterinary medicine,
major advances in pharmacology, including the demonstration of species differences in pharmacokinetics and drug
biotransformation, have been made. This development
created the need to disseminate newly acquired scientific
information and ideas. To meet this need the European
Association for Veterinary Pharmacology and Toxicology was
formed in 1978 and shortly afterwards a few eminent
scientists organized the first congress in 1979 in
Utrecht. About 200 participants attended this first
congress and they came mainly from European countries.
Three years later, in 1982, the second congress was held
in Toulouse and it was primarily devoted to papers on

ruminant pharmacology. Today, 3 years later, we meet again in Ghent, one of the oldest of Flemish and western European cities, for our third congress with the theme "Comparative Veterinary Pharmacology, Toxicology and Therapy".

The main purpose of this Congress is to consider comparative aspects of pharmacology and toxicology in the common animal species belonging to the companion group of animals as well as to the production group of animals. Our aim is to further our understanding and thus to increase the success of veterinary therapy. However, our objectives at this Congress are even broader. The comparative considerations will not be restricted to differences between these animal species, for an attempt has also been made to compare some aspects of human and veterinary pharmacology. In this venture we are pleased to acknowledge the collaboration of the staff members of the Heymans Institute of Pharmacology in the organization of the congress. In addition, some eminent human pharmacologists have been invited to present full papers.

The organizing committee has worked tirelessly to produce a scientific programme which will, I am sure, satisfy even the most critical participant. More than 20 leading scientists have agreed to present, as invited speakers, an up-to-date account of one of the 15 topics which will be incorporated in 22 separate sessions. More than 180 scientific contributions have been accepted for presentation in the form of invited papers, free communications or posters. Speakers and participants representing more than 25 countries are attending the Congress. Most are from Europe, but there are also many delegates from non-European countries. We hope that the exchange of scientific knowledge through the scientific programme as well as through personal contacts will enable you to return to your homes enriched with much new information. We realize that it is not simply the number of participants that makes a congress great. This is important, but I believe that EAVPT congresses have something even more special. They have always been characterized by the spirit of true friendship, constructive criticism and friendly debate. This open-minded approach is certainly necessary for the spontaneous exchange of scientific information. I hope that every participant, and in particular the younger scientists and colleagues amongst us, will make good use of this open-mindedness which characterizes all that we do here in Ghent. I also sincerely hope that every one of us will return to his or her institute and laboratory with a fund of new knowledge and ideas to motivate and to stimulate our own researches.

It is, I believe, true to say that research has always been and will always remain as the pillar on which progress is built. It is of course a continuing process, and this is what progress is all about. I therefore hope that those responsible for funding our research can be made aware that research is the only good investment for the future. Researchers for their part have to realize that only research of the highest quality can expect to be funded in the present economic climate. Sharing progress in the field of pharmacology and toxicology is the purpose of our being here together this week in Ghent. It gives me a particular pleasure to realize that so many scientists, both veterinarians and non-veterinarians, working in the field of pharmacology and toxicology and coming from so many countries will present the results of their research funded from many differing sources. They will moreover communicate their findings and views in a spirit of solidarity. If all this is achieved for the benefit of mankind and the welfare of the animals themselves, then I am sure that organizing this 3rd EAVPT Congress in Ghent will have been worthwhile. We hope that this exchange of knowledge may contribute to the prestige of the EAVPT, to the advancement of veterinary pharmacology and toxicology and to the improvement of clinical veterinary practice.

At the same time, we hope that this Congress will be

the ideal forum for meeting colleagues, renewing old friendships and making new acquaintances. Finally, your stay in our marvellous medieval city of Ghent and the surrounding provinces of Flanders will enable you to enjoy the famous hospitality and the high creativity of the Flemish people in the arts and sciences, and in our architecture.

We must not forget that the organization of this Congress has been made possible by the generous hospitality of the University of Ghent, for which we express our sincere thanks to the Rector of this University. Our thanks are also due for the much appreciated financial support of the Congress sponsors listed on the cover of your programme book.

As Chairman of the organizing committee, I would like to express my personal thanks to all the members of both organizing and scientific committees and all those who have contributed to the organization of this Congress. Their hard work has guaranteed that we shall have an enjoyable and successful Congress.

Thank you for your participation in this Congress. Your presence here in Ghent is much appreciated by the organizers. I know you will help to make this Congress an unforgettable event in the story of the EAVPT.

Inaugural lecture
Comparative pharmacology and toxicology

P. A. JANSSEN

I can think of two, and only two, reasons, why anybody in his right mind would be really interested in pharmacological and toxicological research.

(1) There are those who are fascinated by the purely academic questions about the interaction between non-living and living matter or, more precisely, between inorganic and organic chemical molecules on the one hand and biological systems (enzymes, receptors, cell membranes and organelles, cell cultures, micro-organisms, isolated tissues or a variety of living creatures) on the other.

(2) Then there are those who are fascinated by the idea of trying to find better drugs than those available for the prevention or treatment of the innumerable diseases that afflict man, animals and plants; those who are dreaming of the ideal drugs of the future : immediately and 100% effective, completely free of unwanted side-effects, easy to use and as cost-effective as possible.

As I have stated on previous occasions : drug research is essentially an interdisciplinary endeavour. It is like an orchestra with chemists, pharmacologists, toxicologists, clinicians and many others playing their instruments. Their various disciplines are like the fingers of a hand : of the same origin, but no longer in contact. To make them work in harmony is not an easy task. It requires perception, deep understanding of the problems to be solved together, enthusiasm and, above all, motivation. To those of you who have heard these words before I can only repeat what Bernard Shaw once said : "When a man has anything to tell in this world, the difficulty is not to make him tell it, but to prevent him from telling it too often". But then, as William Shakespeare wrote : "It is not enough to speak, but to speak true".

Let us therefore keep in mind that the human mind is like a parachute, that it works best when it is open, and also this old and wise Chinese proverb :

    I hear and I forget,
    I see and I remember,
    I do and I understand.

Indeed, all we know about pharmacology and toxicology is directly derived from well-conducted and reproducible experiments providing us with the famous "hard data", the experimental facts. Those of you who have been wrestling with pharmacological and particularly toxicological problems long enough know all too well how difficult it is to distinguish fact from fancy, how easy it is for interpretative theories or opinions to come and go, and how sterile and frustrating emotional discussions on these subjects tend to be.

As I said before : the relevant facts constituting the basis of pharmacological and toxicological knowledge have to do with :

    (1) chemical molecules,
    (2) biological systems, and
    (3) their interactions.

The chemical structure of almost 10,000,000 inorganic

and organic molecules can be found in the literature, and something of the order of 1,000,000 new structures are being determined every year. The majority of these new molecules are made by synthetic chemists, the others being purified naturally occurring substances or products made by modern biotechnological methods.

The spectacular advances in the chemical field over the last decades allow us not only to make new organic molecules more efficiently, but also to determine their precise chemical structure with much greater ease as well as to detect impurities, quantitatively and qualitatively, that were undetectable only a few years ago. Information on the three dimensional structure of small and even very large molecules is being published at an ever-increasing rate. The highly complex natural laws determining the correlation between chemical structure and physical properties are being explored by more and more physical chemists as well as the nature and strength of the various types of intermolecular and intramolecular forces.

The colossal amount of chemical data thus generated made it mandatory to invent a new communication system for chemists. Modern and highly efficient computer-aided techniques are now available in an increasing number of chemical centres for online retrieval of structural information of over 6,000,000 stored structures. A "brave new world" is being created in the field of chemical communication.

Before any of these old or new chemical substances can be tested pharmacologically or toxicologically, however, another seemingly trivial but in fact crucial and sometimes very difficult pharmaceutical problem must be solved - that is, how to prepare a stable solution or any other suitable pharmaceutical form that can be added to the biological system. Many discrepancies in the phar- macological literature are the direct result of the deplorable fact that the importance of this pharmaceutical problem has all too often been underestimated.

The simplest biological systems of interest to

"molecular pharmacologists" are biochemically relevant and relatively large molecules such as enzymes or other proteins, haemoproteins, glycoproteins, constituents of cell membranes such as phospholipids, receptors for the classical neurotransmitters or neuromodulators, for many hormones and growth factors, DNA, RNA, etc.

It is to be expected that within the next decades the mode of interaction between organic molecules and their target macromolecules will be better and better understood. Looking into the future this new body of knowledge should then enable the skilled medicinal chemist to design and make so-called "tailor-made" new molecules fitting optimally with their desirable target macromolecules and, in ideal conditions, with no other biochemically relevant structures.

The question is not "whether" this great dream will ever become a reality, but rather "when". And this will quite obviously depend on how well medicinal, analytical, physical chemists and biochemists as well as pharmacologists and toxicologists will learn to work together in harmony.

One often reads and hears these days about SAR-structure activity-relationship, making slow but steady progress. In 1985 even the best rules of this game are understandably almost entirely empirical, but nevertheless increasingly useful in practical terms to the medicinal chemist trying to predict the pharmacological properties of newly designed but not yet synthesized molecules. The more empirical knowledge the chemist accumulates in a given SAR-field, the more likely it becomes that his predictions will turn out to be correct.

Rather than waste your time to enumerate or classify the innumerable number of more complex biological systems, ranging from single cells to whole healthy or sick animals, that are of interest to pharmacologists and toxicologists, I have chosen to elaborate on the problem of the interactions between chemical molecules and these biological systems.

(4) Inadequate bioavailability;

(5) Drug resistance;

(6) Drug interactions;

(7) Deficient nutritional or immunological status;

(8) Genetic polymorphism of oxidative metabolism in humans, as well as other host factors causing large differences in rates of drug metabolism, for example, genetic constitution, age, dietary habits, hepatic, renal, cardiovascular, gastrointestinal and endocrine function, exposure to other drugs and chemicals, etc.

Common and typical dose-related side-effects are detectable in well-controlled clinical trials and many of them, but not all, are predictable from acute and chronic toxicological experiments.

One should of course keep in mind the fact that there are major species differences in pharmacology as well as in toxicology. To simply extrapolate from one species to another is scientifically unacceptable.

One of the major problems with which we are confronted these days is the detection of extremely rare but serious side-effects in human patients. When their incidence is less than 1 in 1000 only carefully conducted post-marketing surveillance studies involving millions of treated patients can tell us whether a certain unwanted effect is drug-induced or not.

To assess the relative safety of drugs is of course much easier in animals than in man.

Those of you who are professionally confronted with the benefit versus risk assessment problems are of course aware of the fact that absolute safety is an utopian dream and that it is much easier to destroy than to build.

As Bernard Shaw once said : "The reasonable man adapts himself to the world; the unreasonable one persists in trying to adapt the world to himself. Therefore all progress depends on the unreasonable man". A few years later he wrote : "He who can, does. He who cannot, teaches".

Maurice Tubiana in his marvellous book, Le refus du Réel, analyses the psychological reasons why so many inhabitants of technologically advanced countries seem to be more attracted by myths than by facts. While the worldwide consumption of tobacco is increasing, an almost mythical importance is attached to minimal or suspected risks. In spite of the irrational society in which we are living, pharmacologists and toxicologists must be able to convince the world that real progress will not be achieved by paying lip service to uncontrollable theories, but by a better understanding of the real world.

Anaesthesia,
Neuroleptanalgesia
and Sedation

1
Influence of halothane anaesthesia, after xylazine premedication, on serum calcium concentration in the horse

F. GASTHUYS, A. DE MOOR AND C. VAN DEN HENDE

ABSTRACT

In 20 horses breathing spontaneously, xylazine premedication followed by 1.5 h of halothane anaesthesia caused a significant decrease of the total serum calcium concentration. The ionized and complexed calcium fraction showed a non-significant increase. A significant decrease in total serum calcium also occurred in another group of ten horses during halothane anaesthesia with automatic artificial ventilation. The ionized and complexed calcium fraction remained at a constant level in these animals. A possible explanation for, and several consequences of, this calcium decrease are discussed. Determination of the serum calcium concentration might be indicated in some horses during halothane anaesthesia.

INTRODUCTION

Inhalation anaesthesia in the adult horse, especially in animals with a relative high body weight, can cause problems when relatively prolonged anaesthesia is undertaken or when certain predisposing factors are present. The main problems are cardiovascular depression and postanaesthetic myopathy or myonecrosis[1,3]. In some problem cases, we have been able to achieve a better recovery by giving a calcium solution intravenously.

It therefore seemed relevant to examine the influence of halothane anaesthesia on the serum calcium concentration. Halothane causes a pronounced cardiovascular depression and this might be intensified in cases of hypocalcaemia.

MATERIALS AND METHODS
Group 1
In 20 horses the concentrations of total ($Ca^{2+}t$) and of ionized plus complexed ($Ca^{2+}i$) calcium in the serum were measured during 1.5 h of halothane inhalation anaesthesia.

The 20 horses (one thoroughbred, 15 standardbreds and four halfbreds, included ten mares, two stallions and eight geldings) were surgically treated by bilateral neurectomy of the nervi digitali palmaris lateralis and medialis because of podotrochleosis. The average age of the horses was 9.2 years (range 4–14 years) and the average weight was 520 kg (range 420–550 kg). Preoperatively, the horses were in good clinical health. Water was withheld for 12 h, and no access to food was allowed for 24 h, before inducing anaesthesia. The horses received atropine (1 mg/100 kg of body weight intravenously), followed by xylazine (40 mg/100 kg of body weight intravenously). After intravenous injection of 10% guaifenesin (glycerol guaiacolate) at a dosage of 8–10 g/100 kg of body weight, the horses were intubated with a cuffed endotracheal tube and connected to a semiclosed anaesthetic circle system, already primed with 10–15 litres of oxygen. Oxygen and nitrous oxide (% of nitrous oxide : beginning 66.6%, after 5 min 50%, after 10 min completely cut off) were the carrier gases for halothane, which was vaporized from a high precision out-of-circuit vaporizer. After partial denitrogenation, produced by three compressions of the reservoir bag, we attempted to obtain a completely closed system using the inspiratory oxygen concentration as a lead (minimum of 50% FiO_2). In some horses, arterial blood samples were taken for blood gas analysis after 0.5 h of anaesthesia. The depth of anaesthesia was regulated using both clinical signs (disappearance of nystagmus, eyelid-reflex slightly positive) and the recorded capnogram. All horses breathed spontaneously. The average duration of anaesthesia was 1 h 39 min. All animals had an uneventful anaesthesia and recovery.

Heparinized venous blood samples were collected and either analysed directly or stored at 4 °C and analysed within 24 h. After centrifugation of the heparinized blood, total serum calcium was measured by atomic spectro-photometry. After centrifugation of the serum through Centriflo Membrane Cones (Type CF 25, Amicon : cut off 25,000 molecular weight), the ionized and complexed calcium fraction was measured in the filtrate using the same procedure.

Group 2

Another group of ten horses (one halfbred, nine standardbreds including three mares, one stallion and six geldings) was submitted to surgery for different reasons. The horses were also in good clinical condition. The same anaesthetic protocol as in group 1 was followed. However, the horses were ventilated automatically to achieve a normal arterial pCO_2 level (5.44-6.80 kPa), which was determined by blood gas analysis. The average age of the horses was 6.2 years (range 2-12 years) and the average weight was 510 kg (range 400-620 kg). Total calcium and ionized plus complexed calcium were determined in the serum as described above.

Statistical analysis of the data was undertaken using the Student t test and the LSD (least significant diffe-rence) test.

RESULTS
Group 1
The mean serum concentrations of $Ca^{2+}t$ and $Ca^{2+}i$ in 20 spontaneously breathing horses are shown in Figure 1.1. Mean values of 2.86 mmol/l and 1.52 mmol/l for $Ca^{2+}t$ and

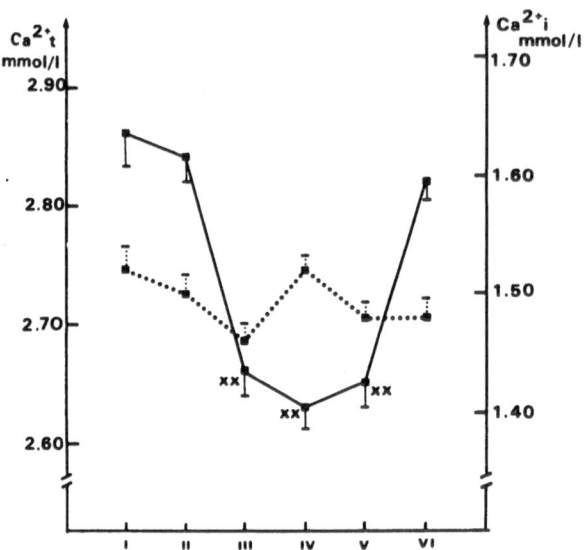

Figure 1.1 Total (Ca²⁺t, ■——■) and ionized plus complexed (Ca²⁺i, ■----■) calcium concentration (mmol/l) in 20 horses before, during and after a halothane anaesthesia of 1.5 h duration (spontaneous respiration, group 1). Mean values plus mean standard error; I : before premedication; II : before induction; III : after 0.5 h of anaesthesia; IV : after 1 h of anaesthesia; V : after 1.5 h of anaesthesia; VI : 0.5 h after disconnection (recovery); xx : significant, P < 0.01, Student t test.

Ca²⁺i, respectively, were found before premedication. Normal range for Ca²⁺t is from 2.8 to 3.3 mmol/l with about 50% of Ca²⁺t in the ionized and complexed form.

The Student t test showed that Ca²⁺t concentrations during anaesthesia were significantly lower (P < 0.01) than the Ca²⁺t concentrations before and after anaesthesia.

The Ca²⁺i concentration did not change significantly; only a slight non-significant increase of the Ca²⁺i concentration was found at the lowest level of Ca²⁺t.

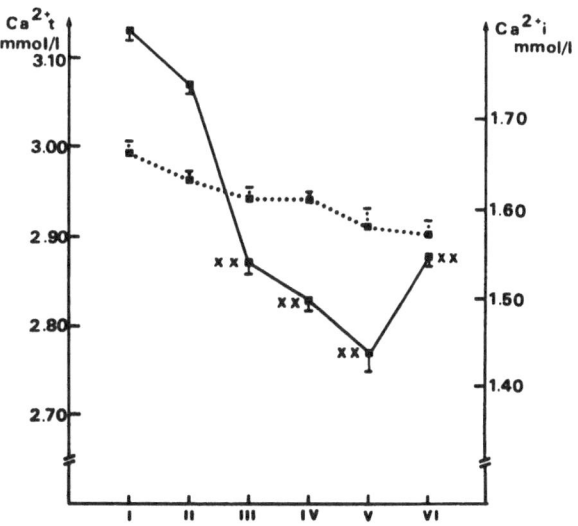

Figure 1.2 Total (Ca²⁺t, ●—●) and ionized plus complexed (Ca²⁺i, ●····●) calcium concentration (mmol/l) in ten horses before, during and after a halothane anaesthesia of 1.5 h duration (automatic artificial ventilation, group 2). Mean values plus standard error; I : before premedication; II : before induction; III : after 0.5 h of anaesthesia; IV : after 1 h of anaesthesia; V : after 1.5 h of anaesthesia; VI : 0.5 h after disconnection (recovery); xx : significant, P < 0.01, Student t test.

Group 2
Figure 1.2 gives the mean serum concentrations of Ca²⁺t and Ca²⁺i (mmol/l) during automatic artificial ventilation in ten horses.   The Student t test showed that in these horses the Ca²⁺t concentrations during anaesthesia were significantly lower (P < 0.01) than the Ca²⁺t concentrations before anaesthesia. The Ca²⁺i concentrations decreased slightly but not significantly.

DISCUSSION
Calcium in the blood consists of a protein-bound and a non-protein-bound fraction. The latter is composed of ionized (free) calcium and calicum complexed with other

ions (such as phosphate, citrate). The free calcium has the highest biological activity. The different fractions remain in equilibrium[7].

During clinical halothane anaesthesia with the horses breathing spontaneously or ventilated automatically, a significant decrease of $Ca^{2+}t$ in the serum without significant changes in the $Ca^{2+}i$ fraction, was obtained. As the latter fraction is the most active biologically, the body attempts to keep this fraction at a constant level.

We noted a difference between the spontaneously breathing and the automatically ventilated horses in the non-protein-bound calcium fraction; in the spontaneously breathing horses a slight non-significant increase in $Ca^{2+}i$ occurred. Acidosis is known to have an influence on the protein-bound fraction : a lower pH decreases this fraction and increases the non-protein-bound calcium. Alkalosis caused the opposite effect[8]. In the first group, the horses were breathing spontaneously with an accumulation of CO_2 in the blood and a respiratory acidosis that was partly metabolically compensated. This might explain the constant and even increased level of $Ca^{2+}i$ in spite of a $Ca^{2+}t$ decrease. In the second group, all horses were automatically ventilated. The arterial pCO_2 level was maintained between 5.44 and 6.80 kPa (40 and 50 mmHg), in order to avoid a respiratory acidosis. The non-protein-bound fraction showed a very slight tendency to decrease in this group, but decrease in the serum $Ca^{2+}t$ cannot be caused by acidosis.

In both groups, total serum calcium concentration decreased while the $Ca^{2+}i$ concentration did not change significantly. Therefore, the protein-bound fraction, which is the difference between $Ca^{2+}t$ and $Ca^{2+}i$, must have decreased. Some hypotheses can be proposed to explain the decrease in this protein-bound fraction. During halothane anaesthesia in the horse, no losses of proteins from the intravascular space occur[9]. It is therefore very unlikely that proteins together with calcium leave the intravascular space. Another unlikely possibility is haemodilution occurring during anaesthesia. If haemodilution was the cause of the decrease in serum calcium, both fractions would have decreased equally. This did not happen; indeed in the spontaneously breathing horses $Ca^{2+}i$ even increased slightly. An explanation for the reduction in protein-bound calcium in the serum during halothane anaesthesia could be "entrapment" of cell membranes by an unknown mechanism. This possibility, however, is entirely speculative.

A loss of the non-protein-bound fraction could also be explained by an increased transport of this calcium into cells, or through an increased excretion (through urine, skin, etc.). The only way to obtain a constant level of the non-protein-bound fraction in this circumstance would be by dissociation of the protein-bound calcium.

Several factors (such as halothane, hormonal imbalance and premedication) could be responsible for the decrease of the total serum calcium during anaesthesia. Halothane has an important influence on homeostasis in horses. Johnson et al.[2] found an elevation of inorganic phosphate and potassium, with a decrease of the total calcium level. These changes were even more pronounced by provoked stress situations before or during anaesthesia. Steffey et al.[10] reported elevated muscle and liver enzymes which persisted for 4 days after anaesthesia, and a small degree of renal depression for, at most, 1 day after anaesthesia. The calcium level did not change after 1 h of anaesthesia.

In vitro experiments have revealed a relationship between halothane and calcium. Price[6] noted that calcium reverses the halothane-induced depressed contractility of the isolated myocardial muscle of cats. Merin[4] described a dose-dependent effect of halothane on cardiac muscle with a diminished uptake of calcium by the sarcoplasmic reticulum caused by a lowered ATPase activity. The effects of halothane in the malignant hyperthermia syndrome have been studied intensively in the pig. Although there is much discussion about the exact mechanism, it seems that only the cell membrane regulation plays a major role in the uncontrolled influx of calcium into the cells[11]. We do not know, however, whether all these processes occur in the horse.

Another possible explanation for the Ca^{2+}t decrease might be a failure of regulation of the hormonal balance during halothane anaesthesia, causing a subsequent hypocalcaemia. After anaesthesia, the rapid normalization of the disturbed hormonal regulation might explain the restoration of serum calcium levels within a short period of time.

Muscle damage (anaesthetic and postanaesthetic myopathy) might also cause a decrease of the serum calcium in the horse[1,12].

Another factor which cannot be discounted is premedication of the horses with atropine and xylazine. Xylazine, a commonly used sedative in horses, has a strong diuretic effect. The actual effect of this agent on serum calcium concentration remains to be determined, however.

Six horses in this study had low total serum calcium levels (2.13–2.78 mmol/l) even before premedication. This might be explained by the preoperative starvation period, which lasted for 24 h[3]. These horses also showed a further decrease in the total calcium during anaesthesia without clinical symptoms, but they must still be considered at risk. In both normal and "low calcium" horses, a rapid postanaesthetic normalization of serum calcium concentration occurred.

Halothane anaesthesia causes in horses marked cardiovascular depression, with a pronounced decrease in cardiac output[11]. In our study, we found a constant hypocalcaemia during halothane anaesthesia but only the total serum calcium was reduced. The animal apparently tried to keep the ionized and complexed calcium concentration at a constant level. We are convinced that in critical patients and possibly in some clinically healthy horses, the low calcium level in the blood must be normalized, before inducing anaesthesia.

CONCLUSIONS

In 20 horses a significant decrease in total calcium concentration in the serum occurred during halothane inhalation anaesthesia (spontaneous ventilation). The same decrease was found in another group of ten horses which were automatically ventilated. Ionized and complexed calcium in both groups showed no significant changes. Although we did not observe clinical symptoms as a result of this hypocalcaemia, complications might occur in critical patients during long-lasting halothane anaesthesia. Preoperative or peroperative determination of the serum calcium concentration might therefore be indicated.

References
1. Friend, S.C.E. (1981). Case report : postanesthetic myonecrosis in horses. Can. Vet. J. 22:367-371.
2. Johnson, B.D., Heath, R.B., Bowman, B., Philips, R.W., Rich, L.D. and Voss, J.L. (1978). Serum chemistry changes in horses during anesthesia : a pilot study investigation of the possible causes of postanesthetic myositis in horses. J. Eq. Med. Surg. 2:109-123.
3. Klein, L. (1979). Post-operative myopathy in the horse-intrinsic and management factors affecting risk. In : Proceedings of the 24th Annual Convention of the American Association of Equine Practice, pp.89-94.
4. Merin, R.G. (1973). Inhalation anesthetics and myo- cardial metabolism. Anesthesiology 39:216-255.
5. Nayler, J.M. (1977). The nutrition of the sick horse. J. Eq. Med. Surg. 1:64-70.
6. Price, H.L. (1974). Calcium reverses myocardial de- pression caused by halothane. Anesthesiology 41:576-579.
7. Simesen, M.G. (1980). Calcium, phosphorus and magne- sium metabolism. In : Clinical Biochemistry of Domestic Animals, 3rd ed., pp.576-635. New York : Academic Press.
8. Stanec, A., Spiro, A.J. and Lent, R.W. (1978). Malig- nant hyperthermia associated with hypocalcaemia. In : Proceedings of the 2nd International Symposium on Malignant Hyperthermia, pp.437-499.
9. Steffey, E.P. and Howlang, D. (1978). Cardiovascular effects of halothane in the horse. Am. J. Vet. Res. 39:611-615.
10. Steffey, E.P., Farver, T., Zinkl, J., Wheat, J.D., Meagher, D.M. and Brown, M.P. (1980). Alternations in horse blood cell count and biochemical values after halothane anesthesia. Am. J. Vet. Res. 41:934-939.
11. Van Den Hende, C., Muylle, E., Vlaminck, K. and Oyaert, W. (1980). Halothaan geïnduceerde maligne

hyperthermie (MH) bij het Belgische Landvarken : enke-
le gegevens in verband met de rol van subcellulaire
fracties. Tijdschr. Diergeneesk. 105:1054-1059.
12. White, K.K. and Short, C.E. (1979). Anesthetic surgical stress-induced myopathy trial. Part II : A postanaesthetic myopathy trial. In : Proceedings of the
24th Annual Convention of the American Association of
Equine Practice, pp.107-115.

2
Pharmacological properties of benzodiazepines in animals

W. F. REHM AND U. SCHATZMANN

ABSTRACT

Benzodiazepines are used in veterinary medicine because of their taming, sedative and skeletal muscle-relaxant effects. The pharmacological properties of benzodiazepines in animals are very species-specific, particularly the reaction of the animal and the duration of action. The effects in ruminants, pigs, dogs and cats are discussed.

INTRODUCTION

In veterinary medicine benzodiazepines are used mainly as drugs for taming aggressive animals, as sedatives and for muscle relaxation. They belong to a large group of psychopharmacologically active compounds which suppress many physiological functions of the animal and reduce both motor activity and aggressiveness. In general, they have no anaesthetic effect. Figure 2.1 lists the most important benzodiazepines relevant for veterinary medicine.

THE MECHANISM OF ACTION OF BENZODIAZEPINES

It is currently believed that the mechanism of action of

* This paper is dedicated to Professor Dr. K. Ammann on the occasion of his 80th birthday.

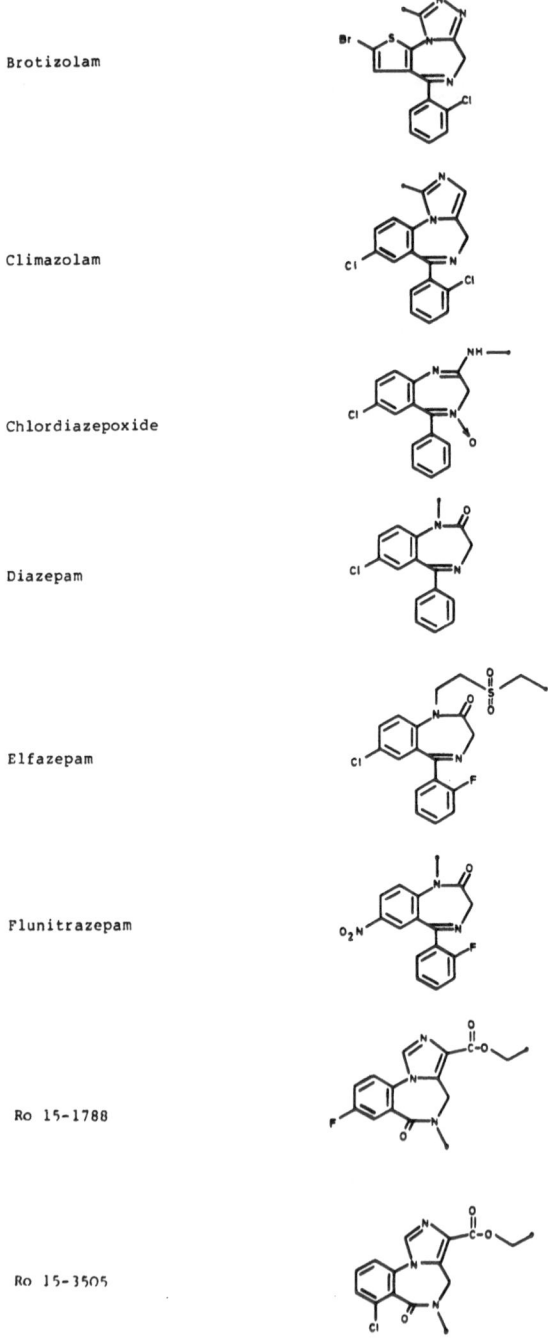

Brotizolam

Climazolam

Chlordiazepoxide

Diazepam

Elfazepam

Flunitrazepam

Ro 15-1788

Ro 15-3505

Figure 2.1   Formulae of benzodiazepines used in animals.

benzodiazepines is the specific enhancement of GABAergic transmission in the CNS. Benzodiazepines modulate, via specific receptors, the coupling mechanism between GABA receptors and their associated chloride channels[3,8,9,14,15,20,21]; Figure 2.2). GABA stimulates the chloride conductance in target neurones. The highest densities of the benzodiazepine receptors occur in the glomerular and external plexiform layers of the olfactory bulb, in the cerebral cortex, islets of Calleja, ventral pallidum, hippocampus, dentate gyrus, superior and inferior colliculi, and cerebellum. The lowest densities are in the corpus callosum, parts of the thalamus, pons and medulla (Figure 2.3). Peripheral binding sites also exist for benzodiazepines. Binding to these sites does not seem to be relevant to the sedative action of these compounds. Unlike benzodiazepines, barbiturates may possibly have a direct effect on the chloride channel. This difference in the mechanism of action may explain why benzodiazepines do not produce (over a wide range of doses) the same intensity of CNS depression as do other sedatives, such as hypnotics and general anaesthetics. The differences in the mechanism of action become evident especially when the dosage is increased. Barbiturates produce surgical anaesthesia and, with "high doses", apnoea and cardiac arrest. Benzodiazepines, on the other hand, are unable to produce complete anaesthesia in animals[8,18].

Benzodiazepines with sedative and anxiolytic properties can be antagonized by compounds which block or displace such benzodiazepine agonists from the receptor. These antagonists were first synthesized by Hunkeler et al.[10] and belong to the imidazobenzodiazepinones. They do not have anxiolytic or sedative properties. Currently, a third group of benzodiazepines that contains compounds which are partly anxiolytic and partly antagonistic (partial agonists) is under development.

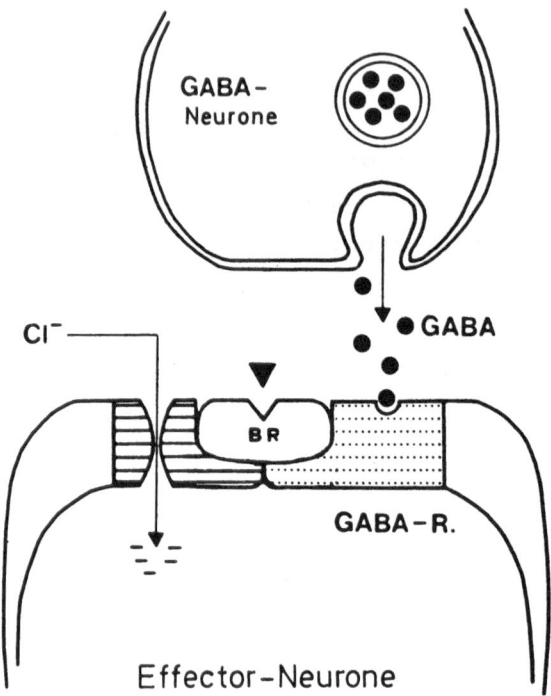

Figure 2.2   Scheme of GABAergic synapse. (From reference[15], with permission).

SOME PHARMACOLOGICAL PROPERTIES OF BENZODIAZEPINES RELEVANT TO THEIR USE IN VETERINARY MEDICINE

Most properties are very species-specific. This particularly pertains to the reaction of the animal and the duration of action. In addition to this, some chemical properties such as the solubility of the benzodiazepines are of importance for their use in animals. The benzodiazepine actions of principal interest for veterinary usage are the taming effect in aggressive animals, the effect of muscle relaxation and sedation. A further property is the influence of benzodiazepines on the intake of feed.

TAMING EFFECT

This psychopharmacological effect is important in the prevention of range fighting during the grouping of

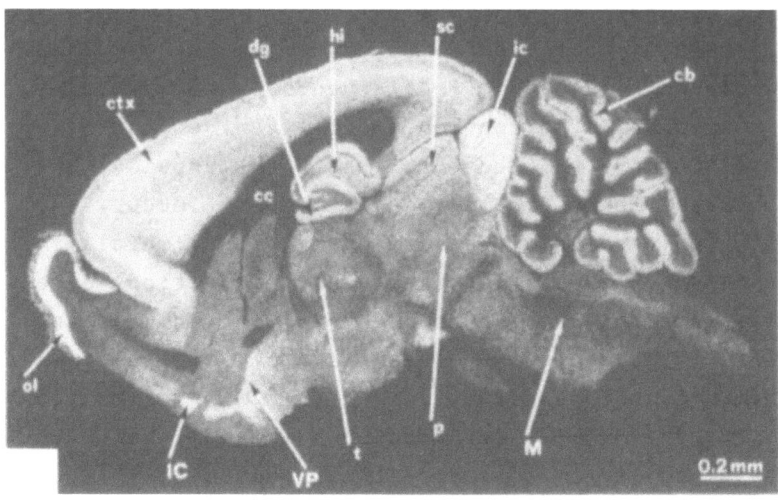

Figure 2.3 Autoradiogram of total binding of [³H]clonaze-
pam in a sagittal rat brain section in vitro. Note the
uneven distribution of receptors : highest densities occur
in the glomerular and external plexiform layers of the
olfactory bulb (ol), in the cerebral cortex (ctx), islets
of Calleja (IC), ventral pallidum (VP), hippocampus (hi),
dentate gyrus (dg), superior and inferior colliculi (sc,
ic), and cerebellum (cb), and lowest densities in the
corpus callosum (cc), parts of the thalamus (t), pons (p)
and medulla (M). (From reference²¹, with permission).

animals, such as before fattening or during transport of
pigs. A benzodiazepine used optimally as a fear-dispel-
ling agent results in the animal appearing to behave
normally without any reaction of fear. The taming effect
of benzodiazepines is also important for use in zoo
animals and pigs. The use of benzodiazepines in zoo
animals is the subject of a recently published review⁷.
The use of benzodiazepines in pigs is referred to in
several recent papers. Our own investigations with
climazolam have shown that doses between 0.05 and 0.1
mg/kg body weight suppress the range fighting of pigs
during grouping and transport. The animals were not
afraid and were able to walk.

MUSCLE RELAXATION AND SEDATION

Whether the sedative or the muscle-relaxant effect of a benzodiazepine appears first depends on the species. In some species a strong muscle-relaxant effect is evident before the onset of sedation; thus, in large animals, such as horses, undesirable reactions may occur. For this reason, chlordiazepoxide, diazepam and climazolam should not be used as single, intravenous injections because of the defence reactions of the horse during casting, and especially because of the risk of marked ataxia. An intramuscular premedication of 0.2 mg/kg diazepam or flunitrazepam 10-20 min before the administration of a xylazine and ketamine combination successfully suppresses ketamine convulsions and allows an induction of anaesthesia free from excitement or other problems. After the intravenous administration of combinations of diazepam, flunitrazepam or climazolam with other anaesthetic agents (xylazine/methadone, ketamine or chloral hydrate) by way of simultaneous injections, or admixed in one syringe, good relaxation and analgesia can be obtained[1,4,6,12,13,16,17]. Our preliminary trials have shown that climazolam in combination with xylazine/methadone or propionylpromazine can be used in the standing, sedated horse to achieve lateral recumbency[18].

USE OF BENZODIAZEPINES IN DIFFERENT SPECIES
Ruminants

In ruminants, optimum sedation can be achieved after intravenous injection of diazepam (0.5 mg/kg body weight) or climazolam (up to 2-4 mg/kg body weight). The cows lie down within 2 min without any complications. Within the first 10 min after high doses there were signs of shallow breathing and a protrusion of the tip of the tongue. The breathing later became quiet and the cow passed into a calm sleep. Approximately 4 h following the injection the animals stood up without difficulty, started to eat and drink and were apparently normal. Intramuscular injections cannot be recommended because of the unpredictable effect[2,11,18]. Problems were encountered with ataxia in the last phase of action and with the large injection volume of the intravenous injection of diazepam. This problem has been solved with a 10% climazolam injection.

Pigs

In pigs, the administration of benzodiazepines for sedation and muscle relaxation has been described for diazepam and climazolam. Diazepam is reported to be useful as a premedicant (0.25 mg/kg diazepam + 0.4 mg/kg azaperone) in the technique of neuroleptanalgesia and to facilitate intubation for nitrous oxide and oxygen anaesthesia, but this method includes a risk of hyperthermia[3,19]. In our trials in pig surgery a good quality of anaesthesia and muscle relaxation could be achieved with a combination of climazolam and metomidate HCl. For grouping before fattening, we found that climazolam alone in dosages between 0.25-0.5 mg/kg body weight should be used; 5 min after administration the animals were unconscious for approximately 15 min and were afterwards sedated for 1-2 h.

Dogs

Dogs alone react to benzodiazepines in a similar way to horses. After intramuscular and intravenous injection of diazepam or climazolam in doses of 1 mg/kg body weight, they show predominantly muscle relaxation with ataxia mainly in the back legs. The sedation is insufficient to keep the animals quiet; on the contrary, they look nervous and sometimes howl. From our experiences with diazepam and climazolam, we were able to use the muscle-relaxant effect of climazolam in combination with methadone and ketamine. The anticonvulsant effect of benzodiazepines suppresses the well-known ketamine convulsions. We recommend that it is preferable to use a combination of 1.5 mg/kg body weight climazolam + 1.0 mg/kg body weight methadone intravenously. This combination can easily be antagonized with a mixture of a benzodiazepine antagonist and an opiate antagonist, for example 0.15 mg Ro 15-1788 + 0.15 mg levallorphan/kg body weight.

Cats
It should be noted that this species should not be excited before the administration of the drug. In excited cats, treatment with either diazepam or climazolam alone may increase the excitation so that useful sedation cannot be achieved. For anaesthesia, diazepam as well as climazolam in doses of 1 mg/kg body weight produce good relaxation in combination with 10-20 mg/kg body weight ketamine.

INFLUENCE OF FEED INTAKE
Benzodiazepines have an appetite-enhancing effect. It is possible for stimulation of appetite to dominate the taming or sedative effect. The mechanism of action of this effect is not fully understood. A direct influence of benzodiazepines on the process of feeding, in particular on hypothalamic GABAergic intrinsic neurones, cannot be totally excluded. On the other hand, it may be that benzodiazepines enhance feed or fluid intake by reducing the inhibitory effect of stimuli of satiation[20]. We assume that benzodiazepines could possibly work as antagonists of CCK (cholecystokinin).

Our investigations[19] showed that the stimulating influence of diazepam, climazolam and certain other benzodiazepines on feed intake is only transient, which does not justify the use of these compounds as so-called growth promoters in animal feed.

ANTAGONISM OF BENZODIAZEPINES
In all our trials, independent of the combination with narcotics or sedatives, it was possible to antagonize the action of benzodiazepine agonists with specific benzodiazepine antagonists. After intravenous injection of the antagonists, the animals in lateral recumbency stood up within 1 min, and sometimes less, without any difficulty.

The specificity of the action of the benzodiazepine

antagonists could be demonstrated when climazolam was administered in combination with ketamine. When the activity of the benzodiazepine was antagonized during ketamine anaesthesia, the ketamine convulsions reappeared[18].

On the basis of our investigations with climazolam we recommend a relationship to the antagonist Ro 15-1788 of 10 to 1. If climazolam is injected in combination with methadone, levallorphan should be used as an opiate antagonist in a ratio of 7.5 parts methadone to one part levallorphan.

CONCLUSIONS

Very few of the large group of benzodiazepines have been developed for use in veterinary medicine.

The most acceptable hypothesis of the mechanism of action of benzodiazepines is the specific enhancement of GABAergic transmission and the indirect action on the chloride channel, via specific receptors. The main pharmacological properties of benzodiazepines are very species-specific; this applies not only to the reaction of the animal but also to the duration of action. For the veterinarian the taming effect, skeletal muscle relaxation and sedation are the principal actions.

The benzodiazepines with sedative and anxiolytic properties can be antagonized by compounds which block or displace the agonists from the receptor. The ability of the specific benzodiazepine antagonists to neutralize the benzodiazepine effect within a very short time makes the use of the muscle-relaxant activity of the benzodiazepines much easier and the well-known long-lasting ataxia resulting from overdosage of benzodiazepines much less dangerous.

Acknowledgements

We thank Dr J.G. Richards for reviewing the manuscript, and Pergamon Press for granting permission to reprint Figure 2.3 from Neuropharmacology.

References
1. Ammann, K., Osman, M.A.R. and Rehm, W.F. (1965).
   Versuche zur Verwendung des Benzodiazepinderivates Ro
   5-2807 als Tranquillizer und Mittel zum medikamentösen
   Niederlegen der Pferde. Schweiz. Arch. Tierheildkd.
   107:59-72.
2. Beglinger, R., Hamza, B., Heizmann, P., Kyburz, E. and
   Rehm, W.F. (1977). Untersuchungen zur Anwendung und
   Antagonisierung von Benzodiazepinen beim Rind. Dtsch.
   Tierärztl. Wochenschr. 89:137-142.
3. Bonetti, E.P., Pieri, L., Cumin, R., Schaffner, R.,
   Pieri, M., Gamzu, E.R., Müller, R.K.M. and Haefely, W.
   (1982). Benzodiazepine antagonist Ro 15-1788 : Neuro-
   logical and behavioral effects. Psychopharmacology
   78:8-18.
4. Butera, T.S., Moore, J.M., Garner, H.E., Amend, J.F.,
   Clarke, L.L. and Hatfield, D.G. (1978). Diazepam/
   xylazine/ketamine combination for short-term anesthesia. Vet. Med. Small Anim. Clin. 73:495-496,499.
5. Conzen, M., Sollmann, H. and Lindner, R. (1984). Erfahrungen mit der Neuroleptanalgesie unter Intubation
   mit einem Lachgas/Sauerstoff-Gemisch für grosse
   neurochirurgische Eingriffe am Hausschwein (Sus
   scrofa). Dtsch. Tierärztl. Wochenschr. 91:396-397.
6. Cronau, P.F., Zebisch, P. and Tilkorn, P. (1980). Aus
   der Praxis : Kurznarkose beim Pferd mit Diazepam —
   Xylazin — Ketamin. Tierärztl. Umsch. 35:393-394.
7. Gutzwiller, A., Völlm, J. and Hamza, B. (1984). Einsatz des Benzodiazepins Climazolam bei Zoo- und Wild-
   tieren. Kleintierpraxis 29:319-332.
8. Haefely, W., Kulczar, A., Möhler, H., Pieri, L., Polc,
   P. and Schaffner, R. (1975). Possible involvement of
   GABA in the central actions of benzodiazepines. Adv.
   Biochem. Psychopharmacol. 14:131-151.
9. Haefely, W., Pole, P., Pieri, L., Schaffner, R. and
   Laurent, J.-P. (1983). Neuropharmacology of benzodia-
   pines : Synaptic mechanisms and neural basis of
   action. In : Costa, E. (ed.). The benzodiazepines,
   pp.21-67. New York : Raven Press.
10. Hunkeler, W., Möhler, H. Pieri, L., Polc, P., Bonetti,
    E.P., Schaffner, R. and Haefely, W. (1981). Selective
    antagonists of benzodiazepines. Nature 290:514-516.
11. Leppert, K. (1967). Das medikamentöse Niederlegen des
    Rindes mit dem Benzodiazepin-Derivat Ro 5-2807 (Hoff-
    man-La Roche). Giessen : Vet. Diss.
12. Marolt, J. (1966). Weitere Erfahrungen mit dem Benzo-
    diazepinderivat Ro 5-2807 bei Haustieren in Kliniek
    und Praxis. Dtsch. Tierärztl. Wochenschr. 73:265-267.
13. Massone, F., Thomassian, A., Hilst, C.L.S., Curi, P.R.
    (1982). Nova associaçao anestésica para cirurgias de
    curta duraçao em equeinos. Rev. Bras. Med. Vet.
    5:14-18.
14. Möhler, H. and Okada, T. (1977). Benzodiazepine re-
    ceptor : Demonstration in the central nervous system.
    Science 198:849-851.
15. Möhler, H. and Richards, J.G. (1983). Benzodiazepine

receptor in the central nervous system. In : Costa,
E. (ed.). The benzodiazepines, pp. 93-116. New York :
Raven Press.
16. Muir, W.W., Sams, R.A., Huffman, R.H. and Noonan, J.S.
(1982). Pharmacodynamic and pharmacokinetic properties of diazepam in horses. Am. J. Vet. Res. 43:
1756-1762.
17. Nowak, M. (1983). Kurzzeit-Narkose mit Diazepam, Xylazin und Ketamin beim Pferd. Hannover : Vet. Diss.
18. Rehm, W.F. and Schatzmann, U. (1984). Benzodiazepines
as sedatives for large animals. J. Assoc. Vet.
Anaesth. of Great Britain and Ireland. No 12:93-106.
19. Rehm, W.F., Beglinger, R., Becker, M., Hamza, B.,
Heizmann, P. and Schulze, J. (1982). Einsatz von
Benzodiazepinen bei Schweinen. Berl. Münch. Tierärztl. Wochenschr. 95:146-151.
20. Thiébot, M.-H. and Soubrié, P. (1983). Behavioral
pharmacology of the benzodiazepines. In : Costa, E.
(ed.). The benzodiazepines, pp.67-92. New York :
Raven Press.
21. Richards, J.G. and Möhler, H. (1984). Benzodiazepine
receptors. Neuropharmacology 23:233-242.

3
Effects of halogenated inhalational anaesthetics on respiration in dogs

L. W. HALL

ABSTRACT

The methods used to assess the respiratory depressant effects of inhalation anaesthetics are illustrated by reference to observations made during halothane and enflurane anaesthesia in dogs. The timing of events of the respiratory cycle, determination of the functional residual capacity with the maximum pressure generated in the occluded airway, ventilation, and the response of these variables to increases in $PaCO_2$ need to be combined to give a complete profile of an agent's effects.

INTRODUCTION

The methods used to study the respiratory effects produced by anaesthetic agents have become more refined with the passage of time. Early observers noted that breathing became more shallow as the depth of central nervous (CNS) depression increased and that it ceased before circulatory arrest occurred. From these observations the characteristics of the breathing pattern came to be used in assessing the depth of anaesthesia and Guedel's classical description of the signs and stages of diethyl ether anaesthesia is characterized by extensive reference to them, but it soon became apparent that respiratory signs must always be related to a particular agent. For

25

example, under halothane anaesthesia respiration may become severely depressed before reaction to painful stimulation is abolished, whereas during ether anaesthesia it is well maintained long after reaction to stimulation disappears. These simple observations suggest that halothane is much more of a selective respiratory depressant than ether but how much greater cannot be deduced.

The introduction of the concept of MAC (minimal alveolar concentration)[5], made direct comparison of the effects of different inhalation anaesthetics much easier and the arrival of simple methods for the determination of blood gases enabled the clinician to determine the influence of anaesthetics and analgesics on oxygenation of the blood and/or the removal of carbon dioxide from the body. Clearly, determination of the blood gases at equivalent levels of CNS depression allows assessment of the respiratory effects of the agents in question, but it gives no indication of how any observed respiratory depression arises.

Other methods of assessing the respiratory effects of drugs centre on the measurement of ventilatory responses to changes in arterial or end-tidal carbon dioxide levels during anaesthesia or after the administration of single doses of analgesics such as the opiates. Many variations of the basic technique have been described in the literature but they all involve measurements of pulmonary ventilation, either as end-tidal carbon dioxide tension is increased or during steady state conditions at different carbon dioxide tensions. The various techniques yield carbon dioxide response curves and there can be little doubt that the determination of these at equivalent levels of anaesthesia has proved to be a useful tool in the comparison of the respiratory effects of the inhalation anaesthetics. The response curve undoubtedly defines the way in which depression of the central chemoreceptor is translated into gaseous exchange, but again, it gives no indication of the mechanism involved.

More recently, a method of studying the activity of the respiratory muscles themselves, which gives a much greater insight into the processes involved in respiration, has been introduced[3]. It involves occlusion of the airway and determination of the pressure decrease within it during the occluded inspiration. If the inspiratory effort begins at the same lung volume on each occasion, then the pressure decrease correlates well with the neural activation of these muscles[2]. There are now numerous published accounts of the use of this technique but it does not appear to have been reported in the veterinary literature.

Valuable clues to the mechanisms involved in the production of respiratory depression can be obtained when all the various techniques are taken into account, as may be illustrated by consideration of studies of the respiratory effects of two halogenated anaesthetics, halothane and enflurane.

MATERIALS AND METHODS

The studies to be described here simulated the conditions prevailing during clinical anaesthesia using a mixture of nitrous oxide and oxygen to volatilize the agents and a non-rebreathing circuit for their delivery (Figure 3.1). All the animals involved were racing greyhounds free from evidence of cardiopulmonary disease. Unconsciousness was always produced with the same short-acting intravenous drugs (alfentanil and methohexitone) before the induction of anaesthesia was completed by administration of the inhalation agent through a face-mask until endotracheal intubation could be performed. Anaesthesia was maintained with 1% halothane or 2% enflurane in the inspired gases, and the body temperature was maintained constant between 37 °C and 38 °C. No observations were made until the dog had been in a stable state of anaesthesia with a constant arterial carbon dioxide tension ($PaCO_2$) for at least 30 min. Differences were considered to be statistically significant when the t-test showed $p < 0.05$.

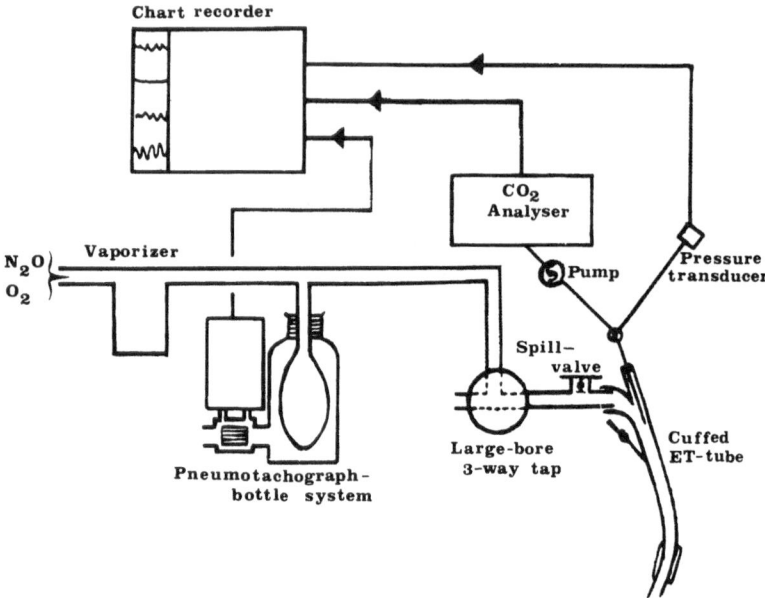

Figure 3.1 Modification of the Magill non-rebreathing circuit used.

RESULTS AND DISCUSSION

During anaesthesia the mean values for arterial blood pressure and heart rate did not differ significantly between halothane and enflurane, while arterial oxygen tension (PaO_2) was always over 26 kPa so there was no hypoxic or hypotensive respiratory drive to complicate the interpretation of results. Mean $PaCO_2$ was always lower under halothane (Table 3.1) but the difference was not significant and thus, by this criterion, the two agents were equally depressant to breathing. The mean slopes of the CO_2 responses, however, differed (Figure 3.2) and consideration of the tidal and minute volume responses show that when end-tidal $PaCO_2$ is increased under halothane the rate is affected more than the tidal volume.

Minute volume (V) was significantly greater under halothane (p = 0.04) but there was no statistical diffe-rence (p = 0.15) between the tidal volumes (V_t). The du-ration of inspiration (T_i) under enflurane was signi-

Table 3.1 Arterial carbon dioxide tension ($PaCO_2$; KPa), inspiratory (T_i), expiratory (T_e) and total (T_{tot}) cycle times (seconds), maximum pressure in occluded airway (P_{max}; cmH_2O), occluded inspiration time (T_{io}; seconds) and tidal volume (V_t; ml/kg) in racing greyhounds under halothane (dog 1-7) or enflurane (dog 8-14) anaesthesia.

Animal	$PaCO_2$	T_i	T_e	T_{tot}	P_{max}	T_{io}	V_t
Halothane							
1	4.93	0.65	2.29	2.94	22.4	1.42	16.8
2	7.33	0.69	5.80	6.49	24.4	1.01	11.0
3	6.67	0.67	2.83	3.50	20.0	1.27	9.3
4	7.73	0.74	4.45	5.19	60.0	0.87	7.6
5	7.07	0.45	3.18	3.63	32.5	0.70	13.0
6	5.47	0.98	2.43	4.14	16.4	0.70	16.4
7	5.47	0.57	3.24	3.80	26.7	0.74	11.9
Enflurane							
8	6.00	0.60	9.40	10.00	29.5	0.60	13.2
9	7.07	1.45	5.64	7.09	19.9	2.18	17.6
10	8.67	1.74	15.60	17.00	17.0	1.74	15.0
11	6.93	1.24	5.54	6.78	29.3	1.42	9.0
12	6.53	1.73	5.15	6.88	11.7	1.48	11.0
13	5.60	0.80	8.19	8.99	31.9	1.01	19.0
14	7.33	1.28	7.19	8.47	30.2	1.86	12.0

ficantly longer than under halothane ($p = 0.006$), and this may permit much better distribution of inspired gas within the lungs thus making gas exchange more efficient at the lower breathing rate associated with enflurane.

Under both anaesthetics section of the vagus nerves increased inspiratory time (T_i) indicating that vagal feedback was involved in the termination of inspiration, but it also increased the inspiratory time of occluded breaths (T_{io}) so that the shorter T_i during halothane cannot be explained solely on the basis of differences of

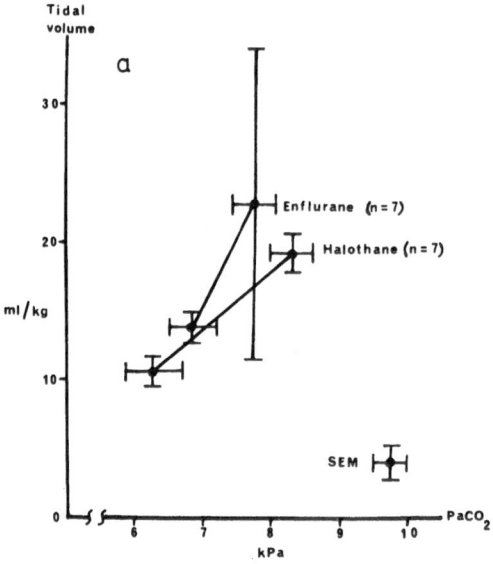

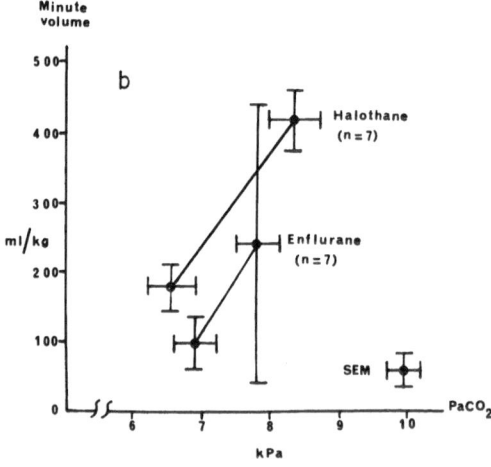

Figure 3.2   CO₂   responses (a) tidal, and (b) minute volumes.

activity in the vagus nerves.

Although   the   difference   was   not   statistically
significant,   the   maximum   pressure   generated   in   the
occluded   airway   (P_max)   was   greater   under   enflurane,
possibly   indicating   the   retention   of more power in the
respiratory muscles   than   during   halothane   anaesthesia.

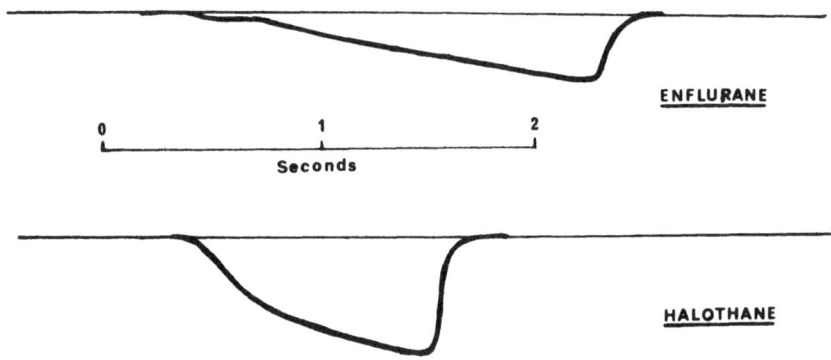

Figure 3.3 Shape of occlusion pressure curves under halothane and enflurane anaesthesia.

However, under enflurane the shape of the occlusion
pressure curve was markedly different (Figure 3.3) in that
the initial rate of decrease in pressure was obviously
less than under halothane but after this initial period
the rates of decrease were not dissimilar. The cause of
this difference is not readily apparent; it may have been
due to weakness of the intercostal muscles or it may
indicate asynchronous activation of the intercostal
muscles and diaphragm during enflurane anaesthesia.

The effective elastance $[P_{max}/V_t]$ was virtually
identical under the two anaesthetics and although not
statistically apparent (probably due to the small number
of animals involved) the effective impedance $[(P_{max}/I_i)/(V_t/T_i)]$ was higher under enflurane, indicating greater
bronchomotor tone and an increase in the work of breathing
under this anaesthetic.

The results support the suggestion that halothane and
enflurane produce respiratory depression in dogs through
different effects on the bulbopontine pacemaker
mechanism[4], but all the observations reported here were
made in the absence of surgical stimulation, and it is
known that measurements made with or without such
stimulation will lead to different conclusions being drawn
about the respiratory depressant effects of an agent such

as isoflurane[1]. Nor were end-tidal concentrations of the anaesthetics monitored, although inspired concentrations of 1% halothane and 2% enflurane administered from a non-rebreathing circuit should produce equivalent levels of depression of the CNS. Also assumed was that the respiratory muscles acted from the same initial fibre length under different anaesthetics, but this would not be the case if the functional residual capacity was not the same and there is some evidence to suggest that under anaesthesia lung volumes depend on the agent used[4].

CONCLUSIONS

It is clear that for the complete assessment of respiratory depressant effects it is necessary to use more than one technique. The timing of events of the respiratory cycle, determination of the functional residual capacity with the maximum pressure generated in the occluded airway, ventilation, and the response of these variables to increases in inspired PCO_2 need to be combined to give a complete profile of an agent's effects.

References
1. Eger, E.I. II (1981). Isoflurane : a review. Anesthesiology 55:559-576.
2. Eldridge, F.L. (1975). Relationship between respiratory nerve and muscle activity and muscle force output. J. Appl. Physiol. 39:567-574.
3. Grunstein, M.M., Younes, M. and Milic-Emili, J. (1973). Control of tidal volume and respiratory frequency in anaesthetized cats. J. Appl. Physiol. 35:463-476.
4. Marsh, H.M., Rehder, K. and Hyatt, R.E. (1981). Respiratory timing and depth of breathing in dogs anaesthetized with halothane or enflurane. J. Appl. Physiol. : Respirat. Environ. Exercise Physiol. 51:19-25.
5. Merkel, G. and Eger II, E.I. (1963). A comparative study of halothane and halopropane anaesthesia. Anesthesiology 24:346-357.

4
Analgesic activity of butorphanol in horses: dosage titration and clinical studies

D. A. GINGERICH, J. E. ROURKE, P. W. STROM, L. L. GORDON
AND M. KALPRAVIDH

ABSTRACT

Butorphanol is a synthetic opiate of the cyclorphan series which possesses both narcotic agonist and antagonist properties. The drug has been characterized pharmacologically and clinically in humans as an analgesic and as a component of balanced anaesthesia, and in dogs it has been used as an antitussive agent.

In order to determine the clinical utility of butorphanol as an analgesic in horses, a clinical and pharmacological evaluation of the agent was undertaken in horses. Analgesic activity was demonstrable in a dose-dependent manner in horses, the intravenous administration of 0.1 mg/kg providing a justifiable clinical dosage. In double-blind clinical studies in horses presenting with acute abdominal pain, the analgesic effectiveness of butorphanol at a dosage of 0.1 mg/kg was confirmed.

INTRODUCTION

In 1680 Sydenham wrote "Among the remedies which it has pleased Almighty God to give to man to relieve his sufferings, none is so universal and so efficaceous as opium"[5]. An extract of the opium poppy Papaver somniferum, opium is now known to be a mixture of alkaloids, the most important of which is morphine.

Although morphine is clinically very effective as an analgesic, respiratory depression, gastrointestinal side-effects, and, most importantly, addiction liability are dangerous attributes of morphine that severely limit its clinical acceptability.

Major scientific developments in this century have led to the synthesis and testing of newer and safer drugs of the opiate type. The observation that N-allyl substitution on the codeine molecule abolished respiratory depression produced by morphine or heroin, gave rise to the concept of narcotic antagonists and structure-activity relationships. The development of opiate receptor theory followed, along with the discovery of endogenous opioids in the brain.

In the search for a safer, more potent analgesic as a replacement for morphine, the narcotic agonist-antagonist class of drugs offered hope. Noting that drugs such as cyclazocine and cyclorphan provided potent analgesia with minimal euphoria, and that drugs containing the 14-hydroxyl group, such as naloxone, showed distinct antagonist properties, scientists at Bristol Laboratories undertook a synthetic programme to pursue the 14-hydroxy cyclorphan series. The 14-hydroxymorphinans had never before been produced through total synthesis and unique chemical procedures had to be devised.

Of the analogues produced, butorphanol proved to be the most promising.

PHARMACOLOGY OF BUTORPHANOL
Chemistry
The chemical structure of butorphanol in comparison with related agents is presented in Figure 4.1. Butorphanol is similar in structure to dextromethorphan but it possesses a N-methylcyclobutyl substitution as well as a 14-hydroxyl group. By comparison, naloxone, which acts as a pure antagonist, is similar in structure to morphine but features an N-allyl substitution and a 14-hydroxyl group.

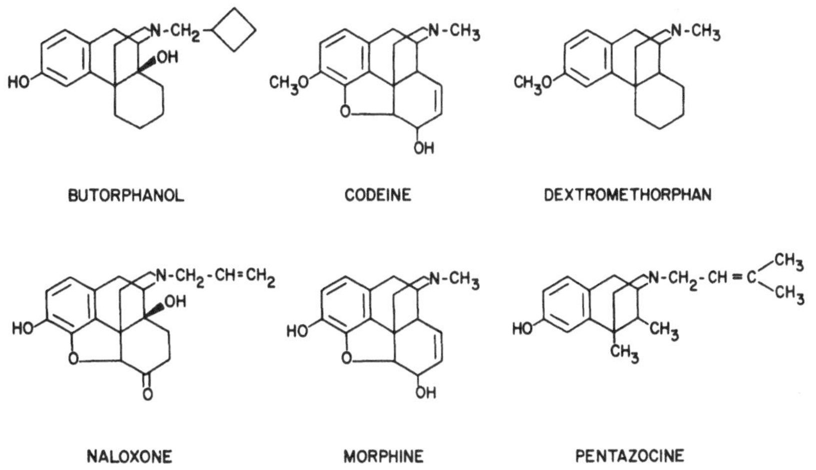

BUTORPHANOL   CODEINE   DEXTROMETHORPHAN

NALOXONE   MORPHINE   PENTAZOCINE

Figure 4.1   Chemical structures of butorphanol and related
agents.

Pharmacokinetics

Butorphanol is rapidly and completely absorbed following
intramuscular or subcutaneous administration. In dogs,
peak concentrations of butorphanol are detected at 0.7 h
after injection[7]. The apparent plasma elimination half-
life (t 1/2) is 1.5-2 h. In horses, intravenous injection
of butorphanol results in a biphasic plasma elimination
curve with a terminal half-life averaging about 2 h as
illustrated in Figure 4.2.

Absorption after oral administration of butorphanol to
dogs is essentially complete. However, oral bioavailability is limited (about 16% in dogs) due to extensive
first-pass metabolism in the liver, primarily to hydroxy-
butorphanol, which is subsequently excreted mainly in
urine[1]. Some biliary excretion, amounting to 11-14% of a
parenteral dosage, also occurs.

Butorphanol readily crosses the placental barrier as
evidenced by studies in both pregnant ewes[6] and women[9].
Butorphanol is measurable in fetal circulation of lambs
within 1 min of parenteral administration to the ewe and
rapidly reaches equilibrium with maternal circulation. In
women, parenterally administered butorphanol crosses the

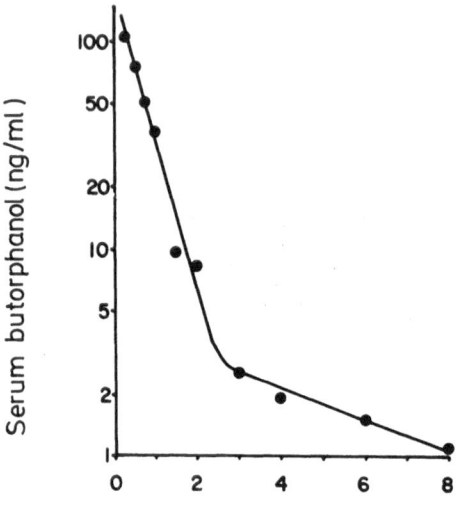

Figure 4.2 Butorphanol serum concentration versus time curve for serum butorphanol in horses (n = 6) following intravenous dosage of 0.1 mg/kg.

placental barrier and is found in neonatal cord serum at concentrations comparable to those in maternal plasma. Butorphanol is also detectable in the milk of lactating women following oral and intramuscular administration, with milk-to-serum ratios ranging from 1.9 (oral) to 0.7 (intramuscular).

Analgesic and antagonist activity
The analgesic activity of butorphanol is demonstrable in rodents using the phenylquinone writing test and the arthritic vocalization test, in which butorphanol has approximately ten and 50 times the subcutaneous potency of morphine and pentazocine, respectively[1]. Naloxone was shown to reverse the analgesic activity of butorphanol in mice, but only at dosages 50 times higher than those required to antagonize morphine.

    The antagonist activity of butorphanol is demonstrable by precipitation of abstinence in non-withdrawn, morphine-dependent mice and by reversal of morphine analgesia. As an antagonist, naloxone was found to be 15 times more potent than butorphanol. The analgesic component of butorphanol is approximately ten times more potent than its antagonistic component.

Antitussive activity

The antitussive activity of butorphanol was demonstrated in guinea-pigs and dogs, utilizing an electrically stimulated cough model[2]. In the dog, butorphanol given subcutaneously was ten and four times more potent than pentazocine and morphine, respectively. Orally, butorphanol was about 15-20 times more potent than codeine as an antitussive.

In clinical studies, butorphanol given subcutaneously at a dosage of 0.055 mg/kg had a rapid onset of antitussive action in dogs with chronic cough due to tracheobronchitis, tonsillitis, pharyngitis, or bronchitis[3]. Follow-up treatment with butorphanol oral tablets at a dosage of 0.55 mg/kg provided antitussive control in dogs for 7-12 h[4].

In horses, amplitude and frequency of experimentally induced cough were markedly suppressed by intravenous butorphanol dosages of 0.1 and 0.01 mg/kg, but less so by dosages of 0.001 mg/kg (Caudle, A.B., personal communication, 1985).

Cardiopulmonary effects

Butorphanol has considerably less potential to produce respiratory depression when compared to morphine, as reflected by comparison of changes in arterial blood pCO_2 and pH in rats and dogs[1]. Clinical dosages of butorphanol cause minimal cardiovascular effects as demonstrated in humans, dogs, and horses[10]. Unlike morphine, butorphanol has no significant effect on venous plasma histamine concentration[11].

Effect on intestinal motility

In contrast to morphine, which decreased intestinal motility, increased duodenal smooth muscle activity, and decreased bile duct flow, butorphanol given at equianalgesic doses had little or no effect on bile duct flow and one-tenth the effect on intestinal motility and smooth muscle activity[1]. In horses, butorphanol given intravenously at dosages of 0.5 mg/kg every 4 h for 48 h had no clinical effect on intestinal motility. In ponies, migrating myoelectrical complex frequencies and spike burst frequencies measured in the distal jejunum and left dorsal colon were not diminished following intravenous administration of butorphanol at the clinical dosage of 0.1 mg/kg (Adams, S.B., personal communication, 1982).

Butorphanol in anaesthesia

As a pre-anaesthetic agent in dogs, butorphanol given intramuscularly at dosages of 0.055, 0.11 or 0.22 mg/kg reduced the dosage of thiamylal sodium required for induction of anaesthesia in a dose-dependent fashion. Ponies premedicated with butorphanol at intramuscular dosages of 0.11 mg/kg, induced with xylazine and ketamine (1.1 and 2.2 mg/kg, respectively), and maintained on halothane, achieved a deeper plane of anaesthesia at comparable halothane flow rates than non-premedicated controls (Short, C.E., personal communication, 1985).

Butorphanol has been used in horses at dosages of 0.05 to 0.1 mg/kg in conjunction with xylazine (1.1 mg/kg) to provide analgesia (particularly in the rear quarters) for minor surgical procedures that do not require recumbency. Under these conditions, transient ataxia is the side-effect most frequently observed.

ANALGESIA IN EQUINE COLIC

Materials and methods

Dosage titration studies

Six healthy adult horses of both sexes and of various breeds were instrumented for measurement of pain threshold

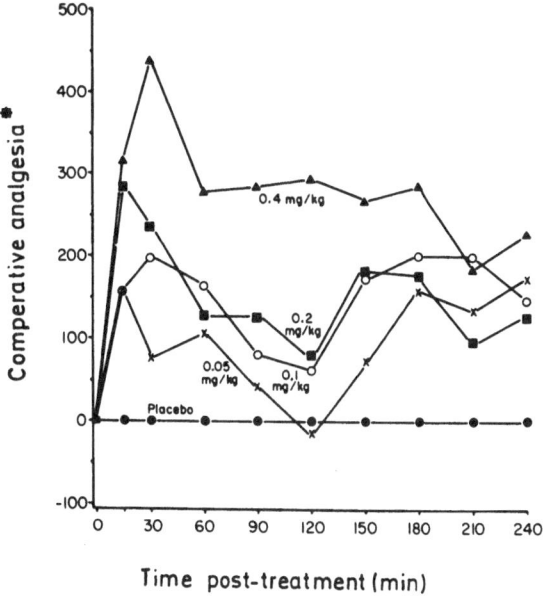

Figure 4.3 Analgesic effects of butorphanol given at various dosages in horses with visceral pain (* = mean change in response time, in sec, to visceral pain stimulus relative to placebo, n = 6).

according to methods described by Pippi and Lumb[8]. The experiments were conducted using a 6 x 6 Latin square design wherein each horse was evaluated with each of the following six intravenous treatments : butorphanol at 0.05, 0.1, 0.2 and 0.4 mg/kg, pentazocine at 2.2 mg/kg (positive control) and saline. A washout period of at least 3 days was allowed between successive treatments.

Pain threshold, defined as the elapsed time between painful stimulus (balloon inflated in caecum [visceral] or quartz lamp focused on blackened skin [superficial]) and purposeful avoidance movement, was measured before drug treatment, 15 to 30 min after treatment and every 30 min thereafter for a total of 4 h. The resulting data were analysed statistically by analysis of variance and linear regression.

Double-blind clinical studies

The analgesic effects of butorphanol (Torbugesic-Bristol Laboratories) at an intravenous dosage of 0.1 mg/kg were compared with those of pentazocine at its approved dosage of 0.33 mg/kg in horses presenting with acute abdominal pain (colic). Pain intensity was determined before treatment and at 15 min intervals after treatment by : (a) a clinical scoring system for individual signs of colic (sweating, kicking, pawing and head and body movement), on a 0-4 scale, 0 being normal and 4 signifying severe signs; (b) monitoring pulse and respiratory rates; and (c) standardized behavioural observations. The attending veterinarians also rated the overall clinical analgesic effect on a poor, fair, good, or excellent basis.

Analgesia scores were calculated for each parameter by subtracting the post-treatment pain score from the pretreatment pain score at each observation time, and compared statistically between treatment groups by Student's t test. Overall clinical effects were compared using the chi square test.

Results

Effect on visceral pain threshold

Measurable increases in response time to visceral pain stimuli were detected within 15 min at all butorphanol dosages. Analgesia persisted throughout the 4 h as illustrated in Figure 4.3. The apparent biphasic shape of the analgesic response curves was an artifact produced by slight increases in placebo response times at 90 and 120 min. No evidence of enterohepatic shunting of butorphanol was encountered (see Figure 4.2). A statistically significant (p less than 0.01) linear relationship was detected between the mean change in response time and the log of the butorphanol dosage (Table 4.1).

Butorphanol at dosages of 0.1, 0.2 and 0.4 mg/kg, but not 0.05 mg/kg, had an effect significantly (p less than 0.05) greater than placebo. The effect of pentazocine, at the exaggerated dosage of 2.2 mg/kg, was also significant-

Table 4.1   Change in response time induced by butorphanol

Butorphanol dosage (mg/kg)	Mean change in response time (sec) relative to placebo
0.05	100
0.1	152
0.2	158
0.4	284

Superficial pain

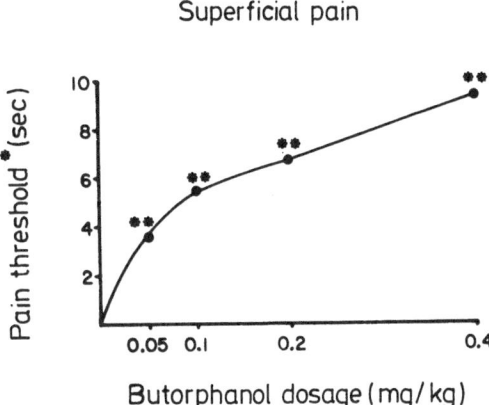

Butorphanol dosage (mg/kg)

Figure 4.4   Dose-response   relationship   of butorphanol in
horses with superficial pain (* = mean change in   response
time,   in   sec,   to   superficial pain stimulus relative to
placebo at 15 min after intravenous injection, n =   6;   **
significantly different from placebo, p less than 0.001).

ly greater than placebo, its activity falling between that
of butorphanol at 0.2 and 0.4 mg/kg.

Effect on superficial pain threshold
Repeated measures analysis of variance across   post-treatment   times   resulted   in   significant   (p less than 0.05)
interaction between treatments and times, such that it was
necessary   to   compare   treatments   at   each   of   the nine
post-treatment times.   All four dosages of butorphanol and

ANALGESIC SCORE

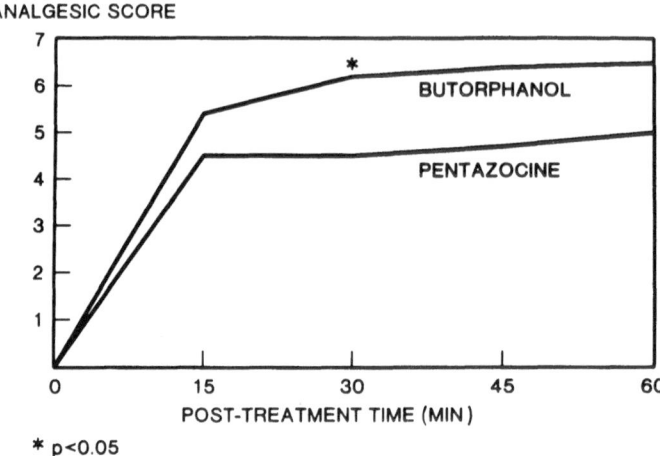

* p<0.05

Figure 4.5 Comparison of analgesic effectiveness of intravenous butorphanol (0.1 mg/kg) and pentazocine (0.33
mg/kg) in horses presenting with acute abdominal pain;
analgesia score refers to pretreatment pain score minus
pain score at indicated post-treatment times (* p less
than 0.05).

also pentazocine were significantly (p less than 0.01)
more effective than placebo at 15 min post-treatment. A
dose-response relationship was detected numerically but
not statistically (Figure 4.4). No significant differences between any treatments and placebo were detected
beyond 30 min post-treatment.

Butorphanol was occasionally associated with side-
effects consisting of restlessness, ataxia, or sedation
while pentazocine (given at an elevated dosage) caused
restlessness, ataxia, and shivering in all cases.

Analgesia in clinical colic
Case reports on a total of 69 horses with acute abdominal
pain associated with intestinal obstruction, excessive gas
or hypermotility were received, of which 34 were treated
with butorphanol (0.1 mg/kg) and 35 with pentazocine (0.33
mg/kg). Marked improvement in the clinical signs of colic

was detected within 15 min following injection of butorphanol or pentazocine. Based on calculated mean analgesic scores, horses of the butorphanol group showed greater improvement in all parameters at all post-treatment times than did the pentazocine group (Figure 4.5). Those differences were found to be statistically significant (p less than 0.05) with regard to sweating, pawing, total score, and reduction in respiratory rate (toward normal). An overall satisfactory clinical rating was given in 88% of the butorphanol cases compared with 59% of the pentazocine-treated horses, a statistically significant difference (p less than 0.05). Side-effects in these studies were limited to slight, transient ataxia and sedation, observed occasionally in both groups.

CONCLUSIONS

The results of these studies indicate that butorphanol is effective as an analgesic in alleviating abdominal pain associated with colic in the horse. Analgesic activity was measurable pharmacologically, a dose-response relationship was detected and analgesia was confirmed in double-blind clinical studies conducted under conditions of veterinary practice.

References
1. Caruso, F.S., Pircio, A.W., Madissoo, H., Smyth, R.D. and Pachter, I.J. (1977). Butorphanol. In : Goldberg, M.E. (ed.). Pharmacological and Biochemical Properties of Drug Substances. Washington DC : American Pharmaceutical Association Academy of Pharmaceutical Sciences, pp.19-57.
2. Cavanagh, R.L., Glylys, J.A. and Bierwagen, M.E. (1976). Antitussive properties of butorphanol. Arch. Int. Pharmacodyn. Ther. 220:258-268.
3. Christie, G.J., Strom, P.W. and Rourke, J.E. (1980). Butorphanol tartrate : a new antitussive agent for use in dogs. Vet. Med. Small. An. Clin. 75:1559-1562.
4. Gingerich, D.A., Rourke, J.E. and Strom, P.W. (1983). Controlling canine cough : clinical efficacy of butorphanol injectable and tablets. Vet. Med. Small An. Clin. 78:179-182.
5. Jaffe, J.H. and Martin, W.R. (1975). Narcotic analgesics and antagonists. In : Goodman, L.S. and Gilman, A. (eds). The Pharmacological Basis of Therapeutics, 5th ed., pp.245-283. New York : Macmillan Publishing

Company.

6. Maduska, A.L., Pittman, K.A., Ahokas, R.A., Anderson, G.D., Lipshitz, J., Morrison, J.C. and Smyth, R.D. (1980). Placental transfer and other physiologic studies with intravenous butorphanol in the anesthetized pregnant ewe. Res. Commun. Pathol. Pharmacol. 29:229-241.

7. Pfeffer, M., Smyth, R.D., Pittman, K.A. and Nardella, P.A. (1980). Pharmacokinetics of subcutaneous and intramuscular butorphanol in dogs. J. Pharmacol. Sci. 69:801-803.

8. Pippi, N.L. and Lumb, W.V. (1979). Objective tests of analgesic drugs in ponies. Am. J. Vet. Res. 40:1082-1086.

9. Pittman, K.A., Smyth, R.D., Losada, M., Zichelboim, I., Maduska, A.L. and Sunshine, A. (1980). Human perinatal distribution of butorphanol. Am. J. Obstet. Gynecol. 138:797-800.

10. Robertson, J.T., Muir, W.W. and Sams, R. (1981). Cardiopulmonary effects of butorphanol tartrate in horses. Am. J. Vet. Res. 42:41-44.

11. Schurig, J.E., Cavanagh, R.L. and Buyniski, J.P. (1978). Effect of butorphanol and morphine on pulmonary mechanics, arterial blood pressure and venous plasma histamine in the anesthetized dog. Arch. Int. Pharmacodyn. 233:296-304.

Teaching Veterinary Pharmacology

5
Postgraduate training in the veterinary pharmacology

D. DROUMEV

ABSTRACT

The system of postgraduate training in veterinary pharmacology adopted in European countries varies — in some
countries it is connected predominantly with intensive
research work and with conferring of scientific degrees
(PhD, DSc); in others it involves attending special courses with formal examinations, optional research work and
receiving certificates (diplomas); in most countries short
postgraduate refresher courses are organized for qualified
veterinarians and pharmacologists. But there are no special postgraduate training courses for pharmacologists in
the pharmaceutical industry.

Proposals are presented for postgraduate training in
veterinary pharmacology within the framework of the EAVPT
— a unified system of courses (both long-term and
short-term) for specialization and training of young
graduates leading to the awarding of scientific degrees.
Some courses, including international ones, for furthering
qualifications and knowledge are proposed for those
working in veterinary pharmacology; there are also courses
organized with the help of eminent guest scientists
invited to particular countries and mutual visits in
institutes and laboratories. A preliminary 2 year basic
academic course for training of candidates is advisable in

the pharmaceutical industry, followed by special training in research laboratories of the pharmaceutical firms. It is preferable that for all courses not only classical education methods such as frontal lectures and practical exercises are used, but also films, videotapes, computer techniques, etc. A permanent committee of the EAVPT should be set up to organize and coordinate the post-graduate training courses in veterinary pharmacology, and also be concerned with preparing methodology instructions, dispatching visual and audiovisual materials, videotapes, printed materials and editing a periodical bulletin.

INTRODUCTION

Postgraduate and specialist training in veterinary pharma-cology is both a national, and an international problem. Each European country strives to educate veterinary pharmacologists for both research and teaching work in universities, research institutes and academies, and also for research work in the pharmaceutical and ecological laboratories, etc.[3]. The system of specialist training in this respect is generally different in the various coun-tries; they need to be unified within the framework of EAVPT, to improve and possibly lead to more effective and speedier education of pharmacologists.

SYSTEMS OF POSTGRADUATE TRAINING IN VETERINARY PHARMACO-LOGY WITHIN THE FRAMEWORK OF EAVPT

Almost every European country has a system of postgraduate training of veterinary pharmacologists. In most cases it is allied to the need for teachers in pharmacology in the universities and colleges. The training is usually car-ried out individually in the institutes and laboratories, and is a matter of personal interest, of diligence and persistence in the candidate, but it also concerns the respective institutions.

POSTGRADUATE TRAINING   IN VETERINARY PHARMACOLOGY LEADING
TO SCIENTIFIC DEGREES
This is used in most of the European countries and is the
main system for creating academic staff - veterinary pharmacologists in the veterinary universities, in colleges,
in agricultural and veterinary academies - but also in
some research institutes, and in many cases in the
pharmaceutical   industry.   It   is based on intensive
research work in the field of pharmacology, and is linked
with scientific theses, dissertations, doctorates and with
awarding of scientific degrees. The training terms vary
depending on the profile of the speciality, on the requirements for depth of knowledge, on mastering of research
methods, on the scientific achievements and the scientific
titles.

For scientific degree Doctor of Philosophy (PhD), lic.
med. vet. (licentiate degree, CSc) it is necessary first
of all to take educational courses to study investigation
methods, and conduct practical exercises by undergraduate
students in some universities, take examinations, then do
research work and write theses (dissertations) or articles
in scientific publications. The duration of this postgraduate training is 2-3 years. The named system (with
some variants) has been introduced in the United Kingdom,
West Germany (a comparable degree is DVM after defence of
the inaugural dissertation), the Netherlands, Denmark
(lic. med. vet.), USSR, East Germany, Czechoslovakia,
Poland, Bulgaria (CSc), Yugoslavia and other countries[2,]
[3,8,9].

The scientific degree Doctor of Science (DSc, DVSc, Dr
med. vet.) is higher than PhD. For preparing the thesis
intensive research work over a 4-5 year period (without
attending training courses and without a supervisor) is
mandatory. The conferring of the DSc degree is linked to
a great extent with the originality of the scientific
contribution, with the discovery of new regularities of
fundamental character and/or of scientific-practical
application. The DSc degree is usually conferred after a

successful public defence, but in some countries it is possible to gain a degree instead by contribution to scientific publications. The DSc postgraduate system is used in the United Kingdom, Norway and Denmark (Dr med. vet.), France (after the doctorate - Doctor of Biology in Pharmacology), USSR, West Germany, Czechoslovakia, Poland, Bulgaria (DSc), Yugoslavia among others[2,6,7,8,9].

For the scientific degree Master of Science (MSc) the candidate must attend a postgraduate course in veterinary pharmacology. Then he works on a (mainly optional) research project and presents a lecture connected with the major subject. The greater part of the practical training programme and the research project is taken by an appointed supervisor. The courses at Master's level in Denmark, for example, are foreseen for postgraduate students in the developing countries, and the degree MSc, is then conferred by the home university[2,8]. The same level degree in Norway is named Dr scient. The postgraduate student must present a thesis in the form of monograph or articles in scientific journals, which must satisfy the standards of the reputed journals. In France the comparable scientific degree is Master in Pharmacology[7].

POSTGRADUATE TRAINING IN VETERINARY PHARMACOLOGY LEADING TO CERTIFICATES (DIPLOMAS)

This exists only in a few countries in the form of special courses lasting 2 years; for example in West Germany (Hanover) the course is "Basic Biological Disciplines" together with theoretical and practical physiology, biochemistry and toxicology; in Israel the course lasts one semester, and is mostly theoretical; in Bulgaria the course lasts 30 days, and is mostly theoretical clinical pharmacology. Postgraduate students in West Germany in addition have to produce a research study, and in all the above-mentioned countries an examination must be passed at the end of the course before a certificate is received[8,10].

POSTGRADUATE TRAINING IN VETERINARY PHARMACOLOGY FOR FURTHER QUALIFICATIONS AND REFRESHER COURSES FOR WORKING VETERINARY PHARMACOLOGISTS

This training lasts 3-6 months and should be renewed for all those qualified every 5 years. It acquaints practising veterinary pharmacologists with new investigation methods, new apparatus and enables them to take part in a research programme[3,4,10]. It is possible for specialists to attend lectures and discussions on review materials in the various fields of pharmacology (in the USSR it is in the Faculty of Postgraduate Training of Veterinary specialists of the Moscow Veterinary Academy). This kind of training is also organized individually in certain pharmacological institutes with an individual work-plan[4].

COMPARING POSTGRADUATE TRAINING

The above types of postgraduate training in veterinary pharmacology are not practised equally in the various countries. Almost all European countries link postgraduate training with scientific degrees. And usually each European country has its own postgraduate basic training, only rarely sending graduates to foreign countries for training.

Postgraduate training leading to certificates (diplomas) can be considered very valuable because of the relatively rapid possibility of specialization, but regrettably it is used to only a limited extent in the different countries of the EAVPT. Postgraduate training for further qualification, with refresher courses for veterinary pharmacologists, is very good, but it is not systematically introduced in all European countries. The above-mentioned postgraduate courses are mainly to create veterinary pharmacologists for research and education.

There is still no specialized way of educating pharmacologists and toxicologists for the pharmaceutical industry linked to the specificity of polyvalent knowledge and to respective research profiles. The need for this kind of specialist is considerable at present because the ratio between chemists and pharmacologists in pharmaceutical research laboratories is 1:2[7].

There is no unified postgraduate training system for veterinary pharmacologists within the framework of the EAVPT which provides planned postgraduate education of equal standards. So at the First Congress in Zeist (1979) the EAVPT was forced to direct its attention to teaching students and specialists in veterinary pharmacology. The problem was discussed at the International Conference on Veterinary Pharmacology, Toxicology and Therapeutics in Cambridge (1980). The Board of the EAVPT considered it expedient to set a unified standard for qualification in veterinary pharmacology and establish compatible education and postgraduate training standards. Some institutes for training of young pharmacologists (with scholarships for 3-6 months) were specified at the Second Congress of the EAVPT in Toulouse (1982). The problem of both postgraduate and undergraduate training in veterinary pharmacology was discussed at the Third Congress of the EAVPT in Ghent (1985).

PROPOSALS FOR POSTGRADUATE TRAINING IN VETERINARY PHARMACOLOGY

Unified systems

It is advisable for a committee to prepare a unified system for postgraduate training of specialists in veterinary pharmacology and toxicology to increase the postgraduate training level in those countries within the framework of the EAVPT. It is important for training profiles to be specified with the view of creating small personnel units for research institutions and academies, for universities and colleges, for the pharmaceutical industry, for ecological institutions, and those concerned with basic pharmacology, clinical pharmacology, toxicology and biopharmacy, etc.

Scientific degrees

Training courses can ensure the comparatively rapid

education of veterinary pharmacologists. Long-term and medium-term courses for each country, with a common basis within the framework of the EAVPT should be organized for studying new achievements in the field of pharmacology, for mastering investigation methods and for doing limited research work, culminating in a certificate (diploma) for particular specialties, and optionally (if the scientific contributions are of greater importance) a scientific degree. The long-lasting courses (8-12 months or more) are convenient for young veterinary graduates to specialize. The medium-term courses (3 months to occasionally, 6 months) are suitable for specialists who need new knowledge and experience in the research work in particular areas of pharmacology or a neighbouring discipline[1].

It is expedient for international specialists to be invited to supervise training and to demonstrate new investigation methods. Both classical and modern training methods should be used: frontal lectures with not only slides and transparencies, but also films, videotapes, television techniques and computer techniques, showing simulation of drug influences on the biological systems, simulation techniques for teaching pharmacokinetics, investigation of pharmacokinetics on healthy and sick animals, specifying optimal doses and the intervals of drug application, determination of withdrawal times, including the minimum to use without killing the animals, multiple choice examination system, etc[3,5,11,12].

The pharmaceutical industry

The postgraduate training of veterinary pharmacologists for the pharmaceutical industry needs a more complicated system[7]. Preliminary training of young graduates with an academic basis (lasting approximately 2 years, and leading to a scientific degree), or a long-term postgraduate course leading to a certificate (diploma) (relatively seldom) should be organized, followed by specialist training in research laboratories of pharmaceutical firms. An ongoing postgraduate education system reflects favourably upon the activity of the pharmacologists in industry. It is advisable for them to be able to work every few years for up to 6 months in the university laboratories.

Short-term courses

For the higher qualifications and refresher courses for working veterinary pharmacologists, short-term training courses for 1-3 months, both national and international, are suitable : these include lectures and demonstrations on new research methods, review material about new achievements in various areas of veterinary pharmacology, and discussions. Other training systems can be used - such as short-term courses organized with guest scientists who have considerable scientific and practical experience, or mutual visits to institutes and laboratories can be arranged for young pharmacologists to acquaint them with the achievements of the respective staffs there. Videotapes can be exchanged for the same purpose.

Creating a permanent committee

For organizing the systems of postgraduate training in veterinary pharmacology mentioned above the creating of a permanent committee may be the answer. The EAVPT Board can utilize a training base, coordinate postgraduate training activities, and deal with the education problems, give regular periodic information to all member countries of the EAVPT, prepare methodology instructions, visual and audiovisual materials, videotapes, and printed material (booklets, technical bulletins, guidelines, monographs, specialist books). It is also advisable to produce a review-type periodical bulletin, presenting up-to-date scientific and research news.

CONCLUSIONS

Three types of postgraduate training in veterinary pharmacology are used, but are not equal in the various European countries mentioned above, mostly those courses

leading to scientific degrees. Proposals are presented
for introducing an unified system within the framework of
EAVPT countries - postgraduate training courses (both
long-term and medium-term), leading to scientific degrees,
higher qualifications and refreshment courses, including
those with invited guest scientists. For postgraduate
training in the pharmaceutical industry, academic-based
training in long-term courses followed by work in pharmaceutical firms, is preferable, using modern methods of
education. Creation of a permanent committee connected to
the EAVPT Board for organizing and coordinating postgraduate activity is advisable.

References
 1. Brien, J.F. and Racz, W.J. (1984). A methodology
    course for graduate students in pharmacology. Trends
    in Pharmacol. Sci. 5:171-173.
 2. Bruhn, K. and Rasmussen, F. (1983). The Royal Veteri-
    nary and Agricultural University, Copenhagen : an
    institute for higher education and its relationship to
    developing countries. Member CRE Inform. 63:153-161.
 3. Brune, K., Ganten, D. and Habermann, E. (1984).
    Teaching of pharmacology, toxicology and clinical
    pharmacology. Trends in Pharmacol. Sci. 5:127-131.
 4. Evdokimov, P.D. (1984). Tasks of clinical veterinary
    pharmacology. Veterinaria (USSR) 9:67-68.
 5. Hughes, I. (1983). Computer club : computers in phar-
    macology teaching. Trends in Pharmacol. Sci. 4:
    251-252.
 6. Knifton, A. (1983). Teaching of veterinary pharmaco-
    logy in the United Kingdom. Vet. Res. Comm. 7: 1-4.
 7. Pekkarinen, A. (ed.) (1976). Contemporary trends in
    the training of pharmacologists. Helsinki : IUPHAR.
 8. The Royal Veterinary and Agricultural University In-
    formation. Copenhagen (1984). 13.
 9. The Royal Veterinary College. University of London,
    Postgraduate Prospectus (1984), 10,14.
10. Sanford, J. (1980). Aims and objectives of teaching
    clinical pharmacology and toxicology. In : van Miert,
    A.S.J.P.A.M., Frens, J. and van der Kreek (eds).
    Trends in Veterinary Pharmacology and Toxicology,
    pp.156-161. Amsterdam : Elsevier.
11. Walaczek, E.J. and Doull, J. (1984). Using computers
    for teaching of pharmacology, toxicology and therapy.
    London : IUPHAR 9th International Congress of
    Pharmacology, Abstracts:E5. London : Macmillan press.
12. Welpton, R. (1984). Simulation technique in training
    pharmacology. London : IUPHAR 9th International Con-
    gress of Pharmacology, Abstracts:E6. London : Macmil-
    lan press.

6
The teaching of veterinary pharmacology and toxicology

J. D. BAGGOT

ABSTRACT

In the teaching of veterinary pharmacology and toxicology it is important that the courses be placed at stages in the curriculum when the students have acquired adequate background in allied disciplines and are enthusiastic about the material presented. The expertise of the faculty and the involvement of its members in basic aspects of clinical veterinary research can greatly influence the attitude of students towards the discipline. Postgraduate training in pharmacology and toxicology is best provided through organized graduate programmes which have a critical mass of faculty specialists in the discipline.

RECENT HISTORICAL DEVELOPMENTS

It is now almost 30 years ago since veterinary pharmacology underwent the major change from materia medica to systemic pharmacology with a bias towards physiology. This change in emphasis took place rather abruptly and, in becoming a basic science, the discipline unintentionally restricted its scope by virtually ignoring its application in clinical veterinary medicine. I cannot but feel that the separation from therapeutics which followed this change must have been a source of disappointment to Professor L. Meyer Jones. It was his textbook of Veterinary Pharmacology and Therapeutics, the first edition of which was written solely by him and published in 1954, that was largely responsible for introducing veterinary pharmacology as it is today[5]. In An Introduction to Veterinary Pharmacology, first published in 1960, Professor Frank Alexander emphasized the principles of veterinary pharmacology and their application in selected therapeutic situations[1]. Prior to these decisive texts, which changed the content and direction of veterinary pharmacology, Wallis Hoare's Veterinary Materia Medica and Therapeutics (first edition, 1895) with the various revisions edited by Professors J. Russell Greig and G.F. Boddie had been the standard textbook for over 50 years[4]. Through his studies on the passage of antimicrobial agents from the systemic circulation into milk, Professor Folke Rasmussen stimulated research on the distribution and elimination of drugs in food-producing animals[6,7]. His paper, published in 1958[6], was the first in a series of research papers that linked basic principles to clinical application.

It was through the combined efforts of Professor Charles R. Short and the late Dr. Andrew T. Yoxall that the Journal of Veterinary Pharmacology and Therapeutics was created in 1978. The introduction of this international journal marked a significant development in the discipline, as it provides a means not only for disseminating recent information to veterinary pharmacologists throughout the world, but also for consolidating the discipline by providing it with an identity. I should like to think that the monograph Principles of Drug Disposition in Domestic Animals[2] has contributed to the development of veterinary pharmacology, particularly in the area of clinical pharmacokinetics.

Veterinary toxicology has developed in quite a different way from the pattern of development in veterinary pharmacology. This can be largely attributed to the diversity of backgrounds of veterinary toxicologists, many of whom have appointments in other major disciplines, such as clinical veterinary medicine or veterinary pathology. For at least the last 25 years the principles of toxicology have been incorporated in pharmacology while applied toxicology is taught much later in the veterinary curriculum. Veterinary Toxicology (originally published as Lander's Veterinary Toxicology) re-written by Professor E.G.C. Clarke and M.L. Clarke (first edition, 1975) has been the standard textbook over the years[3]. In the preface to the first edition (1975) the authors state that since the book was first published in 1912, toxicology has changed out of all recognition. A section entitled Veterinary Toxicology was added to the fourth edition (1977) of Veterinary Pharmacology and Therapeutics.

Since analytical techniques have now been mastered in most diagnostic toxicology laboratories, I feel confident that at least some of these laboratories will in the future participate more fully in research activities. Their sophisticated equipment could be used to advantage in determining the distribution pattern and elimination kinetics of toxic substances in the body, and for projects that would elucidate the biochemical mechanisms of toxicity. Another area of research that is begging the attention of veterinary toxicologists is to outline the pathophysiology of chemical-induced disease conditions and to determine how these physiological alterations affect the dispositon and dosage of drugs that might be used in their presence and/or treatment. I am optimistic that veterinary toxicology is rapidly approaching a threshold, beyond which significant scientific advances will follow in rapid succession.

COURSES IN VETERINARY PHARMACOLOGY AND TOXICOLOGY

There are three features of most courses in the veterinary medical curriculum, including those in veterinary pharmacology and toxicology, that deserve particular attention. The first is the content or syllabus which most delicately blends the basic and applied aspects of the discipline; the second is the stage in the curriculum at which the course is offered, and the third feature is the manner in which the factual material is presented.

The integrated curriculum, in which pharmacology was presented in a fragmented manner and economy of time was an underlying objective, was introduced in some US schools and colleges of veterinary medicine in 1969. Although this curriculum was found to be unsatisfactory and was largely abandoned within a decade, it resulted in a shorter time being assigned to pharmacology than the traditional course had enjoyed. Not only was the number of lectures reduced by about 25%, but the laboratory classes in which students traditionally participated were largely replaced by demonstrations and video tapes. The beneficial outcome from the demise of the integrated curriculum was that an independent course in veterinary pharmacology was re-established. The situation was somewhat different for veterinary toxicology in that it was spared from the humiliation of fragmentation in the integrated curriculum and the subsequent drastic reduction in the time assigned to the course.

CURRICULUM
The curriculum in veterinary pharmacology and toxicology that is presently offered at the University of California, Davis is outlined in Table 6.1.

OBJECTIVES
The objectives of the course in veterinary pharmacology are to introduce the basic principles and general concepts of pharmacology and toxicology and to apply them in a veterinary context. The molecular mechanisms of action and effects of drugs on body systems are presented with attention given to species variations in response. This course provides factual information on the classes of drugs that are of importance in clinical veterinary medicine.

Table 6.1 Professional courses in veterinary pharmacology and toxicology
----

Veterinary pharmacology I; First year-spring
Principles of pharmacology and toxicology (includes
    kinetics, fate processes and mechanisms of drug action)
Eight lectures and one laboratory demonstration
Systemic pharmacology (drugs acting on autonomic and
    central nervous system, including anaesthetic agents
    and neuromuscular blocking drugs)
17 lectures and two laboratory demonstrations
    Total : 25 lectures and three laboratory classes

Veterinary pharmacology II; Second year-autumn
Systemic pharmacology (diuretics, cardiovascular drugs,
    autocoids, hormones and hormone antagonists, non-
    steroidal anti-inflammatory agents (NSAIDS))
Ten lectures and one laboratory demonstration
Chemotherapy (antimicrobial agents and antineoplastic
    drugs)
Eight lectures and one laboratory demonstration
Principles of therapeutics
Two lectures
    Total : 20 lectures and two laboratory classes

Clinical pharmacology (elective course); Third year-winter
Principles of antimicrobial therapy and approach to
treatment of selected infectious disease conditions (9);
treatment of gastrointestinal diseases in dogs and cats
(1); management of congestive heart failure in dogs (2);
selection and use of antiarrhythmic agents in horses (1);
analgesic and non-steroidal anti-inflammatory agents in
the horse (2); drug therapy of respiratory disorders (1);
treatment of skin conditions in small animals (1);
pharmacological basis of drug interactions (1); adverse
reactions to drugs (1); considerations governing the use
of drugs in neonatal animals (1).
    Total : 20 lectures

<u>Veterinary Toxicology</u>: Third year—spring
The prevalence of toxic agents in the environment and exposure of animals to them; the incidence, pathology, pathogenesis, diagnosis and treatment of diseases of animals caused by chemical poisons, organic and inorganic.

Total : 28 lectures

The overall objective of the course in clinical pharmacology is to apply the factors involved in the selection of particular drug preparations for the treatment of infectious diseases and the therapy of disorders of body systems. The message presented is that diagnosis, at least tentative, of the disease and the physiological condition of the animal patient must first be determined and this information be used in the selection of a drug preparation and its dosage regimen. This course encourages students to think about the use of drugs in animals, the limitations imposed by the dosage forms (including veterinary preparations) that are available in relation to the functional and behavioural differences among the animal species with which we are concerned, and the procedures for the clinical evaluation of drugs.

Veterinary toxicology, which is essentially an applied course, has the overall objective of providing factual information on the incidence, pathogenesis, diagnosis, and treatment of diseases in animals caused by poisonous substances.

VETERINARY PHARMACOLOGY
All veterinary students have completed a bachelor's and some a master's degree in science before entering the 4-year DVM degree programme in the School of Veterinary Medicine. With their background in mathematics, chemistry and mammalian physiology, the veterinary students are well prepared to understand the basic concepts of pharmacology and the mechanisms of action of

drugs at the molecular level. It is only because of the strong background of the students and the fact that comprehensive printed lecture notes are provided that the time assigned for the two-part core course in veterinary pharmacology, which consists of a total of 45 lectures and five laboratory classes, is marginally adequate. The assignment of more time to the pharmacology course would enable us to elaborate on and discuss the material presented more fully. It would also enable us to present lectures on topics that are omitted, such as the pharmacology of anthelmintic drugs. In the student evaluations of the course, two comments consistently made are that more lectures should be assigned to the pharmacology course to cater for the amount of material presented, and that the use of video tapes in laboratory classes is not entirely satisfactory. The content and management of the laboratory classes are of particular concern, since they provide the opportunity for students to participate and to gain a "feel" for the discipline. It is an unfortunate fact that no lectures are presented in the pharmacology course on anthelmintic drugs.

CLINICAL PHARMACOLOGY
Clinical pharmacology is an elective course in which an emphasis is placed on drug therapy of diseases in the companion animal species (such as horses, dogs, and cats). This course is offered in the winter quarter of the third year of the veterinary curriculum. Clinical specialists in microbiology and various aspects of internal medicine, and the hospital pharmacist make valuable contributions to this course, and it is largely their input that stimulates constructive discussion regarding the basis for selection and effective dosage of drug preparations in the treatment of disease conditions.

VETERINARY TOXICOLOGY
Veterinary toxicology, which is offered in the spring quarter of the third year, is a component of the core

Table 6.2 Required coursework for MS and PhD degrees

Courses	Quarter units

Core course block

Principles of Pharmacology and Toxicology :

    I. Concepts, fate processes,
       kinetics-dynamics   5

   II. Effects of drugs and toxicants on
       body systems and organs (1); prin-
       ciples of chemotherapy and drug design   5

  III. Effects of drugs and toxicants on
       body systems and organs (2); develop-
       ment and regulation of drugs and
       chemicals   5

Pharmacology-Toxicology seminar   1

Elective course blocks

Experimental statistics   2

Molecular, physiological, and/or morphological
sciences   5

Advanced graduate courses in pharmacology and/or
toxicology   8

Non-block elective courses

Proficiency in one foreign language (French, German, Spa-
nish, or Russian) is a requirement for the PhD degree

Research project for MS/PhD thesis
----

curriculum. This course is largely of an applied nature,
since knowledge of the basic principles of toxicology is
assumed and were presented in veterinary pharmacology.
Since the students are involved in clinical activities at
this stage of the curriculum, there is much less need for
providing laboratory classes in toxicology compared with

their requirement in basic pharmacology. A single 4 h session is provided for small groups of students in the Diagnostic and Clinical Toxicology Laboratory. The purpose of this session is to familiarize the students with the range of service offered by the laboratory, the types of specimens that should be submitted for chemical analysis, and by reviewing selected cases the scope of toxicology will be seen in perspective.

PHARMACOLOGY-TOXICOLOGY GRADUATE PROGRAMME

At UC Davis we have an integrated pharmacology-toxicology graduate programme in which there are 40 faculty members and 45 graduate students. The majority of the graduate faculty is based in one of the three member departments of the programme. These departments are Human Pharmacology (School of Medicine), Environmental Toxicology (College of Agricultural and Environmental Sciences), and Veterinary Pharmacology and Toxicology (School of Veterinary Medicine).

In the autumn quarter of this year (September 1985) a new core curriculum will be introduced into the graduate programme (Table 6.2).

The Principles of Pharmacology and Toxicology is a three-quarter sequence of courses. In each quarter there will be 30 lectures, ten discussion periods, and ten laboratory exercises/demonstrations, which make up five units.

This structured graduate programme provides advanced coursework in both pharmacology and toxicology and the opportunity to conduct research in a variety of specialized areas, including veterinary pharmacology and toxicology.

References
1. Alexander, F. (1960). An Introduction to Veterinary Pharmacology. Edinburgh: E. & S. Livingstone. Presently in 3rd edition (1976). Edinburgh: Churchill Livingstone.
2. Baggot, J.D. (1977). Principles of Drug Disposition in Domestic Animals : The Basis of Veterinary Clinical

Pharmacology. Philadelphia: W.B. Saunders Co.
3. Clarke, E.G.C. and Clarke, M.L. (1975). Veterinary
   Toxicology. London: Bailliere Tindall. Presently in 2nd
   edition (1981), Clarke, M.L., Harvey, D.G. and Hum-
   phreys, D.J. (eds). London: Bailliere Tindall.
4. Hoare, W. (1895). Veterinary Materia Medica and Therapeutics. Sixth edition (1942), edited and revised by
   J. Russell Greig and G.F. Boddie. London: Bailliere,
   Tindall and Cox.
5. Jones, L. Meyer (1954). Veterinary Pharmacology and
   Therapeutics. Ames, Iowa: The Iowa State University
   Press. Presently in 5th edition (1982), Booth, N.H. and
   McDonald, L.E. (eds). Ames, Iowa: The Iowa State
   University Press.
6. Rasmussen, F. (1958). Mammary excretion of sulphonamides. Acta Pharmacol. Toxicol. 15:139-148.
7. Rasmussen, F. (1966). Studies on the Mammary Excretion
   and Absorption of Drugs. Copenhagen: Carl Fr. Morten-
   sen.

Drug Delivery Systems and Bioavailability

7
Design and evaluation of studies on drug delivery systems

A. VAN PEER AND J. HEYKANTS

ABSTRACT

The definition of bioavailability and acceptable procedures to determine bioavailability of drug delivery systems are considered in this chapter. Pharmacokinetic methods to estimate the rate and extent of absorption by drug concentration measurements in plasma and urine are discussed. Principles relevant to the design, statistical analysis and clinical interpretation of bioavailability studies are reviewed.

INTRODUCTION

In the 1970's it was recognized that bioavailability could present practical problems both in safety and effectiveness of drug usage. As a consequence, guidelines and requirements for the design and execution of studies on drug delivery systems were issued by regulatory authorities, first for drugs intended for use in humans[1] and later for drugs to be used in veterinary medicine[2].

DEFINITIONS

The American Food and Drug Administration (FDA) defines bioavailability as "the rate and extent to which the active drug ingredient or therapeutic moiety is absorbed from a drug product and becomes available at the site of action"[1]. Various types of bioavailability experiments exist, such as absolute and relative bioavailability and bioequivalence studies. Common to all studies is the comparative component that is the evaluation of test product(s) versus a reference preparation. The reference in an absolute bioavailability study is intravenous administration of the drug(s) in solution whereas it may be a solution or an approved drug product in a relative bioavailability study. The latter is used to determine the bioequivalence between products. The objective then is to demonstrate that the bioavailability of, for example, a solid dosage form and a solution does not differ significantly, or does not differ more than a certain degree, usually 20%.

PHARMACOKINETIC APPROACH
In practice, all bioavailability studies are based on plasma concentration or urinary excretion-time profiles.

Most studies on drug delivery systems involve a single-dose comparison of the test product(s) and the reference, although multiple-dose steady-state studies may be considered when plasma or urine concentrations are too low for accurate measurement. Other reasons for a study at steady-state are : comparison of a sustained-release formulation to a conventional-release product, or to overcome excessive variability in absorption by dosing drugs admixed with food.

RATE OF ABSORPTION
Methods of estimating absorption rates have serious limitations and depend on the size and choice of sufficient sampling points in the absorption phase. This is why urinary excretion profiles do not allow efficient estimation of this parameter. The easiest approach is the determination of the time to reach the maximal plasma concentration (T_{max}) and the peak concentration (C_{max}) by visual inspection of the plasma concentration-time curve. Other methods are tedious, often complicated and require

time-consuming   curve-fitting.   Examples   are   the
deconvolution methods of Wagner and Nelson and Loo and
Riegelman and direct curve-fitting to well-established
pharmacokinetic models[4]. Moment analysis is a new
approach to absorption, and is simply based on
calculations of the area under the plasma concentration
time-curve[7].

EXTENT OF ABSORPTION

The extent of absorption (F) is expressed as the ratio of
the total area under the plasma concentration-time curve
(AUC) of the test product to that of the reference
product, or as the ratio of the total amount of parent
drug excreted in urine (U), corrected for dose. To
calculate total AUC and U in single-dose studies, plasma
concentrations and urinary excretion should be determined
for at least three to four times the terminal elimination
half-life $(t_{1/2})$. In multiple-dose studies, pre-dose
plasma concentrations on three or more consecutive days
are measured first to establish steady-state, then
comparison of the AUC in a dosing interval gives the
bioavailability of test to the reference product. The
cumulative amount excreted in urine during a dosing
interval at steady-state may also be used.

DESIGN OF BIOAVAILABILITY STUDIES

Crossover design is, in general, preferred because each
animal is subjected to all formulations or drug products
(treatments) and serves as its own control[3]. The simplest
design is the two-way crossover with two treatments (test
and reference product), two periods and two equal groups
of a sufficient number of animals. Assignment of three or
more treatments can occur according to a series of Latin
squares.

    Another type of crossover design is the balanced
incomplete block, where each animal receives a fraction of
the treatments rather than all. When it is impossible to
retain any crossover, a parallel design can be chosen

where each animal receives a single treatment, either test or reference. The latter types of study are considered as valid alternatives when there are extended washout periods in the crossover design, or when frequent sampling of blood or urine is impossible in the target animal species.

In whatever design, a proper number of animals should be studied in order to detect a significant difference of 20% between products at an alpha = 0.05 and power = 0.80 (Power test).

STATISTICAL ANALYSIS

Analysis of variance (ANOVA) on bioavailability data has advantages above simple paired tests. ANOVA enables the exclusion of important sources of variability such as individual differences and effects of periods, groups, sex, etc. from the residual error. However, ANOVA merely indicates whether there are or are not significant differences among treatment averages. Therefore multiple range tests, such as Fisher's least significant difference test, are used to compare a posteriori any pair of treatments for statistical difference. Bioavailability decisions by ANOVA are based on accepting or rejecting the null hypothesis of equivalence between test and reference product. This may result in demonstrating inequivalence of treatments, whereas clinically the difference is small and acceptable (for example, 5%). To overcome these problems, alternative approaches were developed, such as Bayesian methods[3], and parametric and nonparametric confidence intervals [5,6].

CONCLUSIONS

The objective of a bioavailability study is to compare the rate and extent of absorption of an active drug given by different routes or products, and to ensure clinical effectiveness. An appropriate design and reliable pharmacokinetic parameters and statistics are needed to demonstrate bioequivalence of products in the target animal species. However, it is obvious that decisions cannot be based solely on selected pharmacokinetic parameters and pure statistics. The bioavailability approach does not necessarily establish a comparable depletion profile in residues, and there are also economic aspects in product selection, such as cost/benefit considerations and use of convenient drug delivery systems.

References
1. American Food and Drug Administration (1977). Bio-availability and bioequivalence requirements. Fed. Reg. 42:1624-1653.
2. American Food and Drug Administration (1982). Bio-equivalence study guideline. Bureau of Veterinary Medicine.
3. Cochran, W.G. and Cox, G.M. (1957). Experimental Designs, 2nd ed. New York: Wiley.
4. Gibaldi, M. and Perrier, D. (1982). Pharmacokinetics, 2nd ed. New York: Marcel Dekker.
5. Metzler, C.M. and Huang, D.C. (1983). Statistical methods for bioavailability and bioequivalence. Clin. Res. Pract. Drug Reg. Affairs 1:109-132.
6. Steinijans, V.W. and Diletti, E. (1983). Statistical analysis of bioavailability studies : parametric and nonparametric confidence intervals. Eur. J. Clin. Pharmacol. 24:127-136.
7. Yamaoka, K., Nakagawa, T. and Uno, T. (1978). Statis-tical moments in pharmacokinetics. J. Pharmacokin. Biopharm. 6:547-558.

8
Potential of new drug delivery systems in veterinary medicine

D. D. BREIMER

ABSTRACT

New drug delivery systems are characterized by rate-controlled drug release in vivo, which is predictable on the basis of the in vitro release profile. They are capable of producing relatively constant drug concentrations in the body for long periods of time and this may be desirable for many drugs. This is discussed in terms of pharmacokinetic/pharmacodynamic relationships. The potential advantages of rate-controlled drug delivery systems are reviewed, and their use as research tools in pharmacology and toxicology (for example osmotic pumps) is described. The extent of application in animal health care is very much dependent on economic benefit; some examples are given of rumen delivery systems and injectable or implantable systems. The major areas of application include therapy with antibiotic and parasitic agents, the long-term delivery of anthelmintic and/or antibacterial agents for growth promotion, the delivery of hormones to achieve accelerated growth or oestrus synchronization and the long-term administration of trace nutrients.

INTRODUCTION

New drug delivery systems as used in the terminology of

75

this chapter are defined and characterized by rate-controlled drug release in vivo, which is predictable on the basis of the release profile in vitro. There are four principal elements that such systems consist of: a drug reservoir, a rate-controlled device, an energy source that makes the drug leave the system, and a delivery portal or exit. They are often capable of producing relatively constant drug concentrations in plasma or at other sites in the body for long periods of time, whereas conventional dosage forms give rise to far greater fluctuations (peak and valley) in concentration-time profiles. Such new systems have recently been introduced into human clinical practice, for example : infusion pumps (portable or implantable), transdermal devices with nitroglycerine, scopolamine, clonidine or oestradiol, osmotic pump systems for oral therapy with beta-blocking agents, ocular systems for local therapy with pilocarpine, intrauterine systems containing progesterone, etc.[7,12]. Most of these systems have been designed on the premise that constant rate delivery is the desirable rate-programme, and that the longest duration consistent with reproducible (constant) bioavailability-rate is best to achieve optimal therapy. In this chapter some pharmacokinetic/pharmacodynamic principles underlying this concept will be given, although it should be realized that this will not be valid for all drugs or hormones. Subsequently, the potential advantages of rate-controlled drug delivery systems will be discussed as related to both therapeutic practice and research and finally their potential use in veterinary medicine will be outlined.

THEORETICAL CONSIDERATIONS

Rational therapeutic management of disease, both in animals and in man, usually requires that drugs are given for a certain period of time, during which the therapeutic effect is achieved and maintained in the absence of undesirable side-effects. Similar considerations apply in drug prevention of disease. For many drugs the intensity

of the pharmacological effect is related to their
concentration at the site of action (in the biophase near
the receptor) and in the plasma under steady-state
conditions. The therapeutic concentration range
(therapeutic window) is defined as the range above which
unacceptable or undesirable side-effects are encountered
(maximal safe concentration, MSC) and below which the
desired effect is generally not achieved (minimal
effective concentration, MEC). The ratio of these
concentrations is often defined as the therapeutic
concentration ratio or therapeutic index. During therapy
drug concentration should be continuously between MEC and
MSC. It has been shown that the various effects of a drug
(desirable and undesirable) may indeed be dissociated at
different serum concentrations[11]. If this therapeutic
range is small, then a high degree of control over the
plasma concentration must be exerted to maintain the
concentration within this range. When a drug's
elimination half-life is long, this may be possible with
conventional dosage forms at dosage intervals of, for
instance, 1 day. In theory the following relationship
exists between the maximal dosage interval (Δt_{max}), elimination half-life ($t_{1/2el}$; first-order kinetics) and
the therapeutic concentration ratio (the fluctuation in
plasma concentrations should not be larger than this
ratio) :

$$\Delta t_{max} = 1.44 \times t_{1/2el} \times \ln \frac{MSC}{MEC}$$

When the elimination half-life is short, as is the case
for most drugs in many animal species, it is often
impossible or impractical to maintain relatively constant
plasma concentrations without the need of frequent
re-dosing. The latter is often very impractical or even
impossible in veterinary medicine. In such cases it is
desirable to apply rate-controlled input of the drug into
the plasma to compensate for rapid elimination. The

frequency of dosing by systems with such characteristics is, in principle, independent of the kinetics of the drugs, but will depend on factors like transit through the gastrointestinal tract (oral systems), capacity of the system, lifetime of the system, etc. Thereby the duration of action of the drug becomes a design property of the rate-controlled dosage form.

POTENTIAL ADVANTAGES OF RATE-CONTROLLED DRUG DELIVERY SYSTEMS

The advantages of new drug delivery systems with a defined rate of release may be summarized as follows[21] :

(1) Release of drug in vivo is predictable from in vitro test methods and is theoretically independent of the conditions applied in vitro, which in general is not possible with conventional dosage forms or "sustained release" dosage forms. Also the release in vivo is in principle independent of physiological conditions, such as pH, enzymatic environment, food, etc.

(2) The plasma and biophase concentrations of a drug are maintained constant and within the therapeutically desirable range with little fluctuation. Since there exists large variability in the rate of drug elimination between different animal species, it will be necessary to use different release rates in different species.

(3) The selectivity of drug action is optimized, that is, the number of undesirable side-effects in severity and incidence is minimized. The latter may, for instance, be associated particularly with peak levels of conventional dosage forms or a rapid change of plasma concentration.

(4) Predictable and extended duration of drug action is provided.

(5) The inconvenience of repetitive dosing is avoided.

(6) In a single delivery system, the combination of

drugs that have complementary therapeutic actions
but are pharmacokinetically dissimilar, are
rationalized by releasing each drug at its
respective optimum rate for the same period of
time.

(7) The drug systems may be used as research tools in
pharmacology and toxicology : to study in vivo
dose (concentration) response relationships[19]; in
drug toxicity testing[13]; to study certain
time-dependent pharmacodynamic or pharmacokinetic
phenomena, like the development of tolerance or
adaptation, drug-drug interactions, circadian
variation, etc.[3].

The most widely applied drug delivery systems in such
studies are based upon the osmotic pump principle, which
was described almost 10 years ago by Theeuwes and Yum[20].
The systems consist of a flexible drug reservoir which is
surrounded by a sealed osmotic agent with an outer
semipermeable membrane. The osmotic agent imbibes water
and generates a hydrostatic pressure on the flexible
membrane of the reservoir, thereby displacing the drug
solution or suspension through the orifice at zero-order
rate. These systems, which are developed by ALZA (Palo
Alto, California), are available with 0.2 and 2.0 ml
reservoirs and total delivery times between 8 h and 2
weeks. They are widely used as implanted drug delivery
devices in laboratory animals and have thereby opened
novel and previously impractical methods, protocols and
models in drug and hormone research[22]. Also for human
drug research the systems are suitable and may be applied
orally (0.2 ml systems) or rectally (2.0 ml systems)[4,10].

APPLICATIONS OF NEW DRUG DELIVERY SYSTEMS IN VETERINARY
MEDICINE
Recently the potential uses and opportunities of new drug
delivery systems in veterinary medicine have been reviewed
and it was emphasized that there are numerous potential

applications in the entire field of animal health care[6]. Relative to the development of devices (systems) for human use, several differences exist for veterinary application. These include the direct testing and use in the target animal species, the lack of concern relative to cosmetic considerations, the latitude in device design and the fact that the devices need not necessarily biodegrade or be removed upon complete release of drug. Furthermore, many situations exist in which controlled release drug delivery for longer periods of time may be the only rational method to give a drug, for example, in grazing animals. In principle, the same theoretical considerations apply for the use of and the potentials of new drug delivery systems in animals as compared to man. However, economic considerations also play a very important role in the field of animal health care. Therefore the range of therapeutic applications of new systems is likely to be limited to those diseases which lead to an economic loss for the grower and/or to an application in which a cost-effective accelerated growth of the animal is achieved. These include the therapeutic delivery of antibiotic and parasitic drugs, the long-term delivery of anthelmintic and antibacterial drugs for growth promotion, the delivery of hormones to achieve accelerated growth and the long-term delivery of trace nutrients (copper, zinc, cobalt, selenium, vitamins, aminoacids)[6]. In most cases, systems exhibiting a very long duration of drug delivery are required, which limits their use to relatively potent drugs. Some examples of systems which either have reached the market place or are still in the research phase are reviewed briefly.

Rumen delivery systems
The rumen of cattle has proved to be a suitable place to keep drug delivery devices for longer periods of time, provided that a suitable method is found to prevent the device from either being regurgitated or from moving through the remainder of the gastrointestinal tract. This

can be accomplished via either weight or geometry. It has been suggested that a density of about 1.8 is required for retention in the rumen, whereas with a density greater than 2.2 the devices are retained in the reticulum[17]. Similar information on the geometry effects on retention is not available but it seems likely that if the system opens to a diameter which is much greater than that of the oesophagus, then regurgitation should not be a problem. An example of a slowly eroding device with high density has been used by Byford, River and Hair[5] for the long-term delivery of oxytetracycline. This consists of drug, carnuba wax, barium sulphate, polyethylene glycol (PEG) and iron powder and produces a relatively constant release rate for about 50 days. A second example is exemplified by morantel tartrate as administered in a metal cylinder[13]. The ends of the cylinder are capped with two microporous sintered polyethylene discs impregnated with a hydrogel to achieve overall rate control. The device is to be administered at the beginning of the growing season to young cattle upon their first exposure to the field. Depending on the degree of contamination of the field, treated animals may gain about 50 kg or more weight during their first year of growth as compared to controls[2,16]. In the patent literature information is available on a number of devices which were designed to utilize geometry as the retention mechanism. One consists of a cylinder which contains the drug in an erodible core matrix; retention is accomplished via two polyethylene "wings" which fold against the device during insertion, but open upon passage from the oesophagus[18].

Another example of a delivery system of this category is represented by soluble glass containing trace elements (copper, cobalt, and selenium)[1]. Systems can be produced which have an effective lifetime of 1 year and are capable of preventing trace element deficiencies in cattle and sheep.

Injectable or implantable systems

A number of products containing steroidal hormones to achieve growth promotion in cattle are currently used as implants (oestradiol, progesterone, testosterone and/or their esters, either alone or in combination)[14]. Detailed information on the system design is generally not available, but dispersion of drugs into a polymer matrix and the use of coatings to achieve further rate control seem to be a common design property.

Implants are also used for the synchronization of oestrus. The burden of oestrus detection would be greatly relieved and the rate of conception substantially increased if an effective oestrus synchronization treatment could be developed which produces a sexual response so precise that artificial insemination can be carried out at a predetermined time schedule, without the need for oestrus detection in every animal. An example of a system successfully developed for this purpose has been described by Chien[8], which contains norgestomet in a suspension of solid particles in a hydrogel/water polymer. The same group also uses a flurogestone acetate-impregnated vaginal pessary to achieve oestrus synchronization in sheep[9].

CONCLUSIONS

There is considerable potential for new drug delivery systems in the entire field of animal health care, in particular when economic benefit of the treatment regimen can clearly be established. Therefore the major areas of application of such systems include therapy with antibiotic and parasitic agents, the long-term delivery of anthelmintic and/or antibacterial agents for growth promotion, the delivery of hormones to achieve accelerated growth or oestrus synchronization and the long-term administration of trace nutrients[6].

References
1. Algar. B., Irlam, P., Knott, P., Telfer, S. and
   Zervas, G. (1985). The use of soluble glasses to

provide a controlled supply of trace elements to ruminant animals. In: Peppas, N.A. and Haluska, R.J. (eds). Proceedings of the 12th International Symposium on Controlled Release of Bioactive Materials, pp.190-191. Lincolnshire: The Controlled Release Society Inc.

2. Borgsteed, F.H.M. (1983). The effects of morantel sustained release bolus system on calves grazing a highly contaminated pasture in The Netherlands. Vet. Parasitol. 12:251-260.

3. Breimer, D.D., De Leede, L.G.J. and De Boer, A.G. (1984). New drug delivery systems as tools in clinical pharmacology. In: Lemberger, L. and Reidenberg, M.M. (eds). Proceedings of the 2nd World Conference on Clinical Pharmacology and Therapeutics, pp.431-443. Washington: American Society for Pharmacology and Experimental Therapeutics.

4. Breimer, D.D., De Leede, L.G.J. and De Boer, A.G. (1985). Rate-controlled rectal drug delivery. In: Prescott, L.F. and Nimmo, W.S. (eds). Rate Control in Drug Therapy, pp.54-64. Edinburgh: Churchill Livingstone.

5. Byford, R.L., River, J.L. and Hair, J.A. (1981). A sustained release oxytetracycline bolus for ruminants. Bovine Pract. 15:91-94.

6. Cardinal, J. (1985). Controlled drug delivery : veterinary applications. J. Controlled Release 2:393-403.

7. Chien, Y.W. (1982). Novel Drug Delivery Systems. New York: Marcel Dekker.

8. Chien, Y.W. (1985). Implants and depot formulations : subcutaneous controlled oestrus synchronization. In: Prescott, L.F. and Nimmo, W.S. (eds). Rate Control in Drug Therapy, pp.90-102. Edinburgh: Churchill Livingstone.

9. Chien, Y.W. and Kabadi, M.B. (1985). Intravaginal controlled oestrus synchronisation. (II) Intravaginal delivery of flurogestone acetate, in vitro - in vivo correlation and clinical efficacy. In: Peppas, N.A. and Haluska, R.J. (eds). Proceedings of the 12th International Symposium on Controlled Release of Bioactive Materials, pp.353-354. Lincolnshire: The Controlled Release Society Inc.

10. Davis, S.S., Hardy, J.G., Taylor, M.J., Stockwell, A., Whalley, D.R. and Wilson, C.G. (1984). The in vivo evaluation of an osmotic device (OSMET) using gamma scintigraphy. J. Pharm. Pharmacol. 16:740-742.

11. Goldman, P. (1982). Rate-controlled drug delivery. New Engl. J. Med. 307:286-290.

12. Heilman, K. (1982). Therapeutische Systeme. Konzept und Realisation programmierter Arzneiverabreichung, 2nd ed. Stuttgart: Enke Verlag.

13. Jones, R.M. (1983). Therapeutic and prophylactic efficacy of morantel when administered directly into the rumen of cattle on a continuous basis. Vet. Parasitol. 12:223-232.

14. Lambert, S.B. and Davis, G.V. (1983). The effects of Compudose, Ralgro and Synovex-S implants on performance of finishing yearling steers. J. Animal Sci. 57 (Suppl. I), 399.
15. Nau, H. (1983). The role of delivery systems in toxicology and drug development. Pharm. Intern. 4:228-231.
16. Prost, H., Supperer, R., Jones, R.M., Lockwood, P.W. and Bliss, D.H. (1983). Morantel sustained release bolus : a new approach for the control of Trichostrongylosis in Austrian cattle. Vet. Parasitol. 12:239-250.
17. River, J.L., Byford, R.L., Stratton, L.G. and Hair, J.A. (1982). Influence of density and location on degradation of sustained release boluses given to cattle. Am. J. Vet. Res. 43:2023-2030.
18. Simpson, B.E. (1983). Sustained release capsule for ruminants. U.S. Patent 4.416.659.
19. Struyker Boudier, H.A.J. (1982). Rate-controlled drug delivery : pharmacological, therapeutic and industrial perspective. Trends Pharmacol. Sci. 3:162-164.
20. Theeuwes, F. and Yum, S.I. (1976). Principles of the design and operation of generic osmotic pumps for the delivery of semisolid or liquid formulations. Ann. Biomed. Eng. 4:343-353.
21. Urquhart, J. (1981). Performance requirement for controlled-release dosage forms : therapeutic and pharmacological perspective. In: Urquhart, J. (ed.). Controlled-Release Pharmaceuticals, pp.1-48. Washington: American Pharmaceutical Association.
22. Urquhart, J., Fara, J. and Willis, K.L. (1984). Rate-controlled delivery systems in drug and hormone research. Ann. Rev. Pharmacol. Toxicol. 24:199-236.

9
Influence of injection site on the depot effect of procaine penicillin in dogs

E. G. HARTMAN

ABSTRACT

The influence of the site and route of injection on the depot effect of procaine penicillin in dogs was investigated. The drug was administered either intramuscularly (M. longissimus dorsi, M. semitendineus/M. gracilis, M. gluteus medius) or subcutaneously (lateral thorax and neck). The depot effect (> 0.1 IU/ml of serum at 24 h) was found in a higher percentage of cases following injection into the M. longissimus dorsi (77%), than following injection into the other intramuscular sites (33% and 20%, respectively). The probability of a depot effect was highest following subcutaneous injection in the lateral thorax region, whereas subcutaneous injection in the neck resulted in a depot effect in 60% of the cases.

INTRODUCTION

Recent studies both in man and animals have indicated that, in many instances, differences in absorption rates from various intramuscular and subcutaneous tissue sites may be significant[2,3,5-7]. In canine practice penicillin is administered most commonly either intramuscularly in the thigh or subcutaneously in the lateral thorax or neck. Pharmacokinetic properties of new formulations of antimicrobial drugs for dogs need to be tested in the same

animal species before being licensed. However, no
directions are provided with respect to the route and site
of administration.

The aim of the present study was to investigate the
possible influence of the site and route of parenteral
administration on the absorption rate, and the depot
effect achieved with procaine penicillin.

MATERIALS AND METHODS
Adult beagles of either sex weighing 15-20 kg were
injected with a suspension of procaine benzylpenicillin
(Depocillin, Gist-Brocades, The Netherlands) at a dose
rate of 1 ml per 10 kg body weight, which is equivalent to
30,000 IU procaine penicillin per kg body weight.

The sites used were either intramuscular (M.
longissimus dorsi, M. gracilis/M. semitendineus, M.
gluteus medius) or subcutaneous (lateral thorax and the
neck region). The subcutaneous injection sites were
chosen as these are commonly used in veterinary practice,
as is intramuscular injection into the thigh region (M.
semitendineus/M. gracilis). Intramuscular injection into
the M. gluteus medius was chosen as an alternative to
injection into the thigh region, as the latter might
result in an intermuscular injection. Injection into the
M. longissimus dorsi was expected to be intramuscular as
this muscle consists of a solid, easily accessible, muscle
mass. Injection into the M. gluteus medius was chosen
because this site is often used in humans. Blood samples
were drawn from the cephalic vein at 2, 4, 6, 8, 12 and
24 h. Blood was allowed to clot and the serum removed by
centrifugation. Serum was analysed for penicillin by an
agar diffusion technique using plate count agar (Oxoid)
and Bacillus stearothermophilus var. calidolactis as assay
organism[1]. The course of the serum penicillin
concentration in each individual animal was classified
tentatively in one of four groups as follows :

Level (IU) at :	12 h	24 h	group
	> 0.5	> 0.5	1A
	> 0.5	> 0.1	1B
	> 0.5	< 0.1	2A
	< 0.5	< 0.1	2B

RESULTS

Four different patterns of mean serum penicillin curves following intramuscular and subcutaneous injection are depicted in Figure 9.1. These curves are the mean of the individual serum penicillin curves classified as described above. Intramuscular and subcutaneous administration of procaine penicillin resulted in similar types of mean serum penicillin curves.

In Table 9.1 the classification of the course of the serum penicillin concentration is presented according to

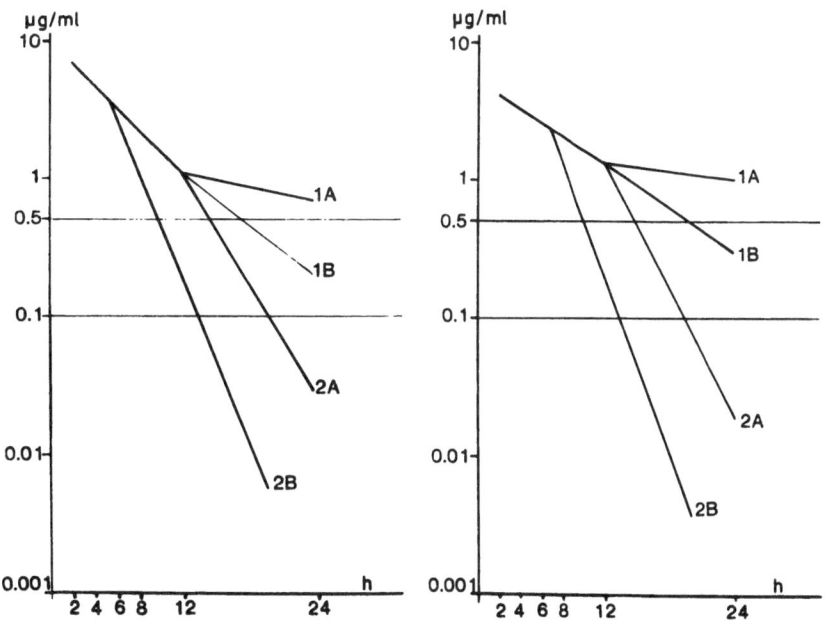

Figure 9.1 Patterns of mean serum penicillin curves following intramuscular (left panel) and subcutaneous (right panel) administration.

Table 9.1   Classification of the course of the serum
penicillin concentration according to the site of
injection

| Injection site | Classification group | | | |
	1A	1B	2A	2B
M. longissimus dorsi	3	7	2	1
M. gracilis/M. semitendineus	–	5	6	4
M. gluteus medius	1	–	2	2
Lateral thorax	9	1	1	–
Neck	2	4	3	1

Table 9.2   Depot effect (> 0.1 IU at 24 h) of procaine
penicillin, expressed as the probability in percentages,
depending on the site and route of injection

Route	Site	Percentage (%)
Intramuscular	M. longissimus dorsi	77
	M. gracilis/M. semi-tendineus	33
	M. gluteus medius	20
Subcutaneous	Lateral thorax	91
	Neck	60

----

the site of injection and the corresponding number of
animals.

The probability of a high serum concentration (above
0.1 IU/ml) at 24 h following administration was
determined by comparing group 1A plus 1B with group 2A
plus 2B. The results according to the different injection
sites and routes are given in Table 9.2.

As procaine penicillin preparations are expected to
produce a depot effect, the best sites of injection are
either subcutaneous in the lateral thorax region or

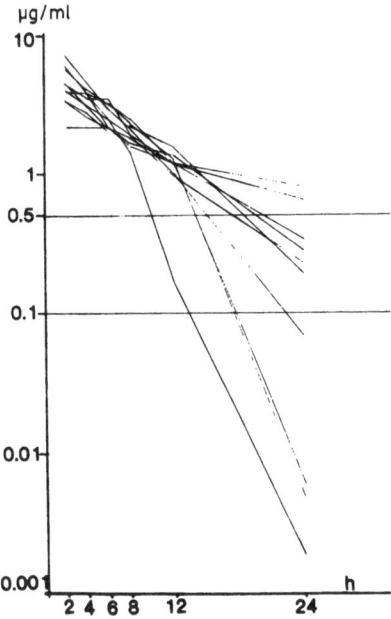

Figure 9.2 Variation of individual curves following subcutaneous injection at the same injection site (neck).

intramuscularly into the M. longissimus dorsi.

DISCUSSION

Procaine penicillin is a poorly water-soluble salt of
penicillin and is for this reason used in depot
preparations with the purpose of obtaining higher serum
levels for an extended period of time. Absorption from
the injection site will depend not only on the solubility
of the compound in water but also on factors such as the
structure of the tissue at the site of injection, blood
flow and spreading of the injected mass which will affect
surface area presented for absorption, as was demonstrated
in several mammalian species including man[4]. The results
obtained in this study indicate that the release of active
substance from the injection depot into the blood stream
may vary considerably.

The M. longissimus dorsi was chosen to enhance the
probability that the injection would be correctly

intramuscular. The other intramuscular sites were expected to give a greater chance of an intermuscular injection. Indeed a depot effect was found in a higher percentage of cases after an injection into the M. longissimus dorsi, thus supporting the conclusion of Palmer[3,6], that there will be a difference in absorption rate following intramuscular and intermuscular injection.

The rapid absorption of penicillin from the thigh and the M. gluteus medius, however, might also be attributable to the contraction of these muscles during exercise. The more pronounced depot effect following injection into the M. longissimus dorsi could be the result of the different activity of this muscle, which is almost restricted to a variation in tension rather than the large contractions seen with limb muscles.

The difference between the neck and the lateral thorax might also be the result of exercise, as the subcutaneous region of the neck will be massaged more intensively during exercise than the lateral thorax at which site movement is almost restricted to excursions of the thoracic wall resulting from breathing. However, the cause of the variation of the individual curves following subcutaneous injection in the neck (Figure 9.2) remains to be established.

CONCLUSION
This study emphasizes that more attention should be paid to the actual sites of injection of drugs. If, as described here, a depot effect is desired the best site for intramuscular injection of procaine penicillin is the M. longissimus dorsi, and for subcutaneous application the lateral thorax site is preferred.

Acknowledgements
The author wishes to express his gratitude to Dr R. Beukers for technical advice and assistance in preparing this paper. Mrs E.C. Bakker-de Koff and Mrs. H.G. van Laar are gratefully acknowledged for their excellent

technical assistance.

References
1. Galesloot, T. and Hassing, F. (1962). A rapid and sensitive paper disc method for the detection of penicillin in milk. Neth. Milk Dairy J. 16:93-95.
2. Groothuis, D.G. and Van Miert, A.S.J.P.A.M. (1979).
   Diergeneesmiddelen en extravasculaire injecties.
   Tijdschr. Diergeneesk. 104:886-887.
3. Groothuis, D.G., Werdler, M.E.B., Van Miert, A.S.J.P.A.
   M. and Van Duin, C.T.M. (1980). Factors affecting the
   absorption of ampicillin administered intramuscularly
   in dwarf goats. Res. Vet. Sci. 29:116-117.
4. MacDiarmid, S.C. (1983). The absorption of drugs from
   subcutaneous and intramuscular injection sites. Vet.
   Bull. 53:9-21.
5. Marshall, A.B. and Palmer, G.H. (1980). Injection
   sites and drug bioavailability. In: Van Miert, A.S.J.
   P.A.M. et al. (eds). Trends in Veterinary Pharmacology and Toxicology, pp.54-60. Amsterdam: Elsevier.
6. Palmer, G.H. (1980). Effect of injection site on bioavailability of aminopenicillins in calves. In: Van
   Miert, A.S.J.P.A.M. et al. (eds). Trends in Veterinary Pharmacology and Toxicology, pp.337-338. Amsterdam: Elsevier.
7. Rutgers, L.J.E., Van Miert, A.S.J.P.A.M., Nouws, J.F.M.
   and Van Ginneken, C.A.M. (1980). Effect of the injection site on the bioavailability of amoxycillin tri-
   hydrate in dairy cows. J. Vet. Pharmacol. Ther.
   3:125-132.

10
Influence of food on absorption of antimicrobial drugs

A. D. J. WATSON

ABSTRACT

Interactions between food and drugs affecting drug absorption are widely recognized in human medicine but have received little attention in the veterinary sphere. The most common outcome of these interactions is reduced or delayed absorption of the drug, although in some instances absorption can be increased or unaffected. The mechanisms responsible are complex and involve both food-induced changes in gut physiology and direct interactions between food components and drugs. The clinical significance of interactions affecting antimicrobial drugs is uncertain. However, impaired absorption is more likely to hinder antimicrobial efficacy than to help it. Accordingly, it seems prudent to fast patients for 2 hours before and 2 hours after administration of those agents whose absorption can be impaired substantially by food, namely most penicillins and tetracyclines, some cephalosporins and certain erythromycin products. A few antimicrobial drugs may not require food restriction (chloramphenicol, erythromycin estolate, hetacillin) and some could be given with food to improve absorption (erythromycin esters, griseofulvin, nitrofurantoin) or reduce gastric irritation associated with dosage (doxycycline, metronidazole. nitrofurantoin).

INTRODUCTION

There is now extensive evidence that the presence of food in the gastrointestinal tract, and particularly in the stomach, can have a profound effect on the absorption of drugs administered by mouth. These effects can result from physiological changes in the gut and from direct physical or chemical interactions between drugs and ingesta. In many cases the mechanism by which food affects the availability of a particular drug is not known precisely, as the various changes induced by food can interact in complex ways.

The interplay of possible effects in man was reviewed by Welling and Tse[12] in the following way. Large fluid volumes tend to increase gastric emptying rate, but solid food has the opposite effect. As most drugs are absorbed mainly in the small intestine, delayed gastric emptying may reduce the rate of drug absorption, and also reduce the efficiency of absorption of drugs which are unstable at low pH. Conversely, prolonged retention in the stomach may enhance the percentage of drug in solution when it eventually passes into the small intestine, thereby enhancing absorption efficiency. For drugs which are absorbed by active and saturable processes, slow stomach emptying may increase the efficiency of absorption due to non-saturation of carrier mechanisms. Large fluid volumes and meals with high fluid content tend to increase the rate and efficiency of drug absorption, apparently related to increased dissolution and faster stomach emptying. The increase in intestinal motility induced by ingesta may aid drug absorption because of faster dissolution and greater exposure of drug to the intestinal epithelium, but it could also reduce absorption because of a quicker transit time. Theoretically, an increase in splanchnic blood flow associated with eating could also influence drug absorption.

Furthermore, the ingestion of food causes increases in gastrointestinal secretions, such as hydrochloric acid, bile and digestive enzymes, which could also influence drug absorption[12]. Gastric acid tends to accelerate dissolution and absorption of basic drugs but causes degradation of acid-labile compounds. Bile secretion may aid dissolution of compounds having poor aqueous solubility and enhance dissolution of waxy drug matrices and lipoidal coatings, causing faster drug absorption. However, bile salts may reduce availability of drugs such as kanamycin and polymyxin through complexation. Proteolytic enzymes will degrade peptide molecules, while esterases of the intestinal lumen and epithelial lining are capable of hydrolysing esterified drug forms.

In addition, direct interactions between drugs and food components can also occur[12]. Food can act as a physical barrier which limits drug access to the absorptive surface of the mucosa. Also, complexing of drugs with certain polyvalent cations or protein can reduce absorption.

The form in which the drug is given can also have an effect on the outcome of a particular food-drug interaction[12]. In general, solutions and suspensions might be less susceptible than solid dosage forms to the effects of ingesta because they are mobile in the gut and pass with relative ease from stomach to intestine. Enteric-coated tablets could be particularly susceptible to food interactions because the presence of food may cause them to remain intact in the stomach for prolonged periods.

HUMAN FINDINGS

Studies in man have shown that the effect of food on drug absorption is dependent upon the type and size of the meal, the chemical and physical form of the drug, the dosage form, and the time relation between eating and drug administration[12]. The outcome of any such interaction is difficult to predict, and, considering the variety of possible effects involved, it is not surprising that simple rules governing food-drug interactions have not been found.

Three possible outcomes of interaction between food and orally administered drugs have been identified : drug absorption may be increased, not affected, or decreased[11,12]. The "decreased" category can be subdivided into those interactions where drug absorption is reduced and those in which absorption is delayed.

With antimicrobial drugs, interactions with food most commonly produce reduced or delayed absorption (Table 10.1). Reduced absorption occurs with most of the penicillins and tetracyclines, although other types of interaction are also seen sometimes with certain penicillins. Most oral formulations of cephalosporins and sulphonamides generally exhibit delayed absorption, in which the rate of absorption is slowed but the overall absorption efficiency is unaffected, as assessed by the area under the curve of plasma drug concentration plotted against time or from urinary excretion data.

By contrast, few food-drug interactions have been reported to increase the systemic availability of antimicrobial drugs or to have no appreciable effect (Table 10.2). Note that amoxycillin availability has been reported variously to be reduced, delayed and unaffected by food (Tables 10.1 and 10.2). This illustrates the complexity of the problem and the undesirability of making general recommendations on the basis of a single study.

Erythromycin is considered separately (Table 10.3) because of the variety of food-drug interactions reported with different erythromycin formulations. As erythromycin base is unstable at low pH, various oral formulations have been developed to improve stability and increase absorption. This has involved formulation of erythromycin base or its salts in tablets with acid-resistant coatings, and the development of relatively acid-stable forms such as the estolate and ethylsuccinate esters of erythromycin. The general picture with erythromycin products is that the coated formulations of erythromycin base are affected to only a small extent by food, the absorption of erythromycine stearate is reduced in most cases (but may increase

when   given   before   meals)   and   the   availability   of
erythromycin esters tends to be improved by concomitant
food intake[12].

Table 10.1 Antimicrobial agents whose systemic availability may be reduced or delayed by food after oral administration in man[*][+]

Reduced	Delayed
Amoxycillin cap, susp	Amoxycillin ns
Ampicillin cap	Cefaclor tab, susp
Cephalexin cap, susp	Cephalexin cap
Demethylchlortetracycline cap	Cephadrine cap
Doxycycline cap[+][+]	Metronidazole tab
Ketoconazole tab	Sulphadiazine susp
Lincomycin cap	Sulphadiazine (Na) sol
Methacycline cap	Sulphadimethoxine ns
Nafcillin tab	Sulphafurazole ns
Oxytetracycline cap	Sulphanilamide susp
Penicillin G tab, susp	Sulphamethoxypyridazine ns
Penicillin V (acid) tab	Sulphasymazine ns
Penicillin V (Ca) tab	
Penicillin V (K) tab, cap, susp	
Phenethicillin tab, cap	
Pivampicillin cap	
Rifampicin ns	
Tetracycline cap	

----

[*]Modified from references [11], [12] and [13], which should be
 consulted for original sources.   Erythromycin data is
 presented separately in Table 10.3.
[+]Dosage forms as follows : cap = capsules, tab = tablets,
 susp = suspension, sol = solution, ns = not stated.
[+][+]Slightly reduced.

SOME VETERINARY DATA
Interactions with food affecting drug absorption are not

Table 10.2 Antimicrobial agents whose systemic availability may be not affected or increased by food after oral
administration in man[**]

Not affected   Increased

Amoxycillin cap   Griseofulvin ns
Ampicillin susp   Hetacillin cap[**]
Penicillin V (acid) tab   Nitrofurantoin tab, cap
Pivampicillin cap   Pivampicillin cap
Spiramycin tab   Sulphamethoxydiazine tab
Sulphaisodimidine tab

---

[*]Modified   from   references[11,12]   and   [13],   which
 should be consulted for original   sources.   Erythromycin
 data is presented separately in Table 10.3.
[+]Dosage forms as follows : cap = capsules, tab = tablets,
 susp = suspension, ns = not stated.
[**]Slightly increased.

confined   to   human   therapy,   but   they   have   not   been
investigated thoroughly in species of veterinary interest.
Although   several   authors   have   suggested guidelines for
timing drug dosage in relation to food   intake   in   animal
patients[2,6,7]   their   proposals   have   been   based,   of
necessity, largely on human data.
    Chloramphenicol   is   one   drug   for   which   there   is
veterinary   information   without corresponding human data.
Chloramphenicol absorption appeared to be faster when   the
drug   was   given   in capsules to greyhounds fed ad libitum
but consumption of canned food immediately   before   dosing
did   not   affect   plasma drug concentrations[3,4].   In cats,
the availability of chloramphenicol from tablets   was   not
affected   by feeding ad libitum, or by administering water
with   the   tablet[5].   With   chloramphenicol   palmitate
suspension,   however,   drug   availability   was   poorer   in
fasted cats than in the same cats   when   fed   ad   libitum.
Thus these findings suggest that food does not impede (and

Table 10.3 Influence of food on systemic availability of erythromycin[*]

Compound	Dosage form	Effect
Erythromycin base	Capsules	Reduced
	Tablets	Reduced
	Coated tablets	Delayed or unaffected[+]
Erythromycin stearate	Coated tablets	Reduced[**]
Erythromycin estolate	Capsules	Increased
	Suspension	Unaffected
Erythromycin ethyl-carbonate	Suspension	Unaffected
Erythromycin ethyl-succinate	Coated tablets	Increased
	Film tablets	Delayed
	Suspension	Increased or unaffected

[*]Modified from reference[12], which should be consulted for original sources.

[+]Different effects reported by various workers, also reduced absorption in one report.

[**]Reduced absorption when administered after food, one report of improved bioavailability when given immediately before food.

may even enhance) the systemic availability of chloramphenicol from solid dosage forms, and that reduced bioavailability might occur with administration of chloramphenicol palmitate suspensions in fasting animals, at least in cats.

Data concerning interactions between food and amoxycillin are conflicting in dogs as in man. In

Table 10.4   Provisional suggestions on feeding and oral administration of antimicrobial drugs in small animals

---

Administer on an empty stomach*	Cephalosporins
	Erythromycin stearate
	Lincomycin
	Penicillins (except hetacillin)
	Sulphonamides (except sulpha-
	    isodimidine, sulphamethoxy-
	    diazine)
	Tetracyclines (except doxycy-
	    cline)

Food restriction not necessary	Chloramphenicol Erythromycin coated formulations Hetacillin Spiramycin Sulphaisodimidine Sulphamethoxydiazine
Possibly administer with food	Doxycycline+ Erythromycin esters Griseofulvin Metronidazole+ Nitrofurantoin+

---

*Administer at least 2 hours before or 2 hours after food.

+Drugs which are often irritant when taken on an empty stomach and whose absorption is not inhibited significantly by food, so should be given after food.

greyhounds, amoxycillin absorption seemed to be little affected by food, whether given as dry food ad libitum or as a single meal immediately before drug administration[10]. In recent experiments with dogs of various breeds, however, the absorption of amoxycillin was reduced and delayed when food was eaten just before drug dosage. The decrease in bioavailability was evident with both tablet and suspension formulations of amoxycillin and was of similar magnitude to that seen with ampicillin tablets[9]. Food-drug interactions causing reduced absorption of penicillin V, phenethicillin and cloxacillin were also demonstrated in this study.

THE TIME FACTOR

The effect of the time interval between food consumption and drug dosage has not been studied extensively. Welling and Tse[12] recommend giving those drugs whose absorption is reduced by food at least 1 hour before food whenever possible. On the other hand Welling[12] states that "if a drug is taken shortly before a meal, its absorption is likely to be either increased or unaffected". With post-prandial administration, the extent to which drug absorption is affected is said to be inversely proportional to the elapsed time between eating and dosing, being maximal when the drug is taken immediately after food and negligible when the drug is administered 2 hours after eating[13].

Experiments with penicillin V in children[1] and dogs[8] support the suggestion that a fasting period of 1-2 hours before, and 1-2 hours after, drug administration may be advisable for drugs at risk. In dogs, the systemic availability of penicillin V was reduced when food was given immediately before drug dosage, and there was a clear trend for availability to improve as the fasting period before and after dosing was increased. The optimum fasting period might depend on the animal, the drug, type of food and other factors; however, fasting for 2 hours before and 2 hours after drug administration seems a reasonable starting point and should be possible in most patients.

CLINICAL RELEVANCE

It is difficult to assess the clinical importance of food-drug interactions as studies comparing the clinical efficacy of antimicrobial therapy under fasting and non-fasting conditions have not been reported. This may be an area where veterinary and human clinical pharmacologists could cooperate usefully, as studies of this type could be difficult to perform in human patients.

Of main concern are interactions which reduce or delay drug absorption. When circulating drug concentrations are close to the minimum inhibitory concentration for the offending pathogen, then reduced absorption may well be clinically significant. Thus the risk of therapeutic failure may be high in these circumstances with drugs whose absorption is reduced markedly by food, such as most penicillins and tetracyclines, some cephalosporins, and some erythromycin products[12]. On the other hand, there might be little risk if the same drugs are given well in excess of requirements against susceptible microbes.

Absorption which is delayed but not reduced adversely affects tissue penetration by the drug and might be deleterious whenever immediate antimicrobial activity is required. In a few instances, however, delayed absorption might be advantageous, by permitting drug concentrations to be maintained in vivo more effectively between doses.

The enhancement of drug absorption by food, as seen with griseofulvin, nitrofurantoin and erythromycin esters, could conceivably improve the clinical efficacy of antimicrobial therapy, but this has yet to be proven.

CONCLUSIONS

It is apparent that food-drug interactions occur in domestic animals and that veterinarians need to consider them when prescribing antimicrobial agents for enteral administration in their patients. At the present time recommendations must be based mainly on human data. Although this might be satisfactory for species whose physiology and feeding do not differ greatly from those of man, such as dogs and cats, it could prove unsuitable for other species.

As the most common outcome of food-drug interactions

seems to be decreased (that is, reduced or delayed) absorption, administration on an empty stomach should be the
general rule: exception can be made for a few drugs which
cause gastric irritation, and those whose absorption is
known to be not affected adversely by food. Provisional
suggestions are made in Table 10.4; these may need to be
modified   as   additional   information   on   food-drug
interactions in domestic animals becomes available.

References
1. Finkel, Y., Bolme, P. and Eriksson, M. (1981). The
   effect of food on the oral absorption of penicillin V
   preparations   in   children.   Acta Pharmacol. Toxicol.
   49:301-304.
2. Green, C.E., O'Neal, K.G. and Barsanti, J.A. (1984).
   Antimicrobial chemotherapy. In: Green, C.D. (ed.).
   Clinical Microbiology and Infectious Diseases of the
   Dog and Cat. pp.144-188. Philadelphia: W.B. Saunders.
3. Watson, A.D.J. (1974). Chloramphenicol in the dog :
   observations   of   plasma   levels   following   oral
   administration. Res. Vet. Sci. 16:147-151.
4. Watson, A.D.J. (1977). Effect of concurrent drug
   therapy and of feeding on plasma chloramphenicol
   levels after oral administration of chloramphenicol in
   dogs. Res. Vet. Sci. 22:68-71.
5. Watson, A.D.J. (1979). Effect of ingesta on systemic
   availability   of   chloramphenicol   from   two   oral
   preparations in cats.   J. Vet. Pharmacol.   Ther.
   2:117-121.
6. Watson, A.D.J. (1979). Some factors affecting bioavailability of antimicrobial drugs given by mouth in small
   animals. In: Grunsell, C.S.G. and Hill, F.W.G. (eds).
   Veterinary Annual, 19th issue, pp. 217-222. Bristol :
   Scientechnica.
7. Watson, A.D.J. (1983). Effects of food on absorption
   of antibacterial drugs. In: Grunsell, C.S.G. and
   Hill, F.W.G. (eds). Veterinary Annual, 23rd issue,
   pp.241- 243. Bristol : Scientechnica.
8. Watson, A.D.J. (1985). Effect of time between feeding
   and dosing on systemic availability of penicillin V in
   dogs (abstract).   Proceedings, Voorjaarsdagen 1985.
   Post Academisch Onderwijs, publikatie no 85-6:24-25.
9. Watson, A.D.J. (1985). Food impairs systemic availability of penicillins administered orally in
   dogs.   In: Van Miert, A.S.J.P.A.M., Bogaert, M.G. and
   Debackere, M. (eds).   Comparative   Veterinary
   Pharmacology, Toxicology and Therapy. Proc. 3rd EAVPT
   Congress. Part I, Abstracts, p.53. Utrecht : EAVPT.
10. Watson, A.D.J. and Egerton, J.R. (1977). Effect of
    feeding on plasma antibiotic concentrations in
    greyhounds given ampicillin and amoxycillin by mouth.
    J. Small An. Pract. 18:779-786.

11. Welling, P.G. (1984). Interactions affecting drug absorption. Clin. Pharmacokin. 9:404-434.
12. Welling, P.G. and Tse, F.L.S. (1982). The influence of food on the absorption of antimicrobial agents. J. Antimicrob. Chemother. 9:7-27.
13. Welling, P.G. and Tse, F.L.S. (1984). Factors contributing to variability in drug pharmacokinetics. 1. Absorption. J. Clin. Hosp. Pharm. 9:163-179.

Smooth Muscle Pharmacology

11
Pharmacology of the (fore)-stomach smooth muscles

L. A .A. OOMS, A. WEYNS, A. DEGRYSE AND Y. RUCKEBUSCH

ABSTRACT

A short review is presented on the pharmacology of the (fore)-stomach smooth muscles. Detailed information is given on the smooth muscle pharmacology of the lower oesophageal sphincter, the oesophageal groove, the reticulum, the rumen, the omasum, the abomasum and the pylorus.

CONTRACTION OF SMOOTH MUSCLES

Smooth muscle membrane permeability changes usually affect membrane potential by allowing one or more ions to pass through the membrane more freely. Since none of the ions in smooth muscle cells is in equilibrium at a membrane potential of −50 to −60 mV, there will be a net flow of ions into and out of the cells, tending to move the membrane potential closer to equilibrium. Membrane depolarization usually results in a contraction, although a change in potential is not a prerequisite for induction of contraction in all smooth muscle cells[9]. Contraction of smooth muscles can be initiated by changes in membrane permeability either after binding of agonists to their receptors or after exposure to high K^+ concentrations[5,45]. In either instance, electrical or chemical cell membrane signals indirectly activate contractile elements by releasing membrane-bound Ca^{2+}, or increasing Ca^{2+} influx, or

both. Three sources of Ca can be distinguished : the free
Ca in the extracellular fluid, the Ca bound to the surface
membrane and the intracellular Ca in endoplasmic reticulum
and mitochondria. Ca influx during receptor activation
seems to be different from Ca influx induced by membrane
depolarization[15]. Two pathways of transmembrane flux of
Ca^{2+} exist : a voltage-dependent Ca^{2+} channel, activated
by changes in membrane potential, and a receptor-linked
channel, activated by binding of agonists to their receptors. The plasma membrane of vascular, intestinal and
myometrial smooth muscle seems to be equipped with the exchange system to regulate intracellular Ca^{2+} concentration[51]. A $(Ca^{2+}-Mg^{2+})$-ATPase was demonstrated in pig stomach muscle, which could be purified on a calmodulin affinity column and is calmodulin-dependent[53,54]. This protein is able, when incorporated into lipid vesicles, to
transport Ca^{2+} in an uphill fashion if ATP is present in
the medium[52].

Receptor agonists also induce contraction without changing membrane potential in smooth muscles that do not generate action potentials, or in depolarized smooth muscles[45]. All eukaryotic cells contain inositol lipids.
Phospholipase C catalyses the breakdown of phosphatidylinositol 4,5-biphosphate, a multiple-charged anion that
has a very high affinity for Ca^{2+} (greater than that of
EDTA) and exhibits a rapid turnover in vivo. Its hydro-
philic/hydrophobic solubility partition coefficient is
markedly altered when Ca^{2+} replaces monovalent phosphate
counterions[6,11]. The receptor-mediated breakdown of phospholipids is not mediated by an increase in cytosol Ca^{2+}
but is closely coupled to receptor occupation. Inositol
triphosphate (IP₃) and also the lipid-soluble product of
phoshatidylinositol 4,5-biphosphate breakdown, 1,2 diacylglycerol (DAG), act as second messengers in the cells[25].
The phosphoryl groups, covalently attached to IP, turn
over extremely rapidly. The rise in IP₃ may be the means
whereby the intracellular (non-mitochondrial) pools of
calcium are mobilized[46]. The less Ca^{2+} bound to inositol

1,4,5-triphosphate, the stronger the attraction of Ca^{2+}. Diacylglycerol acts in its own right and activates a specific, calcium-activated, phospholipid-dependent protein kinase, C-kinase, which catalyses the phosphorylation of a specific group of protein substrates. Diacylglycerol is one of the sources of arachidonic acid (liberated by phospholipase A_2) which serves as the substrate for prostaglandin, leukotriene and/or thromboxane synthesis[30,47].

A group of organic Ca^{2+} antagonists or Ca^{2+} channel blockers (including verapamil, methoxyverapamil [D600], nifedipine, diltiazem and flunarizine) are specific inhibitors of Ca^{2+} influx through voltage-dependent Ca^{2+} channels[30,55,56]. Nitrocompounds, especially sodium nitroprusside, are selective inhibitors of the receptor-linked Ca^{2+} channel[23]. Tetraethyl-ammonium (TEA) increases spike activity of many spike generating smooth muscles and induces spike potentials in spontaneously inactive guinea-pig fundic muscles[22,32]. No effect was observed on the spontaneously inactive ruminal preparations by micromolar TEA. Acetylcholine (10^{-6} g/ml) applied to TEA (3×10^{-3} to 10^{-2}M) pretreated ruminal preparations produced no spike-free tonic contraction but spike activity and phasic contractions[29].

Unphosphorylated and dephosphorylated myosin cannot be activated by actin, but the phosphorylated and rephosphorylated myosin can be activated by actin. The same relationship between phosphorylation and enzymatic activity was found for a chymotryptic peptide of myosin, smooth muscle heavy meromyosin[1].

Many hormones and neurotransmitters (for example, glucagon, adrenaline [acting through beta-adrenoceptors]) trigger the activation of adenylate cyclase (AC). Stimulation of AC results in an elevation of the intracellular concentration of cAMP, which transmits the hormonal signal by activating cyclic AMP dependent protein kinase (PK). This enzyme phosphorylates a number of intracellular proteins and thereby regulates their activities, for example, serine (and occasionally threonine) residues C-terminal to pairs of adjacent basic amino acids : Arg-Arg-X-Ser and Lys-Arg-X-Y-Ser[10]. Some hormones inhibit adenylate cyclase (including enkephalins and adrenaline [acting through the alpha-2-adrenoceptor]) and activate the GTPase activity of a guanine nucleotide binding protein converting it from a GTP-liganded form (Gs-GTP) that stimulates adenylate cyclase to an inactive GDP-liganded form (Gs-GDP). Hormones that activate adenylate cyclase exert their effect by promoting the conversion of Gs-GDP to Gs-GTP[8]. Indeed, adenylate cyclase consists of a recognition component (a stimulatory receptor unit and an inhibitory receptor unit) and a catalytic unit; Mg^{2+} stimulates activity to levels approaching that observed with hormones. Ca^{2+} at physiological concentrations can stimulate as well as inhibit smooth muscle adenylate cyclase activity. The stimulation of adenylate cyclase activity is mediated by calmodulin. The level of calmodulin associated with smooth muscle adenylate cyclase may modulate the response (both stimulatory and inhibitory) of the enzyme to Ca^{2+}[33]. Forskolin, a steroid-like compound, stimulates the activity of all animal cell cyclase systems, but acts on a component distinct from the 45,000 or 55,000 dalton unit through which GTP acts[44]. Sodium nitroprusside, nitroglycerine and related smooth muscle relaxants were reported to increase smooth muscle levels of cGMP[41]. Nitroprusside is unstable in aqueous solutions and releases nitric oxide. Nitric oxide is a potent activator of guanylate cyclase. cGMP stimulates the activity of the sarcolemmal Ca^{2+} extrusion ATPase in a concentration dependent manner. Through this mechanism cGMP seems to be involved in the relaxing effect of AC stimulation.

In particular, the smooth muscles of the sphincter regions and also of the stomach (reservoir function) are equipped with both voltage-linked and receptor-linked channels. The first regulates the phasic contractions while the second is involved in the tonic contractions. In some muscles overlapping between the different systems is observed. The same is true for the different channel blockers in these muscles.

LOWER OESOPHAGEAL SPHINCTER (LES)

Muscles of the LES show both phasic and tonic contractions. Circular muscle strips from the LES develop a
spontaneous active tension, much higher compared to circular muscle from the body of the oesophagus. LES spike activity was not correlated with basal sphincter pressure.
A decreased muscle tone in muscle strips was observed in
the sphincter region of the opossum oesophagus when it was
exposed to calcium-free solution[19,21]. Intravenous injection of $CaCl_2$ partially restores the LES pressure depressed by verapamil. Sodium nitroprusside causes marked lo-
wering of the resting LES pressure[13].

Innervation of the LES is mediated by both inhibitory
and excitatory autonomic nerves. Alpha-adrenergic
agonists increase LES pressure while alpha-adrenergic
blockers decrease it. Also cholinergic mechanisms appear
to maintain some of the resting LES pressure because
atropine and other anticholinergics have been shown to
lower the pressure. Gastrin receptor activation causes
LES excitation. Motilin, bombesin and substance P are
known to cause contraction of the smooth muscle of the
LES. Morphine significantly reduces while naloxone
increases LES pressure[20]. Studying the identification and
localization of opioid receptors in the opossum LES, it
was shown that mu, kappa, sigma and delta opioid receptors
were present. Mu and kappa inhibitory receptors are
present on the sphincter muscle[34]. Direct inhibition of
the LES muscle was observed by vasoactive intestinal
polypeptide (VIP), gastric inhibitory polypeptide (GIP)
and secretin[4,14,35,39].

Indirect evidence for the involvement of serotonin in
the development of bloat resulted from the observation
that pretreatment with a serotonin-2 blocker resulted in
an increased volume of gas eructated[39]. In vitro
experiments on circular muscle of the LES of cattle
demonstrated that serotonin (10^{-4}M) increased muscle tone

and also the phasic contractions, if present.   Ritanserin
and sodium nitroprusside (10^{-6}M) reduced muscle tone (Ooms
et al., unpublished observations).   Sodium nitroprusside
induced a short-lasting inhibition of all types of activity. Acetylcholine induced a contraction followed by an
increased muscle tone.

   In vivo, the phasic contractions of the reticulum are
under vagal control[38]. The number of phasic reticular
contractions were increased in milk-fed calves when ritanserin, cisapride or both substances were added to the milk
(0.2 mg.kg^{-1} b.i.d.; Ooms et al., unpublished observations). Increasing the release of acetylcholine is important for induction of phasic contractions, but substances
acting directly on the muscles (to decrease tone) also
seem to be useful, for increasing the number of phasic
contractions. In vitro, the majority of the muscle contractions are of the phasic type. Acetylcholine (10^{-6}M)
only induces phasic contractions. Serotonin (10^{-4}M) increases phasic contractions but also muscle tone of the
circular muscle (Ooms et al., unpublished observations).
SP had no direct effect on the muscles, suggesting in vivo
action on the local cholinergic neurones.

OESOPHAGEAL GROOVE
In young and adult animals, oesophageal groove closure can
be evoked by oral application of bicarbonate solutions,
but especially with copper. On smooth muscles of the
oesophageal groove of calves and cattle, both phasic and
tonic contractions were observed in vitro. Sodium
nitroprusside (10^{-6}M) and PGE$_2$ (10^{-6}M), but not verapamil
(10^{-5}M), inhibited all type of activity in the oesophageal
groove of cattle in vitro (Ooms et al., unpublished observations).

RETICULUM
Xylazine, an alpha-2-agonist, reduced the frequency of reticular contractions. Reticular contractions were restored with tolazoline, an alpha 2-blocker[49]. Histamine inhi-

bits reticular contractions. This effect is inhibited by H_1-antagonists, while the H_2-antagonist oxmetidine had no protective action[37].

RUMEN

On the ruminal smooth muscles, phasic and tonic types of activity were observed both in vitro and in vivo. The tone was completely eliminated in Ca^{2+}-free solutions and also by sodium nitroprusside[29] (also Ooms et al., unpublished observations). Verapamil and D600 did not essentially influence the spontaneous tone[29]. In vivo, the motor events occur in cycles (starting on the reticulum to the dorsal and ventral sac of the rumen) lasting about 1 min. and in about 40-60% of the cycles they are followed by a retrograde contraction (Maas, Van Duin and Van Miert, unpublished observations). Substances such as dopamine (20 μg/kg/min for 15 min) and apomorphine (2 μg/kg/min for 10 min) cause inhibition of extrinsic ruminal contractions. Domperidone (0.5 mg/kg), but not naltrexone (0.1 mg/kg), prevented these effects. Naltrexone itself induced a rapid increase in the frequency of extrinsic ruminal contractions. Ruminal strips all reacted with an increase in muscle tone after exposure to apomorphine (2.5 and 5. 10^{-6}M). This rise in tone could be blocked by domperidone (5.10^{-7}M), but not by naltrexone (5.10^{-6}M)[16]. Morphine depressed both frequency and amplitude of ruminal contractions, while naltrexone and naloxone significantly increased the frequency of ruminal contractions. Expulsion of acidic abomasal contents back into the preabomasal compartment was the cause of acidification of the rumen after apomorphine injection[3].

The fetal bovine rumen is highly sensitive to 5-hydroxytryptamine (5-HT) and sensitivity to 5-HT increases until 5 month fetuses, when the magnitude stabilizes[48]. The effect on bovine rumen is not mediated by autonomic nervous structures, but is a direct one on the muscle. Also presynaptic stimulation of cholinergic neurones is observed after addition of serotonin[48]. Intravenous administration of serotonin (6 µg/kg expressed as the base) in sheep resulted in a short-lived contraction followed by a sustained and long-lasting increase in muscle tone and a concomitant inhibition of the extrinsic reticulorumen contractions. The short-lived contraction was probably due to neural stimulation (blocked after morphine and atropine) and the long-lasting increase of muscle tone seemed to be due to a direct smooth muscle action (blocked by the 5-HT antagonists, R 50970 and methysergide)[36]. In sheep, a specific serotonin-2-antagonist (ketanserin; 0.05 mg/kg) significantly increased the volume of eructated gas, when the intraruminal pressure was maintained at 2 mmHg, and increased the frequency of primary and secondary contractions of the rumen by 41.5 and 24.3%, respectively. At an intraruminal pressure of 4 mmHg, ketanserin at a dose level of 0.1 mg/kg, significantly increased the volume of eructated gas and also the frequency of both primary (23.6%) and secondary contractions (23.7%). From these results it seems that specific serotonin-2-antagonists offer the ability to treat bloat in ruminants[18]. In another study, ritanserin (S_2-antagonist) not only prevented bloat during the ruminal stasis induced by hypocalcaemia in sheep and continuous insufflation in cattle, but increased the eructated volume[39].

OMASUM

In the omasum, a significant uptake of fluid and electrolytes occurs. The mucosal area is increased by the fold present in the omasum. For efficient absorption, the mucosa needs time. Rapid transport from reticulum to abomasum seems possible by the omasal groove (limited by particle size). The main activity, as observed in vitro, was of the tonic type (Ooms et al., unpublished observations).

ABOMASUM AND STOMACH OF MONOGASTRIC ANIMALS

The primary control of motility of the stomach of monogastric animals and the abomasum of ruminants is of myogenic origin. Receptors (mechanoreceptors, chemoreceptors and

osmoreceptors), neurones and also hormones influence stomach motility by a direct action on the muscles or by influence on the release of neurotransmitters and hormones.
The proximal part (stomach fundus) has a receptive function while the distal part (stomach antrum) functions as a
cyclic pump.

Dopamine has an inhibitory effect on the stomach fundus
and also reduces the contractile amplitude. The dopamine
inhibitory effect on the rat stomach fundus can be explained by interaction with postjunctional beta-receptors on
the smooth muscle cells and prejunctional alpha-receptors
on the intramural cholinergic neurones. No evidence for
the existence of specific dopamine receptors was found.
The inhibition by dopamine is largely indirect, through
uptake in sympathetic nerve endings and liberation of endogenous noradrenaline. The findings with alpha-agonists
and antagonists suggest that the alpha-receptors on the
intramural cholinergic neurones combine the characteristics of both subtypes of alpha-receptors, or that the
receptor population consists of a mixture of alpha-1 and
alpha-2-receptors[26]. The alpha-adrenergic mechanisms
through which dopamine and noradrenaline are able to relax
and contract the circular smooth muscle from the body region of guinea-pig stomach are of the alpha-1 and alpha-2
types, respectively[40].

Specific desensitization of ganglionic receptors for
5-HT reduced the vagal relaxation. The vagal inhibitory
effect was completely abolished only when competitive
block of acetylcholine receptors was combined with desensitization of 5-HT receptors. The fact that 5-HT is contained within preganglionic nerve fibres in the myenteric
plexus is consistent with the hypothesis that 5-HT, with
acetylcholine, may be a neurotransmitter in the vagal inhibitory innervation of the stomach[31]. While acetylcholine appears to be the sole preganglionic and postganglionic transmitter in the excitatory portion, both 5-HT and
acetylcholine appear to participate as preganglionic
transmitters in the inhibitory portion of the vagal path-

way.   5-HT produces a long-lasting stimulation of inhibitory responses, so strong as to suppress the excitatory
component of the vagal effect. It should therefore be
possible to reduce inhibitory vagal responses by 5-HT
antagonists without reducing responses to nicotinic compounds, just as the non-depolarizing antagonists of acetylcholine reduce vagal responses without affecting responses to 5-HT.

The electrical activity of the pyloric antrum is characterized by slow waves (SW), usually followed by spike
potentials. In cattle, about 80% of the antral SW are
superimposed with spike bursts and half of them pass aborally to the duodenum. The percentage of contractions
running from the antrum to the duodenum seems to depend on
the intensity of the spike bursts (contraction) on the antrum[7]. The peripheral dopamine antagonists domperidone
and metoclopramide improve coordination of antroduodenal
motility both in vivo and in vitro[42]. Metoclopramide also
increases the release of the cholinergic neurotransmitter[24]. In dogs, it was shown that domperidone and cisapride, and to a lesser extent metoclopramide, but not
betanechol, effectively improved antroduodenal coordination indicating that both dopaminergic and cholinergic
pathways modulate antroduodenal coordination[43].

Antroduodenal coordination is important for the control
of gastric emptying. Morphine significantly inhibited
gastric emptying of both solids and liquids while naloxone
results in a non-significant acceleration of solid food
emptying[17]. Intramural cholinergic neurones are activated
by substance P[39]. Substance P is a neurotransmitter
involved in the gastric excitatory motor responses elicited by antidromic activation of thin afferent fibres in
the vagal and splanchnic nerves[12]. The antidromic activation mechanism was present only in the stomach, not in the
pylorus[28]. The contractile effects of substance P were
sensitive to atropine or local infusion of a substance P
analogue (D-Pro[2],D-Trp[7,9])-substance P. Acetylcholine
induces phasic contraction with each slow wave. Betanechol

also increases the contractile activity of the antrum and duodenum. However, the coordination is not enhanced. Nicotine agonists and also hexamethonium inhibit antroduodenal coordination by reducing the amplitude of antral and duodenal contractions. Cholecystokinin, secretin and glucagon decrease the antral contractions. This antroduodenal coordination is reduced by motilin and also by neurotensin.

PYLORUS

The pylorus sphincter is build up on circular muscles (majority) and longitudinal muscles connecting the antrum with the duodenum. In most animal species, the underlying mucosa is not closely attached to the muscular layers. In physiological conditions, the pylorus contracts after application of duodenal stimuli and relaxes during strong peristaltic contractions of the antrum running to the duodenum. Vagal nerve stimulation causes a release (through beta-adrenergic receptor activation) of 5-HT from enterochromaffin cells to the portal circulation and to the gut lumen[2]. The contractile pyloric responses to 5-HT were antagonized by peripheral blockade of 5-HT$_2$ receptors. Such blockade did not influence the motor responses to extrinsic nerve stimulation, suggesting that 5-HT is not essential for the mediation of these responses. In vitro, on antral and pyloric strips from the rat, the responses to substance P and 5-HT were antagonized by antagonist substance P analogue or substance P tachyphylaxis and peripheral blockade of 5-HT$_2$ receptors, respectively. The responses were not reduced by tetrodotoxin, indicating principally activation of muscular receptors. However, the contractile responses were reduced by atropine or hexamethonium, except the substance P-induced pyloric contraction, which was atropine-sensitive but hexamethonium-resistant. Blockade of 5-HT$_2$ receptors reduced the substance P-induced motor responses, indicating an interaction between substance P and 5-HT$_2$ receptors at the muscular level. This may be important since substance P and

5-HT seem to coexist in gut neurones[27]. Substance P may mediate part of the vagally induced pyloric and gastric contraction, the latter probably by axon collaterals on fine cholinergic neurones.

References
1. Adelstein, R.S., Sellers, J.R., Conti, M.A., Pato, M.
   D. and de Lanerolle, P. (1982). Regulation of smooth
   muscle contractile proteins by calmodulin and cyclic
   AMP. Fed. Proc. 41:2873-2878.
2. Ahlman, H. and Dahlström, A. (1983). Vagal mechanisms
   controlling serotonin release from the gastrointestinal tract and pyloric motor function. J. Aut. Nervous
   Syst. 9:119-140.
3. Arias, J.L., Zurich, L. and Bastias, J. (1980). Motor responses to 5-HT of the bovine rumen wall in
   vitro during fetal development. Pharmacol. Res. Comm.
   12:975-985.
4. Behar, J., Field, S. and Marin, C. (1979). Effect of
   glucagon, secretin and vasoactive intestinal polypeptide on the feline lower esophageal sphincter : mechanisms of action. Gastroenterology 77:1001-1007.
5. Bolton, T.B. (1979). Mechanisms of action of transmitters and other substances on smooth muscle.
   Physiol. Rev. 59:606-718.
6. Brockeroff, H. and Ballou, C.E. (1961). The structure
   of the phosphoinositide complex of beef brain. J.
   Biol. Chem. 236:1907-1911.
7. Bülbring, E. and Gershon, M.D. (1967). 5-Hydroxytryp-
   tamine participation in the vagal inhibitory innerva-
   vation of the stomach. J. Physiol. 192:823-846.
8. Burns, D.L., Hewlett, E.L., Moss, J. and Vaughan, M.J.
   (1983). Pertussis toxin inhibits enkephalin stimula-
   lation of GTPase of NG108-IS cells. J. Biol. Chem.
   258:1435-1438.
9. Casteels, R. and Droogmans, G. (1982). Membrane potential and excitation-contraction coupling in smooth
   muscle. Fed. Proc. 41:2879-2882.
10. Cohen, P. (1980). Interaction between chemoreceptive
    modalities of odour and irritation. Nature 1:255-268.
11. Dawson, R.M.C. (1965). Phosphatidopeptide-like com-
    plexes formed by the interaction of calcium triphos-
    phoinositide with protein. Biochem. J. 97:134-138.
12. Delbro, D., Fändriks, L., Rossel, S. and Folkers, K.
    (1983). Inhibition of antidromically induced
    stimulation of gastric motility by substance P
    receptor blockade. Acta Physiol. Scand. 118:309-316.
13. Dent, J., Dodds, W.J. and Arndorfer, R.C. (1978).
    Effect of nitroprusside and verapamil in esophageal
    smooth muscle contractility in the opossum. Gastro-
    enterology 74:1119.
14. Domschke, W., Lux, G., Domschke, S., Strunz, U., Bloom
    S.R. and Wünsch, E. (1978). Effects of vasoactive in-
    testinal peptide on resting and pentagastrin stimula-

ted lower esophageal sphincter pressure.   Gastroenterology 75:9-12.
15. Edman, A.P. and Schild, H.O. (1962).   The need for
    calcium in the contractile responses induced by ace-
    tylcholine and potassium in rat uterus.   J. Physiol.
    (Lond.) 161:424-441.
16. Eiler, H., Lyke, W.A. and Johnson, R. (1981). Inter-
    nal vomiting in the ruminant : effect of apomorphine
    on ruminal pH in sheep. Am. J. Vet. Res. 42:202-204.
17. Fändriks, L. and Delbro, D. (1983).   Neural stimula-
    tion of gastric bicarbonate secretion in the cat.   An
    involvement of vagal axon-reflexes and substance P.
    Acta Physiol. Scand. 118:301-304.
18. Fioramonti, J., Buéno, L., Ooms, L. and Ruckebusch, Y.
    (1982).   Effects of ketanserin on rumino-reticular
    motility and eructation in sheep : a possible appli-
    cation as an anti-bloating substance. J. Vet. Pharma-
    col. Ther. 5:213-215.
19. Fox, J.E. and Daniel, E.E. (1979).   Role of Ca^{2+} in
    the genesis of lower esophageal sphincter tone and
    other active contractions. Am. J. Physiol. 237:E163-
    E171.
20. Frank, E.B., Lange, R., Plankey, M. and McCallum, R.W.
    (1982). Effect of morphine and naloxone on lower
    esophageal sphincter pressure and gastric emptying in
    man. Dig. Dis. Sci. 27:651.
21. Goyal, R.K. and Rattan, S. (1980). Effects of sodium
    nitroprusside and verapamil on lower esophageal sphin-
    cter. Am. J. Physiol. 238:640-644.
22. Ito, Y., Kuriyama, H. and Sakamato, I.K. (1970).
    Effects of tetraethylammonium chloride on the membrane
    activity of guinea-pig stomach smooth muscle. J.
    Physiol. (Lond.) 211:445-460.
23. Karaki, H. and Weiss, G.B. (1984).   Calcium channels
    in smooth muscle. Gastroenterology 87:960-970.
24. Kilbinger, H., Kruel, R., Pfeuffer-Friederich, I. and
    Wessler, I. (1982). The effects of metoclopramide on
    acetylcholine release and on smooth muscle response in
    the isolated guinea-pig ileum. N.S. Arch. Pharmacol.
    319:231-238.
25. Kirk, C.J., Bone, E.A., Palmer, S. and Michell, R.H.
    (1984).   The role of phosphatidylinositol 4,5 biphos-
    phate breakdown in cell-surface receptor activation.
    J. Receptor Res. 4:489-504.
26. Lefebvre, R.A., Blancquaert, J.P., Willems, J.L. and
    Bogaert, M.G. (1983). In vitro study of the inhibi-
    tory effects of dopamine on the rat gastric fundus.
    N.S.Arch. Pharmacol. 322:228-236.
27. Lidberg, P. (1985).   On the role of substance P and
    serotonin in the pyloric motor control. An experi-
    mental study in cat and rat.   Acta Physiol. Scand.
    Suppl. 538.
28. Lidberg, P., Dalhlström, A., Lundberg, J.M. and Ahl-
    man, H. (1983). Different modes of action of
    substance P in the motor control of the feline stomach
    and pylorus. Regulatory Peptides 7:41-52.

29. Milanov, M.P., Stoyanov, N. and Boev, K.K. (1984). Electro-mechanical coupling in the complex stomach smooth muscles. Gen. Pharmacol. 15:99-105.
30. Mishizuka, Y. (1983). A receptor-linked cascade of phospholipid turnover in hormone action. In : Shizume, K., Imura, H. and Shimizu, N. (eds). Endocrinology. International Congress Series 598:15-24. Amsterdam : Excerpta Medica.
31. Ooms, L. and Oyaert, W. (1978). Electromyographic study of the abomasal antrum and proximal duodenum in cattle. Zbl. Vet. Med. Reihe A. 25:464-473.
32. Osa, T. and Kuriyama, H. (1970). The membrane properties and decremental conduction of excitation in the fundus of guinea-pig stomach. Jap. J. Physiol. 20: 626-639.
33. Piascik, M.T., Babich, M. and Rush, M.E. (1983). Calmodulin stimulation and calcium regulation of smooth muscle adenylate cyclase activity. J. Biol. Chem. 258:10913-10918.
34. Rattan, S. and Goyal, R.K. (1982). Identification and localization of opioid receptors in the opossum lower esophageal sphincter (LES) : evidence for a distinct meperidine receptor. Dig. Dis. Sci. 27:651.
35. Rattan, S., Said, S.I. and Goyal, R.K. (1977). Effect of vasoactive intestinal polypeptide (VIP) on lower esophageal sphincter pressure (LESP). Proc. Soc. Exp. Bio. Med. 155:40-43.
36. Ruckebusch, Y. and Ooms, L. (1983). Selective blockade of the responses of reticulo-ruminal muscle to 5-HT in sheep. J. Vet. Pharmacol. Ther. 6:127-132.
37. Ruckebusch, Y. and Soldani, G. (1983). H_1 and H_2 receptors in the ovine digestive tract. Vet. Pharmacol. Therap. 6:229-232.
38. Ruckebusch, Y. and Tomov, T. (1973). The sequential contractions of the rumen associated with eructation in sheep. J. Physiol. 235:447-458.
39. Ruckebusch, Y., Ooms, L.A.A., Degryse A.-D. and Allal, C. (1985). Alleviation of excessive gas accumulation in the ruminant stomach by ritanserin. Am. J. Vet. Res. 46:434-437.
40. Sahyoun, H.A., Costall, B. and Naylor, R.J. (1982). Catecholamines act at alpha-2-adrenoceptors to cause contraction of circular smooth muscle of guinea-pig stomach. J. Pharm. Pharmacol. 34:381-385.
41. Schultz, K.D., Schultz, K. and Schultz, G. (1977). Sodium nitroprusside and other smooth muscle relaxants increase cyclic GMP levels in rat ductus deferens. Nature (Lond.) 265:750-751.
42. Schuurkes, J.A.J. and Van Nueten, J.M. (1981). Food-stimulated gastric acid secretion inhibited by hormones and drugs. Scand. J. Gastroenterol. 16 (Suppl. 67):33-36.
43. Schuurkes, J.A.J. and Van Nueten, J.M. (1984). Control of gastroduodenal coordination : dopaminergic and cholinergic pathways. Scand. J. Gastroenterol. 19 (Suppl. 92):8-12.

44. Seamin, K.B. and Daly, J.W. (1981). Activation of adenylate cyclase by the diterpene forskolin does not require the guanine nucleotide regulatory protein. J. Biol. Chem. 256:9799-9801.
45. Somlyo, A.V. and Somlyo, A.P. (1968). Electromechanical and pharmacological coupling in vascular smooth muscle. J. Pharmacol. Exp. Ther. 159:129-145.
46. Streb, H., Irvine, R.F., Berridge, M.J. and Schulz, I. (1983). Release of Ca^{2+} from a non-mitochondrial store of pancreatic acinar cell by inositol-1,4,5-triphosphate. Nature (Lond.) 306:67-69.
47. Takai, Y., Kishimoto, A., Kawahara, Y. et al. (1981). Calcium and phosphatidylinositol turnover as signalling for transmembrane control of protein phosphorylation. Adv. Cycl. Nucleotide Res. 14:301-313.
48. Taneike, T. (1979). 5-Hydroxytryptamine potentiates contraction mediated by the intramural cholinergic nerve in the longitudinal smooth muscle of the ruminant forestomach. J. Vet. Pharmacol. Ther. 2:59-68.
49. Toutain, P.L., Zingoni, M.R. and Ruckebusch, Y. (1982). Assessment of 2 adrenergic antagonists on the central nervous system using reticular contraction in sheep as a model. J. Pharmacol. Exp. Ther. 223:215-218.
50. Triggle, D.J. (1981). Calcium antagonists : basic chemical and pharmacological aspects. In : Weiss, G.B. (ed.). New Perspectives on Calcium Antagonists, pp.83-94. Baltimore : Williams and Wilkins.
51. Van Breemen, C., Aaronson, P. and Loutzenhiser, R. (1979). Sodium-calcium interactions in mammalian smooth muscle. Pharmacol. Rev. 30:167-208.
52. Wuytack, F., de Schutter, G., Verbist, J. and Casteels, R. (1983). Antibodies to the calmodulin-binding Ca^{2+}-transport ATPase from smooth muscle. FEBS Lett. 154:191-195.
53. Wuytack, F., de Schutter, G. and Casteels, R. (1981). Partial purification of (Ca^{2+}-Mg^{2+})-dependent ATPase from pig smooth muscle and reconstitution of an ATP-dependent Ca^{2+}-transported system. Biochem. J. 198:265-271.
54. Wuytack, F., de Schutter, G. and Casteels, R. (1981). Purification of (Ca^{2+}-Mg^{2+})-ATPase from smooth muscle by calmodulin affinity chromatography. FEBS Lett. 198:265-291.
55. Weiss, G.B. (1977). Calcium and contractility in vascular smooth muscle. In : Narahashi, T. and Bianchi, C.P. (eds). Advances in General and Cellular Pharmacology, pp.71-154. New York : Plenum.
56. Weiss, G.B. (1981). Sites of action of calcium antagonists in vascular smooth muscle. In : Weiss, G.B. (ed.). New Perspectives on Calcium Antagonists, pp.83-94. Baltimore : Williams and Wilkins.

12
Smooth muscle pharmacology of the large intestine

Y. RUCKEBUSCH, T. BARDON, C. CHERBUT, M. PAIRET AND J. P. FERRÉ

ABSTRACT

The distinction between tonic and phasic activity occurring in the isolated colon corresponds to the localized versus propagated colonic activity recorded in the conscious dog. The myogenic activity of the circular muscular layer, unaltered by atropine and adrenergic antagonists in vitro, seems equivalent to the localized spike burst (LSB) activity enhanced by prostaglandin synthetase inhibitors in vivo. The phasic activity of the longitudinal muscular layer, coupled to that of the circular layer via myenteric cholinergic neurones, is similar to the propagated spike bursts (PSB) either isolated or in series (MSB) under the control of a permanent inhibitory sympathetic innervation.

The ubiquitous secretory effects of prostanoids and the prostaglandin-mediated motor effects of several peptides indicate a possible interspecific therapeutic value of anti-inflammatory drugs in several cases of motor or secretory disturbances of the colon.

INTRODUCTION

In carnivores, the colon is a simple tube with a proximal segment where digesta are similar in consistency to the ileum and the antiperistaltic motor activity (that is, retrograde versus antegrade propagated spike bursts - PSB) is predominant. In the middle segment, the contents become firm enough to be solid due to movements of the circular muscle layer, also identified as localized spike bursts (LSB). The contents are moved aborally by PSB in series termed herein migrating spike bursts (MSB) and these are only inhibited by stimulation of the lumbar colonic (sympathetic) nerves. The canine colonic electrical activity consists of two components : one from the longitudinal muscle layer occurring as periods of 13-35 oscillations, and the other arising from the circular muscle layer as an omnipresent myogenic slow-wave activity unaltered by atropine or adrenergic antagonists. Superimposed spikes are associated with contractions which are enhanced by indomethacin (IDM); this suggests inhibition of the circular muscle layer via the release of prostanoids and by tetrodotoxin (TTX), indicating a permissive effect against a permanent neural inhibitory input, and a facilitation of the cholinergic prepotential activity at the longitudinal muscle layer.

The patterns of contractions of the "simple" colon involve :

(1) in vivo sphincteric relaxation by non-adrenergic inhibitory nerves in response to rectal distension, its absence leading to a diagnosis of aganglionosis;
(2) colocolonic reflexes consisting at the ganglionic level of sympathetic inhibition at one end of the colon in response to mechanoreceptor excitation at the other end[10];
(3) the colonic response to eating.

This response in dogs is more pronounced on the proximal colon, including the ileocolonic junction (ICJ), than on the distal colon, is in part mimicked by neurotensin and is decreased after prostaglandin synthetase inhibitor pretreatment[2].

In fact, species variability in colonic structure and

development, especially the enlargement of the large bowel in the horse[13], and caecotrophy in the rabbit[12], may be at the origin of species-specific effects of drugs. The formation of pellets in sheep and in rats[6], the increased transit rate in response to bulk contents in carnivores or omnivores[4], despite a reduced motility index, are other aspects of species variations. Four aspects are emphasized in this chapter :

(1) the importance of spinal sympathetic inhibition of colonic motility;
(2) the role of the cholinergic nerves in relation to the effects of stimulation of the pelvic nerves;
(3) the effects on colonic motor and secretory functions of opiate agonists;
(4) the physiological significance of colonic motility stimulation by prostaglandins (PGs) and serotonin (5-HT).

SPINAL SYMPATHETIC INHIBITION

Following removal of the spinal cord between T9 and L5, the frequency of contractions of the transverse colon was increased by 30% (1.8 versus 1.4/min) without disappearance of the colonic motor cycles. The motility of the transverse colon was likewise stimulated by intrathecal administration of propranolol (10 $\mu g.kg^{-1}$) and to a lesser extent by domperidone (5 $\mu g.kg^{-1}$) and indomethacin (25 $\mu g.kg^{-1}$). The cycles of more intense activity lasting 20 min and 40 min on the proximal and distal colon, respectively, only disappeared during the increased propulsive activity evoked by laxatives[6].

The role of supraspinal and spinal outflow on colonic motility is still unclear[7]. Tolazoline, an alpha$_2$-adrenergic blocking agent (10 $\mu g.kg^{-1}$ intrathecally) is a potent stimulant of colonic motility. The mechanism of this excitatory effect is a blockade of the alpha$_2$-adrenergic receptors acting presynaptically on Auerbach's plexus to inhibit acetylcholine release.

Tolazoline and yohimbine can prevent the gastrointestinal propulsive activity reduced in mice by xylazine or amitraz[9]. The use of amitraz in the horse as an insecticide/ascaricide has an adverse effect : it causes impaction of the colon. Tolazoline (0.5 mg.kg intravenously) is able to antagonize the effects of amitraz, just as it is able to prevent the effect of xylazine in the pony[15], suggesting a similar mediation by alpha$_2$-adrenergic receptors.

CHOLINERGIC STIMULATION

Cooling the cervical vagi to less than 4 °C has been shown to cause a marked reduction of colonic activity[5]. A direct vagal effect is shown by persistence of the inhibition induced by cooling after spinal section. A large number of enkephalin-immunoreactive nerve fibres has been observed in the circular smooth muscle layer, the myenteric plexus and the submucous layer of the feline colon. The enkephalins hyperpolarize myenteric neurones and inhibit action potentials by a reduced release of acetylcholine from myenteric neurones. In addition, enkephalins have a direct contractile effect on smooth muscle devoid of all neural elements. The action is thus unchanged in the presence of tetrodotoxin and blocked by naloxone. A postganglionic enkephalinergic neurone mediates the non-cholinergic contraction of the colon, since naloxone in a dose that blocked the effects of exogenously applied enkephalins also blocked the non-cholinergic activity due to pelvic nerve stimulation under atropine[16].

Among anticholinergics, atropine has long been thought to affect colonic motility. However, clinical experience does not suggest much response to doses of these drugs that are used in practice. The inhibition is, at best, transient and incomplete in carnivores. In the horse, the spiking activity (PSB) at the pelvic flexure level ceases for 30 min after injection of atropine (0.1 mg/kg) with a concomitant increase in the baseline (mechanical activity tracing), suggesting either an increase of smooth muscle tone and/or the absence of any propulsion.

ROLE OF OPIATES

A colonic origin for the constipating effects of morphine is likely, since the retention time of digesta, even in the canine colon, represents more than two-thirds of the total transit time. That these effects result more from the stimulation of colonic LSB than from an increased electrolyte and fluid absorption is questionable.

Motor effects

Mu and delta opiate agonists, administered intrathecally, show a tendency to modulate the activity of the whole colon in a similar way — that is, stimulation followed by inhibition[3]. In contrast to the inhibitory and delayed effects on the small intestine of D-Ala$_2$-D-Leu$_5$-enkephalin administered intracerebroventricularly in rats[14], the effects on the colon are excitatory and not delayed[6]. In both dogs and ponies, the stimulatory component lasted a few minutes and disappeared at the expense of inhibitory effects for 1 or 2 h.

Three opiate agonists : meperidine (Demerol), butor-phanol (Stadol) and pentazocine (Talwin) have only trivial motor effects on the equine pelvic flexure[1]. In fact, opiate-agonists stimulate the tonic (LSB) rather than the phasic (PSB) component of the motility, indicating that the constipating effects of opiate agonists on the colon could not be interpreted in terms of motility. In addition, a decrease in the motility index has been found to be associated with a higher propulsive activity when the bulk content of the colon was increased[4].

We recently found that the injection of naloxone in the pony consistently increases the MSB patterns of motility (Figure 12.1). The effects also obtained with methylnalo-xone, suggest that a local opioid system may be operative to slow the propulsion of contents at the equine colonic level[13]. In the pig, the intraluminal administration of

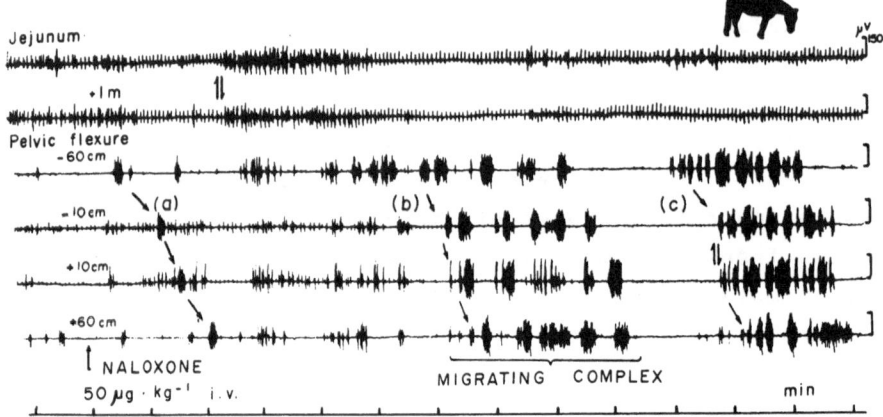

Figure 12.1 Enhancement by naloxone of the electrical activity (direct record) of the jejunum and the colon in the pony; note the high velocity of propagation of spike bursts (a) and of migrating complexes (b, c) recurring at 3 to 5 min intervals.

loperamide, a locally acting opiate agonist, enhances the frequency of cycles on the small and large intestine (Figure 12.2). ACTH(1-24) is able to antagonize such cyclic activity and immunoreactivity since both ACTH and endorphin-related peptides are present in the colon, suggesting the physiological role of a melanocortin-opioid homeostatic system in gut cycling activity.

Effects on fluid transport
The antidiarrhoeal effect of opiates is related to an enhanced absorption of water and electrolytes by the mucosa. Enkephalin and morphine were also shown to block the PGE_2 but not the VIP-stimulated adenylate cyclase activity, hence their efficacy in the prevention of diarrhoea induced by PGs and choleratoxin. Where there is acute diarrhoea and severe depletion of body water, the colon responds homeostatically by a state of secondary hyperaldosteronism, assisting the organism in the Na^+ conservation. The two known factors which increase

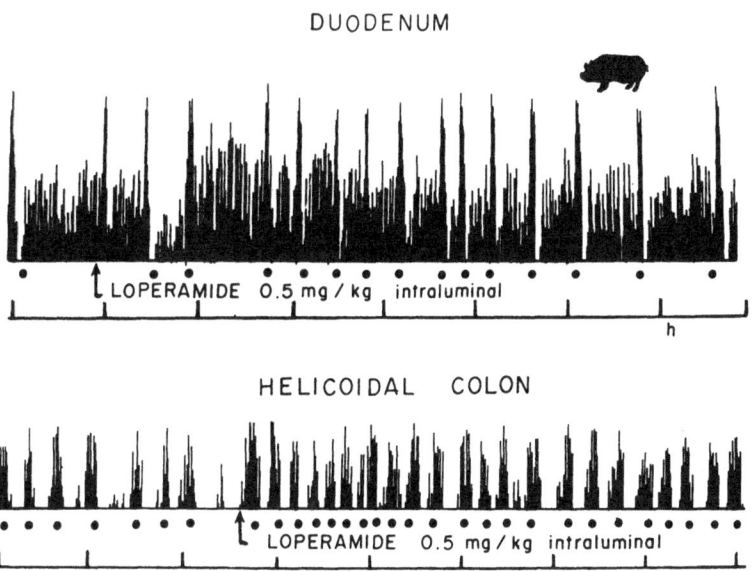

Figure 12.2 Long-lasting enhancement by locally administered loperamide of the cyclical myoelectrical events
(integrated records) of the duodenum and of the helicoidal
colon in the pig.

aldosterone secretion, angiotensin II and dopamine
antagonists like metoclopramide (0.5 mg/kg twice daily for
2 weeks in the rabbit) stimulate the motility of the
intestine. The marked inhibitory effects of dopamine on
the distal colon in vitro are better prevented by beta-
adrenergic antagonists like propranolol or sotalol[8] than
by dopamine antagonists, suggesting a major role for
dopamine in fluid transport rather than in motility.

PROSTAGLANDINS VERSUS SEROTONIN STIMULATION
The first biological effect of prostaglandins to be
described was their ability to induce intestinal smooth
muscle contraction[17]. Defaecation, without emesis, can be
induced selectively in the dog by PGF_2 at the dose level
of 0.15 mg/kg intramuscularly, the response occurring a
few minutes after the injection and the effects persis-

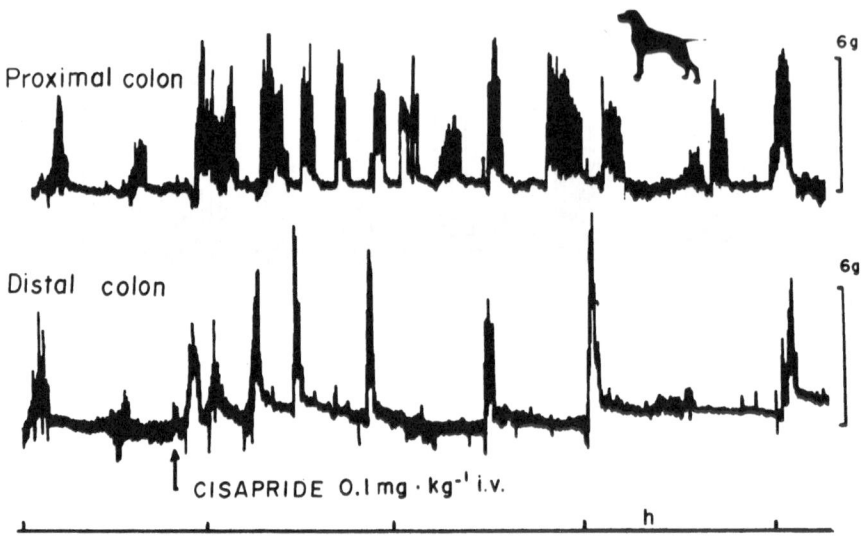

Figure 12.3   Increased propulsive colonic motility (strain gauges) following the intravenous administration of cisapride in the dog.

ting long enough to empty the rectum. The only significant side-effect observed is the increase in respiratory rate, related to the potent bronchoconstrictor effects of $PGF_{2\alpha}$.

A role for endogenous prostaglandins in colonic soft faeces formation by the rabbit has been demonstrated[12]. The inhibition of the proximal colon and the stimulation of the spiking activity of the distal colon during the formation of soft faeces is mimicked by the infusion of both PGE_2 and $PGF_{2\alpha}$. After indomethacin the soft:hard faeces ratio of 1.45 is reduced to 0.92, suggesting a role for prostaglandins. The effects of several neuropeptides, for example, inhibition of gastric acid secretion by somatostatin, drinking behaviour elicited by angiotensin, increased colonic activity or stimulation of borborygmi and defaecation by neurotensin are prostaglandin-mediated. Accordingly, stimulation by neurotensin of the proximal colon in dogs was reduced by aspirin or ketoprofen pretreatment[2]. In horses, the large number of peptides

which   may   be   involved in colonic motor changes supports
the therapeutic value of antiprostaglandins in addition to
their   anti-inflammatory   effects, for example, in ulcerative colitis.

The role of 5-HT and the related peptide, substance P,
in large intestinal motor patterns has not yet been
elucidated[15], except for substances like cisapride, which
has been reported to enhance gastrointestinal transit and
motility via an interaction with 5-HT on myenteric
neurones[11] rather than by a release of acetylcholine.
Figure 12.3 shows that its stimulatory effects on the
canine colon involve primarily enhanced cyclical activity.

References
1. Adams, S.B., Lamar, C.H. and Masty, J. (1984). Motility of the distal portion of the jejunum and pelvic
   flexure in ponies : effects of six drugs. Am. J. Vet.
   Res. 45:795-812.
2. Bardon, T. and Ruckebusch, Y. (1985). Neurotensin-
   induced colonic motor responses in dogs : a mediation
   by prostaglandins. Regul. Peptides 10:107-114.
3. Bardon, T. and Ruckebusch, Y. (1985). Comparative effects of opiate agonists on proximal and distal colonic motility in dogs. Eur. J. Pharmacol. 110:329-334.
4. Cherbut, C. and Ruckebusch, Y. (1985). The effect of
   indigestible particles on digestive transit time and
   colonic motility in dogs and pigs. Br. J. Nutr.
   53:549-557.
5. Collman, P.I., Grundy, D. and Scratcherd, T. (1984).
   Vagal influences on large intestinal motility in the
   anaesthetized ferret. J. Physiol. 348:35-42.
6. Ferré, J.P. and Ruckebusch, Y. (1985). Myoelectrical
   activity and propulsion in the large intestine of fed
   and fasted rats. J. Physiol. 362:93-106.
7. Glick, M.E., Meshkinpour, H., Haldeman, S., Hoehler,
   F., Downey, N. and Bradley, W.E. (1984). Colonic
   dysfunction in patients with thoracic spinal cord
   injury. Gastroenterology 86:287-294.
8. Grivegnée, A.R., Fontaine, J. and Reuse, J. (1984).
   Effect of dopamine on dog distal colon in vitro. J.
   Pharm. Pharmacol. 36:454-457.
9. Hsu, W.H. and Lu, Z.X. (1984). Amitraz-induced delay
   of gastrointestinal transit in mice : mediated by
   alpha$_2$-adrenergic receptors. Drug Devel. Res. 4:
   655-660.
10. King, B.F. and Szurszewski, J.H. (1964). Mechanore-
    ceptor pathway from the distal colon to the autonomic
    nervous system in the guinea-pig. J. Physiol.
    350:93-107.
11. Nemeth, P.R., Ort, C.A., Zafirov, D.H. and Wood, J.D.

(1985). Interactions between serotonin and cisapride on myenteric neurons. Eur. J. Pharmacol. 108:77-83.

12. Pairet, M., Bouyssou, T. and Ruckebusch, Y. (1986). Colonic formation of soft feces in rabbits : a role for endogenous prostaglandins. Am. J. Physiol. (in press).

13. Roger, T., Bardon, T. and Ruckebusch, Y. (1985). Colonic motor responses in the pony : relevance of colonic stimulation by opiate antagonists. Am. J. Vet. Res. 46:31-35.

14. Ruckebusch, Y., Ferré, J.P. and Du, C. (1984). In vivo modulation of intestinal motility and sites of opioid effects in the rat. Regul. Peptides 9:109-117.

15. Sellers, A., Lowe, J.E. and Cummings, J.F. (1985). Trials of serotonin, substance P and alpha$_2$-adrenergic receptor effects on the equine large colon. Cornell Vet. 75:319-323.

16. Sjoqvist, A., Hellstrom, P.M., Jodal, M. and Lundgren, O. (1984). Neurotransmitters involved in the colonic contraction and vasodilatation elicited by activation of the pelvic nerves in the cat. Gastroenterology 86:1481-1487.

17. Thor, P., Konturek, J.W., Konturek, S.J. and Anderson, J.H. (1985). Role of prostaglandins in control of intestinal motility. Am. J. Physiol. 248:G353-G359.

13
Recent advances in the pharmacological control of the intestinal and colonic motor profiles

J. FIORAMONTI, L. BUÉNO AND M. J. FARGEAS

ABSTRACT

Recent studies of the intestinal and colonic motor profiles led to a new approach of digestive pharmacology, based on long-term changes in the pattern of gastrointestinal contractions. Basically the pattern of the small intestine is cyclic and is disrupted for several hours after a meal, while that of the colon consists of phases of contractile activity with a frequency modified by meal ingestion. Opiate drugs are among the most active in modifying this pattern but each drug is characterized by its own effect and involves peripheral and/or central pathways. Endogenous opioid peptides play a role in the control of the motor profile at the level of the central nervous system, since they are able to block the postprandial disruption of the cyclic intestinal pattern and enhance the colonic motor response to feeding. Other peptides are involved in the central control of intestinal motility, but each of them involves its own mechanisms. Several adrenergic, serotoninergic and dopaminergic agonists and/or antagonists are able to modify the occurrence of the cyclic phases of small intestinal activity. These data indicate new effects of classical compounds and the development of new drugs for long-lasting and specific modifications of digestive motility has now commenced.

Most of the pharmacological data on digestive smooth muscle have been obtained under in vitro conditions or in vivo over short time periods. These studies investigated the effects of drugs in terms of increases or decreases in basal or stimulated intestinal motility. Other data have been obtained by determining drug action on intestinal transit time but in view of the complex relationships between digestive motility and the propulsion of digesta no conclusions about the effects of drugs on intestinal contractions can be drawn from these studies. During the last decade the motor profile at various levels of the digestive tract has been established over relatively long periods. Consequently, a new approach to digestive pharmacology, based on the long-term changes in patterns of intestinal motility, has been developed.

SMALL INTESTINAL AND COLONIC MOTOR PROFILES

The use of electrodes or strain gauge transducers chronically fixed to the serosa permitted investigation of the patterns of intestinal and colonic motility. The fundamental pattern of small intestinal contractions is cyclic and was initially described in dogs by Szurszewski in 1969[22]. It consists of a period of quiescence (phase 1) followed by a period of irregular activity (IA or phase 2) and by a period of regular activity (RA or phase 3). These cyclic phases of activity are first seen on the duodenum and are then propagated along the jejunum and the ileum, as a "migrating myoelectric (or motor) complex" (MMC) which occurs every 90 min in dogs and is disrupted for several hours after a meal in many species (Figure 13.1).

A fundamental pattern, analogous to that observed for the small intestine, has not been found for the large bowel. However, in the dog a clearly defined colonic motor profile has been described[11]. It consists of phases of contractile activity, 5-10 min in duration and occurring cyclically at 20-30 min intervals. Ingestion of a daily meal induces three consecutive changes in colonic

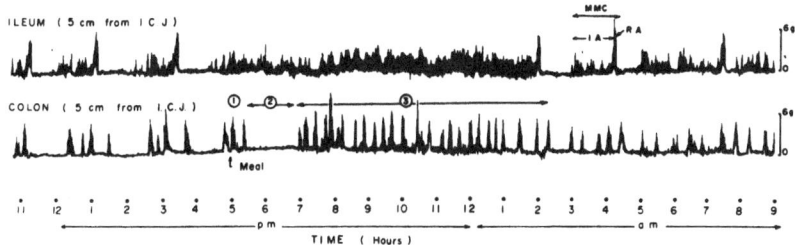

Figure 13.1 Typical intestinal and colonic motor profiles in the conscious dog. The 22 h strain gauge recording of the ileum and the proximal colon shows intestinal MMCs disrupted for several hours after a meal and a triphasic colonic motor response to a meal (1, short lived stimulation; 2, inhibition; 3, long-lasting stimulation). ICJ : ileocolonic junction; IA : irregular activity; RA : regular activity; MMC : migrating motor complex (From reference[11]).

motility : a shortlived stimulation comprising a supplementary phase of contractile activity, inhibition lasting 1-2 h and a long-lasting (8-10 h) increase in the frequency of the cyclic activity phases (see Figure 13.1).

OPIATES

Opiate-like drugs are particularly potent in their effects on digestive motility. However, the existence of multiple opiate receptors, the possible action of opiates on both central and peripheral receptors and differences between the motor profiles at different levels of the digestive tract lead to very heterogeneous responses after opiate administration.

The action of morphine itself on digestive motility involves multiple pathways. It inhibits small intestinal propulsion in rats through central and peripheral pathways[17]. On intestinal motility, intravenous administration of morphine induces a supplementary phase of regular activity (phase 3). This effect was first described in sheep[9] and then confirmed in dogs[20].

Intracerebroventricular administration of morphine to dogs
induces disruption of the cyclic MMC pattern for 5-6 h
instead of an additional phase 3[1 3].

At the colonic level, a stimulatory effect of morphine
has been known for a long time[1] but the effects on the
cyclic pattern of colonic contractions in dogs were only
recently described[8]. They last 3-4 h for a dose of 0.1
mg/kg intravenously and they comprise an increase in the
motility index associated with an increase in the
frequency of the phases of contractions and the occurrence
of periods of continuous contractile activity. These
effects of intravenously administered morphine involve
both central and peripheral opiate receptors, since they
are abolished by a previous intravenous or intracerebroventricular administration of naloxone or of methyllleval-
lorphan, a quaternary compound which does not cross the
blood-brain barrier (unpublished results). Moreover, a
central serotoninergic mechanism is probably involved in
the stimulatory effects of intravenous morphine on colonic
motility, since they are blocked by a previous
intracerebroventricular administration of methysergide[6].
However, the central component of the action of intravenous morphine on colonic motility is not reproduced by
intracerebroventricular administration of morphine, which
induces an unusual pattern of short and frequent phases of
contractions, an effect which is probably mediated through
non-opiate receptors (unpublished results).

Not all opiates have the same effects on the digestive
motor profile. Comparison of the effects of the prototype
mu agonist morphine to those of cyclazocine, a supposed mu
antagonist and mixed kappa and sigma agonist was the first
example given[1 3]. Cyclazocine when given intravenously,
induces disruption and inhibition of the jejunal cyclic
activity instead of a supplementary phase 3 as observed
after morphine. However, cyclazocine and nalorphine,
another mu antagonist and a kappa and sigma agonist,
induce similar stimulatory effects as morphine on colonic
motility[8,13]. Another typical example of the specific

action of an opiate compound is provided by the effect of loperamide. Orally administered at a dose rate of 0.1 mg/kg, loperamide stimulates the motility of the entire digestive tract for a 5-6 h period and induces an unusual pattern of activity never described for any other opiate compound. The cyclic activity of the stomach was replaced by patterns of continuous contractions appearing at about 2 min intervals. The cyclic jejunal MMCs are replaced by continuous irregular activity and the frequency of the phases of colonic contraction is increased. These effects are mediated peripherally since they are not modified by the previous intracerebroventricular administration of a quaternary narcotic antagonist. However, they are probably not local actions since they can be reproduced by subcutaneous administration at the same dosage (unpublished results).

Opiates also modify the pattern of intestinal and colonic contractions in the postprandial state. Morphine given intravenously after a meal consistently induces a phase 3 contraction propagated along the small intestine[20] but the most important effect is probably a control of the small intestinal and colonic patterns of motility by endogenous opiate peptides at the central level. A synthetic analogue of metenkephalin, (D-Ala^2-Met^5)enkephalinamide, when administered intracerebroventricularly just after a meal strongly reduces the duration of the postprandial disruption of the jejunal motor profile and induces cyclic MMCs instead of a continuous irregular activity[7]. Central administration before a meal of the enkephalinase inhibitor, tiorphan, enhances the colonic motor response to feeding, the postprandial colonic motility being increased almost three-fold by comparison to a meal given alone[12].

Finally, the effects of opiates on the digestive motor profile are not unequivocal, and endogenous opiates may play a role in the intestinal and colonic motor response to feeding. However, the data presented here concern the jejunum and the proximal colon of the dog. Another peculiarity of opiates, first described in 1982[15], concerns species differences and the colonic segment considered. For example, morphine stimulates colonic motility in dogs but inhibits it in horses, the effects being more intense on the proximal than on the distal colon.

ADRENERGIC, SEROTONINERGIC, DOPAMINERGIC DRUGS

Alpha-adrenergic agonists are known for their inhibitory effects on intestinal motility. For example, clonidine, an alpha$_2$-agonist inhibits small intestinal propulsion through a central pathway[16]. In contrast, adrenergic antagonists such as phentolamine and dihydroergotamine strongly increase the frequency of MMCs[2]. Beta-adrenergic agonists such as isoprenaline have been found to initiate a phase 3 contraction in both fasted and fed states, through the release of somatostatin[21].

In dogs, serotonin infusion during a period of quiescence, induced an irregular pattern of activity. The serotonin antagonist, methysergide, stimulates jejunal motility and disrupts the cyclic MMC pattern[18]. However, an atypical effect of methysergide has been described in sheep. In this species, contrary to the response in dogs, methysergide increases the frequency of the phase 3 contractions[19].

Dopamine given intravenously induces a premature phase 3 in fasted dogs and sheep, and in fed dogs it restores a fasted pattern of intestinal motility when given intra-cerebroventricularly[14]. Dopamine administered by intra-venous infusion in dogs inhibits the proximal colon and stimulates the distal colon, the inhibitory effect being partially mediated through alpha$_1$-adrenoceptors, the stimulation of the distal colon being mediated through specific dopamine receptors[3]. In contrast, bromo-criptine, a potent dopamine agonist, stimulates both proximal and distal colon, these effects being blocked by dopaminergic, but not adrenergic, antagonists.

PEPTIDES

Biologically active peptides comprise a new sphere of interest in pharmacology and some neuropeptides of the brain-gut axis have been found to modify digestive motility through their central actions. In 1982[9] it was shown for the first time that two peptides centrally administered in fasted rats were able to modify the cyclical pattern of intestinal motility : CCK octapeptide decreased the frequency of MMCs and at higher doses it disrupted the cyclic pattern, while somatostatin increased the frequency of MMCs.

In dogs, two groups of peptides, effective on small intestinal motor activity through a central pathway, have been identified. The first category includes calcitonin, neurotensin, metenkephalin and growth hormone releasing factor (GRF), which induce a cyclic pattern during the postprandial state. It has been shown, initially in rats[10] and then in dogs[4], that the effects of calcitonin are mediated through the release of prostaglandins since they are abolished by indomethacin and reproduced by central administration of PGE_2. However, despite the similarities of the final effects, there is no common mechanism in the action of these peptides. The effects of calcitonin and neurotensin are mediated through a release of prostaglandins, while those of GRF involve central dopaminergic receptors. None of these compounds seem to act through opiate receptors since naloxone does not block the action of these four peptides, even that of metenke-phalin. Other peptides such as corticotropin releasing factor, oxytocin and vasopressin disrupt the cyclic motor profile when administered intracerebro- ventricularly to fasted animals.

Finally, studies of the central actions of some peptides indicate that the digestive influences which induce a postprandial pattern of intestinal motility involve a central pathway which can be inhibited by several peptides.

PERSPECTIVES AND CONCLUSIONS

Knowledge of the patterns of small intestinal and colonic motility permits the development of new compounds, selected for their specific modifications of the digestive motor profile. This is exemplified by cisapride, a non-antidopaminergic and non-cholinergic compound which stimulates the irregular (propulsive) activity of the small intestine and the phasic activity of the colon. According to the relationships between the pattern of digestive motility with the transit of digesta, the absorption of nutrients and the control of the intestinal flora, the therapeutic value of compounds active on this pattern seems promising. However, an accurate diagnosis of digestive motor disturbances is not easy and can limit the use of such future therapy.

References
1. Adler, H.F. and Ivy, C.A. (1940). Morphine-atropine antagonism on colon motility in the dog. J. Pharmacol. Exp. Ther. 70:454-459.
2. Altaparmakov, I. and Wienbeck, M. (1983). Alpha-adrenergic control of the interdigestive migrating electrical complex (IDMEC). In : Labo, G. and Bortolotti, M. (eds). Gastrointestinal Motility, pp.3-7. Verona : Cortina International.
3. Buéno, L., Fargeas, M.J., Fioramonti, J. and Hondé, C. (1984). Effects of dopamine and bromocriptine on colonic motility in dog. Br. J. Pharmacol. 82:35-42.
4. Buéno. L., Fargeas, M.J., Fioramonti, J. and Primi, M.P. (1985). Central control of intestinal motility by prostaglandins : a mediator of the actions of several peptides in rats and dogs. Gastroenterology 88:1888-1894.
5. Buéno, L. and Ferré, J.P. (1982). Central regulation of intestinal motility by somatostatin and cholecystokinin octapeptide. Science 216:1427-1429.
6. Buéno, L. and Fioramonti, J. (1982). A possible central serotonergic mechanism involved in the effects of morphine on colonic motility in dog. Eur. J. Pharmacol. 82:147-153.
7. Buéno, L., Fioramonti, J., Hondé, C., Fargeas, M.J. and Primi, M.P. (1985). Central and peripheral control of gastrointestinal and colonic motility by endogenous opiates in conscious dogs. Gastroenterology 88:549-556.
8. Buéno, L., Fioramonti, J. and Ruckebusch, M. (1981). Comparative effects of morphine and nalorphine on colonic motility in the conscious dog. Eur. J. Pharmacol. 75:239-245.

9. Buéno, L., Ruckebusch, Y. (1978). Origine de l'action excito-motrice de l'intestin par la morphine. C.R. Soc. Biol. 172:972-977.
10. Fargeas, M.J., Fioramonti, J. and Buéno, L. (1984). Prostaglandin E_2 : a neuromodulator in the central control of gastrointestinal motility and feeding behavior by calcitonin. Science 225:1050-1052.
11. Fioramonti, J. and Buéno, L. (1983). Diurnal changes in colonic motor profile in conscious dogs. Dig. Dis. Sci. 28:257-264.
12. Fioramonti, J., Buéno, L. and Fargeas, M.J. (1985). Enhancement of colonic motor response to feeding by central endogenous opiates in the dog. Life Sci. 36:2509-2514.
13. Fioramonti, J., Fargeas, M.J. and Buéno, L. (1984). Comparative effects of morphine and cyclazocine on gastrointestinal motility in conscious dogs. Arch. Int. Pharmacodyn. Ther. 270:141-150.
14. Fioramonti, J., Fargeas, M.J., Hondé, C. and Buéno, L. (1984). Effects of central and peripheral administration of dopamine on pattern of intestinal motility in dogs. Dig. Dis. Sci. 29:1023-1027.
15. Fioramonti, J., Niemegeers, C.J.E. and Awouters, F. (1983). Diarrhoea and antidiarrhoeal drugs. In : Ruckebusch Y., Toutain P.L. and Koritz, G.D. (eds). Veterinary Pharmacology and Toxicology, pp.307-320. Lancaster : MTP Press L.
16. Galligan, J.J. and Burks, T.F. (1983). Effects of centrally and peripherally administered clonidine on small intestinal transit in the rat. Proc. West. Pharmacol. Soc. 26:387-391.
17. Manara. L. and Bianchetti, A. (1985). The central and peripheral influences of opioids on gastrointestinal propulsion. Ann. Rev. Pharmacol. Toxicol. 25:249-273.
18. Ormsbee, H.S., Silber, D.A. and Hardy, F.E. (1984). Serotonin regulation of the canine migrating motor complex. J. Pharmacol. Exp. Ther. 231:436-440.
19. Ruckebusch, Y. and Bardon, T. (1984). Involvement of serotonergic mechanisms in initiation of small intestine cyclic motor events. Dig. Dis. Sci. 29:520-527.
20. Sarna, S., Northcott, P. and Belbeck, L. (1982). Mechanism of cycling of migrating myoelectric complexes : effect of morphine. Am. J. Physiol. 242: G588-G595.
21. Summers, R.W., Flatt, A., Yanda, R.J. and Yamada, T. (1984). Isoproterenol induces activity fronts in fed dogs through somatostatin release. Gastroenterology 87:999-1003.
22. Szurszewski, J.H. (1969). A migrating electric complex of the canine small intestine. Am. J. Physiol. 217:1757-1763.

14
Cholinergic-like effect of the H_2-receptor antagonist ranitidine on the rabbit small intestine

G. KOUNENIS, M. KOUTSOVITI-PAPADOPOULOU AND V. ELEZOGLOU

ABSTRACT

The histamine H_2-receptor antagonist ranitidine was tested for its effect on the rabbit small intestine. Preparations of isolated segments of duodenum, jejunum and ileum of adult animals were used. Ranitidine possessed a significant stimulant action on these preparations, the action being strongest on the duodenum and weakest on the ileum. The maximum response to ranitidine was about 62% of the maximum response to acetylcholine. Ranitidine produced a dose-dependent potentiation of acetylcholine-induced contractions and the stimulant action of ranitidine was prevented by atropine. These findings suggest that ranitidine's stimulant action is associated with the cholinergic system and it occurs in descending degree of intensity from the duodenum to the ileum.

INTRODUCTION

Histamine H_2-receptor antagonists are usually devoid of both cholinergic and anticholinergic properties, although it was reported that under experimental conditions some of them (metiamide, cimetidine and oxmetidine) may inhibit the contractions induced by cholinergic agents on isolated smooth muscle preparations[2,7,10]. It was also reported that the H_2-receptor antagonist ranitidine has no anticholinergic activity[1,8,9], but that it exerts a stimulant effect on the isolated muscular strips of the lower oesophageal sphincter, the gastric fundus and the colon of the rat, as well as on isolated muscle strips of the pylorus of the guinea-pig[4,6]. On the other hand, comparable stimulant effects of ranitidine on isolated heart preparations of the guinea-pig[3] were never observed.

On the basis of these findings we decided to investigate the action of ranitidine on the rabbit small intestine (duodenum, jejunum and ileum) and its possible interactions with acetylcholine and atropine. The findings obtained provide evidence for a cholinergic-like effect of ranitidine on the rabbit small intestine.

MATERIAL AND METHODS

Rabbits of both sexes, weighing approximately 1500 g, were killed by a blow on the back of the neck and exsanguinated. The abdomen was opened and sections of duodenum, jejunum and ileum were removed and placed in beakers containing warm (37 °C) Tyrode solution (millimolar : NaCl 136.80, KCl 2.68, CaCl$_2$ 1.08, MgCl$_2$ 0.49, NaHCO$_3$ 11.90 and glucose 5.56). A segment of 10-15 cm ileum, closest to the caecum, was discarded. After expelling the contents by gently passing Tyrode solution at 37 °C through the lumen, the tissue was placed in clean Tyrode solution and cut in to 1 cm long segments, which were set up in isolated organ baths at 37 °C and bubbled with 95% oxygen and 5% carbon dioxide. The isotonic muscle contractions of the preparations were recorded via a Physiograph (desk model, type DMP-4A, Narco Co., U.S.A.). A resting tension of 2 g was applied to the preparations and they were allowed to stabilize for a period of 30 min.

The following compounds were used : ranitidine hydrochloride (Glaxo, England), acetylcholine chloride (E. Merck, Darmstadt) and atropine sulfate (Chropee, Greece). Drug solutions were added in a cumulative manner at time intervals of 1 min to give molar concentrations from 3.2 x 10^{-6} to 10^{-3}M for ranitidine and 10^{-8} to 10^{-5}M for

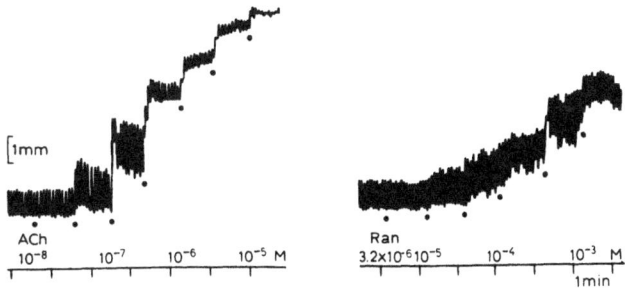

Figure 14.1   Responses to acetylcholine (ACh) and ranitidine (Ran) on the isolated rabbit jejunum, drug doses are
expressed as final molar (M) bath concentrations.

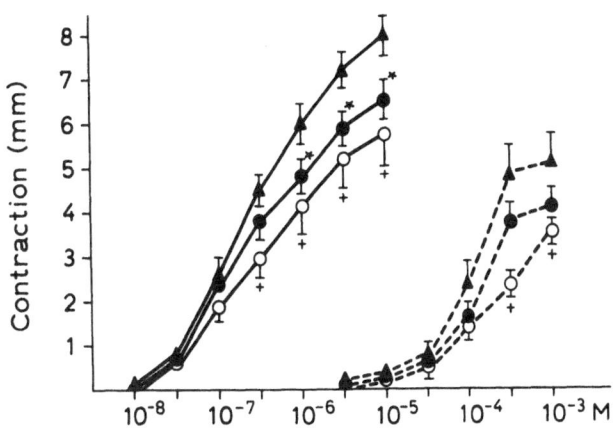

Figure 14.2   Dose-response curves to acetylcholine (solid
lines) and ranitidine (broken lines) on the isolated rabbit duodenum (▲), jejunum (●) and ileum (o). Each point
represents the mean value (n = 10-15) and the vertical
lines indicate the SEM. Asterisks and crosses indicate
the significance of the values (* = Duodenum compared with
jejunum, p < 0.02 - p < 0.05, + = duodenum compared with
ileum, p < 0.01 - p < 0.02).

acetylcholine.   After the maximum concentrations of each
compound had been achieved the preparations were washed
and rested for 10 min. Then acetylcholine was added to
the organ bath fluid 2 min after the treatment with either

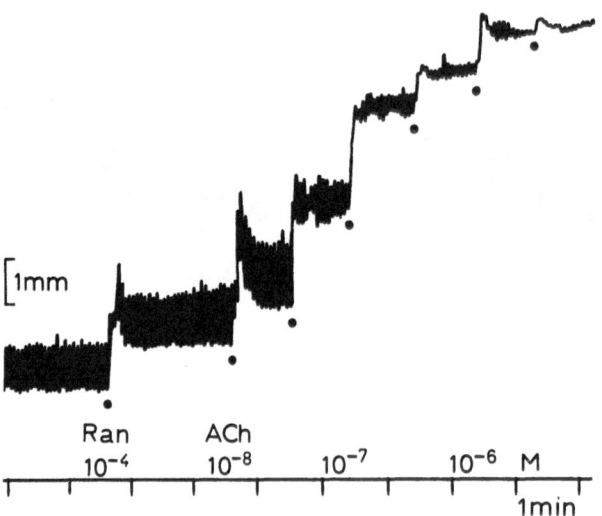

Figure 14.3 The potentiation of the acetylcholine (Ach)-
induced contractions by ranitidine (Ran) on the isolated
rabbit jejunum.

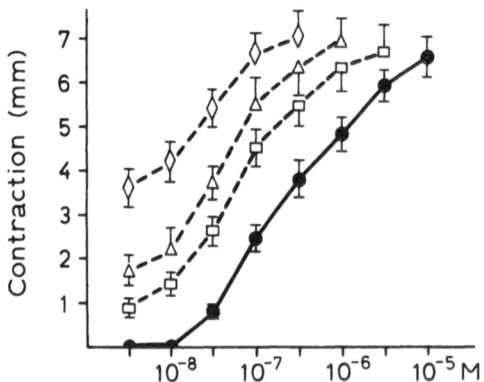

Figure 14.4 Dose-response curves to acetylcholine (solid
line) on the isolated rabbit jejunum and the potentiation
of the acetylcholine-induced contractions by ranitidine
(broken lines) at the concentrations of 3.2×10^{-5} (□),
10^{-4} (▲) and 3.2×10^{-4}M (◊). Each point represents the
mean value (n = 5–15) and the vertical lines indicate the
SEM (all potentiated values were significant, p < 0.001 –
p < 0.05).

Table 14.1 Effect of ranitidine (Ran) and atropine (Atr) on acetylcholine (Ach)-induced contractions (mm) on isolated rabbit jejunum

ACh	ACh			ACh
ACh	Plus Ran 3.2×10^{-5} M	Plus Ran 10^{-4} M	Plus Ran 3.2×10^{-4} M	Plus Atr 10^{-8} M
3.2×10^{-9} M	0.88±0.22	1.67±0.28	3.66±0.43	
10^{-8} M	1.43±0.27	2.16±0.49	4.14±0.44	
3.2×10^{-8} M 0.81±0.11	2.60±0.28	3.73±0.34	5.38±0.41	
10^{-7} M 2.45±0.23	4.50±0.39	5.51±0.59	6.58±0.49	0.11±0.06
3.2×10^{-7} M 3.79±0.37	5.46±0.47	6.37±0.61	7.01±0.62	0.41±0.19
10^{-6} M 4.81±0.35	6.33±0.55	6.88±0.51		1.29±0.33
3.2×10^{-6} M 5.87±0.36	6.67±0.65			3.61±0.42
10^{-5} M 6.55±0.47				4.66±0.62

Values are means ± SEM; n = 5-15.

ranitidine or atropine; ranitidine was also added 2 min after the treatment with atropine.

Statistical evaluation of the data was performed using the Student's t-test for paired or unpaired data.

RESULTS

Ranitidine exerted a significant stimulant effect on the isolated rabbit duodenum and jejunum at concentrations of 10^{-5} to 10^{-3} M and on the ileum from 3.2×10^{-5} to 10^{-3} M. This stimulant effect was stronger on the duodenum and

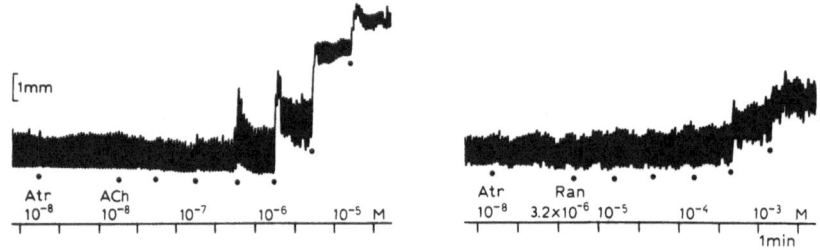

Figure 14.5   The prevention of the acetylcholine (ACh) and ranitidine (Ran)-induced contractions by atropine (Atr) on the isolated rabbit jejunum.

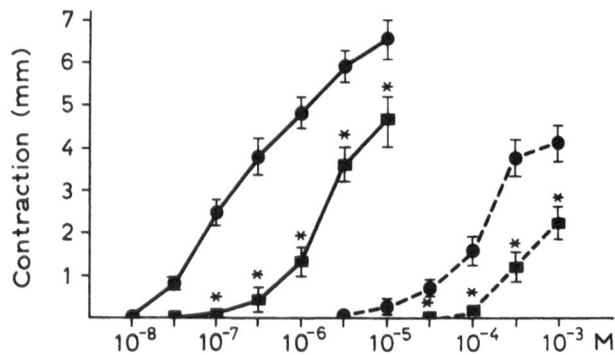

Figure 14.6   Dose-response curves to acetylcholine (solid line,●) and ranitidine (broken line,●) on the isolated rabbit jejunum and the prevention of the acetylcholine and ranitidine-induced contractions by atropine at the concentration of 10^{-8} M (■). Each point represents the mean value (n = 5–15) and the vertical lines indicate the SEM. Asterisks indicate the significance of the values ($p < 0.001 - p < 0.05$).

weaker on the ileum. Similar effects were obtained with acetylcholine at concentrations ranging from 3.2×10^{-8} to 10^{-5} M. The average maximum contractions (mean ± SEM) caused by ranitidine were found to be 5.09 ± 0.62 mm for the duodenum, 4.09 ± 0.37 mm for the jejunum, and 3.49 ± 0.32 mm for the ileum. The above mean values were

Table 14.2 Effect of atropine (Atr) on ranitidine (Ran)-
induced contractions (mm) on isolated rabbit jejunum

	Ran	Ran plus Atr 10^{-8} M
10^{-5} M	0.25 ± 0.08	
3.2×10^{-5} M	0.69 ± 0.14	
10^{-4} M	1.57 ± 0.28	0.14 ± 0.07
3.2×10^{-4} M	3.76 ± 0.41	1.21 ± 0.20
10^{-3} M	4.09 ± 0.37	2.26 ± 0.26

Values are means ± SEM; n = 5-15.

obtained from 10 to 15 separate preparations and were
about 62% of the maximum activity of acetylcholine (8.01 ±
0.45 mm, 6.55 ± 0.47 mm and 5.77 ± 0.72 mm respectively)
(Figures 14.1 and 14.2). Ranitidine potentiated the
acetylcholine-induced contractions on the isolated rabbit
jejunum significantly (Figures 14.3 and 14.4). The mean
results obtained in 5-15 separate preparations are
summarized in Table 14.1. The potentiation of the
acetylcholine-induced contractions depended on the
ranitidine concentration (3.2×10^{-5} to 3.2×10^{-4} M). The
stimulant effects of ranitine and of acetylcholine on the
isolated rabbit jejunum, at concentrations of 10^{-5} to
10^{-3} M for ranitidine, and 3.2×10^{-8} to 10^{-5} M for acetylcholine, were significantly inhibited by atropine 10^{-8} M
(Figures 14.5 and 14.6). The mean values obtained in 5-15
separate preparations are represented in Tables 14.1 and
14.2.

DISCUSSION

The histamine H_2-receptor antagonist ranitidine exerted a strong stimulant effect on rabbit isolated small intestine (duodenum, jejunum and ileum). This stimulant effect became progressively weaker from the duodenum to the ileum. The maximum activity of ranitidine was about 62% of the maximum activity of acetylcholine. In addition ranitidine causes a stimulant effect on isolated muscle strips of the lower oesophageal sphincter, the gastric fundus and the colon of the rat, as well as on isolated muscle strips of the pylorus of the guinea-pig[4,6]. On the other hand, no stimulant action of ranitidine could be demonstrated on isolated heart preparations of the guinea-pig[3]. These data suggest that the stimulant effect of ranitidine is limited to some animals and to some tissues. Also, ranitidine produced a dose-dependent potentiation of acetylcholine-induced contractions on the isolated rabbit jejunum and the stimulant effect of ranitidine was prevented by atropine. The ranitidine stimulant effects are therefore associated with the cholinergic system. The cholinergic effects of ranitidine on the small intestine may modify intestinal motility. They may also explain the diarrhoea and constipation that have been reported in a very small percentage of patients treated with ranitidine[3].

CONCLUSION

Ranitidine exerted a stimulant effect on the isolated rabbit small intestine in descending degree of intensity from the duodenum to the ileum. This stimulant effect was prevented by atropine. Ranitidine potentiated the stimulant effect of acetylcholine. These findings lead us to the conclusion that the ranitidine stimulant effect appears to be associated with the cholinergic system.

References
1. Bertaccini, G. and Dobrilla, G. (1980). Histamine H_2-receptor antagonists : old and new generation. Pharmacology and clinical use. Ital. J. Gastroenterol.

   12:309-314.
2. Bertaccini, G. and Coruzzi, G. (1981). Azione dei
   bloccanti dei recettori istaminici H₂ sullo sfintere
   esofageo inferiore (LES) isolato di ratto. Il Farmaco
   36:129-134.
3. Bertaccini, G. and Coruzzi, G. (1981). Effect of some
   new histamine H₂-receptor antagonists on the guinea-
   pig papillary muscle. Naunyn-Schmiedeberg's Arch.
   Pharmacol. 317:225-227.
4. Bertaccini, G. and Coruzzi, G. (1982). Cholinergic-
   like effects of the new histamine H₂-receptor
   antagonist ranitidine. Agents Actions 12:168-171.
5. Bertaccini, G. and Coruzzi, G. (1984). H₂-receptor
   antagonists : side effects and adverse effects. Ital.
   J. Gastroenterol. 16:119-125.
6. Bertaccini, G., Poli, E., Adami, M. and Coruzzi, G.
   (1983). Effect of some new H₂-receptor antagonists on
   gastrointestinal motility. Agents Actions 13:157-162.
7. Black, J.W. and Spencer, K.E.V. (1983). Metiamide in
   systematic screening tests. In : Wood, C.J. and
   Simkins, M.A. (eds). International Symposium on
   Histamine H₂-Receptor Antagonists, pp.23-26. London :
   Deltakos.
8. Bradshaw, J., Brittain, J.W. , Clitherow, M.J., Daly,
   M.J., Jack, D., Price, B.J. and Stables, R. (1979).
   Ranitidine (AH 19065) : a new potent, selective
   histamine H₂-receptor antagonist. Br. J. Pharmacol.
   66:464.
9. Daly, M.J., Humphray, J.M. and Stables, R. (1981).
   Some "in vitro" and "in vivo" actions of the new
   histamine H₂-receptor antagonist, ranitidine. Br. J.
   Pharmacol. 72:49-54.
10. Voutsas, D., Kokolis, N., Kounenis, G. and Elezoglou,
    V. (1982). Effect of cimetidine (Tagamet) on rabbit
    jejunum "in vitro" and antagonistic action of it with
    acetylcholine, arecoline and pilocarpine. Proceedings
    of the 6th Greek Gastroenterology Congress (1981), pp.
    480-488. Thessaloniki : University Studio Press.

Comparative Pharmacokinetic Studies

15
Comparative pharmacokinetics: introductory remarks

M. G. BOGAERT

ABSTRACT

When comparing the pharmacokinetics of a drug in different species, conclusions can only be drawn from carefully conducted studies and the basic principles of pharmacokinetics should be taken into account. Such comparisons are for example only meaningful if presence of linear kinetics has been ascertained; absorption in different species can only be compared if intravenous plasma concentration data are also available. In these introductory remarks, attention is drawn to a number of possible problems in that regard, as a guide for the systematic discussions of comparative pharmacokinetics which will follow.

INTRODUCTION

Pharmacokinetics is the study of the time course of drug concentrations in the organism, these concentrations depending upon absorption, distribution and elimination.

Measurable concentrations in the organism are attained only after absorption unless the drug is given by the intravenous route. Distribution through the body is influenced by factors such as protein binding in the plasma, and tissue binding. Elimination takes place as excretion in unchanged form, mainly in the urine but also in the bile, or as biotransformation to one or more metabolites.

PRELIMINARY CONSIDERATIONS

There is considerable interest in interspecies differences
in absorption, distribution and elimination. In order to
compare pharmacokinetics in different species, it is necessary to be aware of a number of possible variables,i.e.

1. intraspecies variability;
2. influence of disease states;
3. interactions between drugs;
4. biopharmaceutical factors;
5. presence of non-linear kinetics.

Intraspecies variability

The most important factor is intraspecies variability.
Indeed, interspecies differences can only be evaluated in
the light of intraspecies differences, because of considerable animal-to-animal variations. Hence, to make valid
comparisons between species, large numbers of animals of
each species must be used.

Disease states and drug interactions

The possible presence of disease states should be considered. Pharmacokinetic studies are often carried out in un-
healthy animals. This may lead to misleading and incor-
rect pharmacokinetic data. This also applies to drug interactions : drugs given concomitantly can alter the kinetics of the agent being studied.

Kinetics

Formulation may also significantly affect drug kinetics.
Comparative studies can only be made if the kinetics are
linear. Linearity of the kinetics means that there is
proportionality between the dose given and the plasma
concentrations obtained : if one doubles the dose given,
the concentrations at any given time will also be double.
Linearity is only obtained if absorption, distribution and
elimination follow first order-kinetics. In recent years
it has become apparent that for a number of drugs this

proportionality does not occur, particularly when high doses are given. This can be due, for example, to protein binding with saturation at higher concentrations, or to capacity-limited biotransformation. When the dose is increased, for example by a factor 2, in case of non-linearity within a certain dose-range, the concentrations will increase by much more than that.

ABSORPTION STUDIES

Absorption after oral administration in different species is often compared. Absorption after oral administration involves transfer of the drug from within the gastrointestinal tract into the plasma of the portal vein; from the portal vein the drug reaches the systemic circulation after passing through the liver (so-called first-pass). Every drug given by the oral route and absorbed from the stomach or intestine undergoes the hepatic first-pass effect; some drugs are extracted considerably at that time. By just looking at plasma concentrations, one cannot distinguish between absorption in the strict sense and first-pass effects.

What can be learned from plasma concentration-time relationship after oral administration of a drug ? Peak plasma concentration, the time at which this is obtained, and the area under the plasma concentration-time curve can be estimated. It is important to realize that comparing the oral curve in one species with that in another can be very misleading unless the plasma concentrations after intravenous administration in both species are known. Indeed, the shape of the plasma concentration-time curve after oral administration is not only determined by absorption characteristics, but also by distribution and elimination of the drug. If the latter show interspecies differences, the oral absorption curves will also show differences, even if the absorption pattern is similar. Even the time at which the peak concentration is obtained is influenced to a large degree by the speed of elimination.

DISTRIBUTION AND ELIMINATION

After absorption the drug is distributed throughout the body. Distribution is influenced by factors such as binding of the drug in the plasma, and tissue binding. Difficulties in comparing serum binding in different species are extensively dealt with in chapter 18.

A drug may be eliminated in unchanged form, i.e. excreted (for example, renal excretion) or biotransformed to one or more metabolites. Biotransformation is of particular interest in comparative studies because variability of biotransformation is often the main determinant of the variability of the pharmacokinetics of a drug.

From the plasma concentration-time curve after intravenous administration, the volume of distribution and the elimination parameters can be calculated. It is only after distribution has taken place, that the elimination phase can be studied; in many studies it is not easy to distinguish between distribution and elimination phases. The elimination half-life is the time necessary for the plasma concentrations to fall by 50%. Often, data are expressed as "elimination constant" (k_{el}) which bears a very simple relationship to half-life ($t_{1/2}$) – in other words, $k_{el} = \dfrac{0.693}{t_{1/2}}$.

Clearance is the amount of plasma cleared per unit of time. Some drugs are only cleared by the kidney; others are completely cleared by the liver – that is, by biotransformation – and no unchanged drug leaves the organism. In many instances, however, the drug is cleared both by renal excretion and by biotransformation in the liver, and sometimes by other organs and routes as well. In this case, the "total body clearance" (Cl_{el}) is the sum of the plasma clearances by different organs. "Total body clearance" is also called "plasma clearance", and it can be calculated from the intravenous plasma concentration time-curve by obtaining the volume of distribution and the half-life, where $Cl_{pl} = \dfrac{k_{el}\,0.693}{Vd}$.

Clearance reflects how well the clearing organs are performing, while half-life is not only dependent upon clearance, but also on the volume of distribution. This distinction is important. When a human patient receives digoxin and gentamicin, both are cleared mainly by the kidney, and the plasma clearance of both compounds is rather similar. However, the half-life of digoxin is more than 1 day, whereas the half-life of gentamicin is approximately 2 h. This is because digoxin has a very large volume of distribution, while for gentamicin it is very small.

Evaluation of elimination in two species, involves therefore consideration not only of the half-life but also of the clearance, so that one is not misled by differences in half-life which could be due to differences in volume of distribution.

Species differences in plasma clearance of a substance can be due to several factors. The clearance of a drug by either kidney or liver, depends on three main factors : the intrinsic capacity of the clearing organ, the plasma or blood flow to the organ, and the degree of binding of the drug in plasma.

The intrinsic ability of the liver to metabolize drugs can differ widely from species to species, both in terms of the overall rate and metabolic pathways involved. The way the kidney handles the drug, for example, reabsorption and active secretion in the tubuli, shows interspecies differences. Blood flow to liver and kidney and the extent of binding of the drug in plasma can also differ from one species to another.

It is important to know that the effect on clearance, of changes in the intrinsic abilities of the clearing organs, in flow and in plasma binding, depends upon the drug studied. The hepatic clearance of most drugs will be influenced by changes in the intrinsic state, for example, enzymatic induction; for these same drugs, the hepatic clearance is restricted to drugs which are free in plasma, and changes in flow have only a minor influence : this is the so-called "restrictive, non-flow dependent" hepatic clearance. For some drugs however, such as lidocaine and propranolol, the hepatic clearance depends mainly on flow to the organ and is not restricted to the free fraction. It is less influenced by changes in enzymatic activity; this is the so-called "non-restrictive, flow dependent" clearance.

CONCLUSION

Studies of interspecies differences in pharmacokinetics should be performed in a systematical fashion. Conclusions from occasional observations or from studies made in different circumstances should be viewed with caution; the plasma concentrations should be interpreted on the basis of a correct understanding of pharmacokinetic principles.

16
Comparative neonatal pharmacokinetics

P. DE BACKER

ABSTRACT

Postnatal development can affect the disposition and pharmacokinetics of drugs in man and animals. Factors such as gastric pH, gastrointestinal motility, mucosal absorbing area, microbial population and milk feeding are major determinants in the absorption process of drugs in the neonate. Postnatal evolution in body composition can lead to important alterations in distribution pattern of drugs in newborns. Differences in maturity at birth and in the rate of postnatal development of the renal and hepatic functions are present in the various species. Therefore, important variations in pharmacokinetics and pharmacodynamics between mammalian newborns can be expected for the same drug.

INTRODUCTION

Age is one of the factors which modify the disposition and the actions of a drug. Therefore in the last decade there has been a growing interest in the actions and fate of drugs in neonatal man and animals.

In all species, neonates undergo continuous anatomical and functional changes. Differences between animal species in both the degree of maturity at the time of birth and the rate of postnatal development have been reported. Differences in the disposition of a foreign compound and in its pharmacodynamics between young animals of different species can, therefore, be expected.

The present study deals with the influence of postnatal growth on absorption, distribution and elimination of drugs in animals and man in the neonatal period. These factors will be discussed in the light of anatomical, physiological and biochemical developments.

ABSORPTION

Absorption of drugs from the gastrointestinal tract of the newborn is determined by a variety of continually changing factors[3]. Some of these factors are listed in Table 16.1.

Gastric pH

In the human neonate, gastric pH is between 6.5 and 8.0 at birth, and it fluctuates considerably thereafter and takes several months to reach adult levels[13]. In newborn calves, the abomasal pH is 7.5, but it drops in a few hours to 4.0; on changing to solid food in the following weeks, the average pH of the abomasum is 3.6[12]. A diminished breakdown of, for example, penicillins, with a higher bioavailability can therefore be expected, and has been found in very young humans and calves[10,24].

Gastrointestinal motility

Another major determinant in the drug absorption process is the development of gastrointestinal motility. It is generally accepted that, in the newborn, a lack of propulsive activity affects the transfer of orally administered drugs and leads to delayed absorption. In neonates, it takes 6-8 months before the gastric emptying time approximates to adult values[13]. In dogs also, a foetal pattern of propulsive activity in the intestine is present in the first weeks of postnatal life. Adult patterns of motor activity were registered in the small bowel of the newborn lamb[20]; the development of functional reticuloruminal activity however only starts after birth

Table 16.1 Drug absorption affecting characteristics of
the gastrointestinal tract in the neonate

Gastric acid secretion   low
Gastrointestinal motility   immature
Gastrointestinal anatomy   not fully developed
Microbial population   low
Intestinal enzymatic activity   low
Mucosal absorbing area   small
Blood perfusion   variable

----

and several weeks are needed to achieve a fully developed
forestomach function in this species[13]. The postnatal
anatomical development of the forestomachs can have an
important influence on the absorption process of certain
drugs in the young ruminant.   In the case of sulphonamides, a delayed absorption was noticed in developing
lambs and kids[1,16].

Microbial population
The establishment of a ruminal microbial population in the
forestomachs of young ruminants can interfere with the
absorption of drugs. This can lead to a decreased bioavailability with age as reported for chloramphenicol[6] and
trimethoprim[17] in developing ruminants.

Mucosal area and blood perfusion
In general, at birth the intestinal mucosal absorbing
area is limited while the postnatal development of the
regional blood perfusion in the different parts of the
gastrointestinal tract is variable.   Both factors are
capable of substantially modifying the absorption of
drugs.

Milk feeding and absorption
Finally, it should be added that the feeding of milk, an
important food component in the first period of life, also

affects the absorption of drugs. In calves, a lower bioavailability was found for tetracyclines, penicillin, chloramphenicol and trimethoprim after a meal containing milk components[10].

First pass extraction

In addition to absorption, first pass extraction can also affect the bioavailability of certain drugs. To our knowledge, however, no studies dealing with the evolution of the first pass phenomenon in neonates have been conducted.

DISTRIBUTION

Extracellular and intracellular water

From the plasma, drug is distributed to the tissues. Binding in serum and in tissues can occur and affect the distribution of a foreign compound. The continuous changes in body composition which occur in newborn mammals can alter the distribution pattern of a drug. The most important changes in body composition in the very young animal are listed in Table 16.2. In most mammals, total body water content is initially elevated but decreases during foetal growth and continues to diminish postnatally, although at a slower rate. Concomitantly, extracellular water volume decreases, while intracellular water tends to increase. Therefore a higher volume of distribution at birth can be expected for polar drugs such as penicillin, antipyrine, salicylates, sulphonamides and aminoglycosides.

Adipose tissue and skeletal mass

The changes in adipose tissue and skeletal mass can also lead to a different distribution pattern of a drug during postnatal growth. Experimental data on this subject are limited however.

Blood-brain barrier permeability

The changes in blood-brain barrier permeability in the

Table 16.2 Neonatal body composition, differences in comparison with the adult

---

Total body water	higher
Adipose tissue	lower
Skeletal mass	lower
Cardiac output	lower
Blood-brain barrier permeability	higher
Plasma protein concentration (albumin)	lower

---

neonate are of particular interest. A number of events take place during brain maturation. These include, for instance, modification in the lipid content, a changing rate of production of cerebrospinal fluid, a change in the permeability of the brain capillaries and a tightening of the junction between the choroid plexus epithelial cells and the endothelial cells[1]. As a result, it is possible that antibiotics such as penicillin which normally penetrate this barrier poorly, have an enhanced effectiveness in the brain of young animals[2,3]. On the other hand, elevated concentrations of anaesthetics and anticonsulvants in the CNS of neonatal animals could lead to toxic effects.

Serum protein binding
An important factor in the distribution of drugs is serum protein binding. In general, serum protein concentrations in the newborn are low, mainly the albumin fraction. A low serum binding of usually highly bound drugs such as salicylates and sulphonamides has been reported in the newborn goat, sheep, cow, dog, pig and human[2,3]. A high volume of distribution was reported for these drugs in the first period of life. In the case of sulphamerazine a positive linear correlation was found between plasma binding and albumin concentration in developing lambs and calves[7]. A plasma protein binding of 45% was seen for trimethoprim in newborn piglets during the first week of

life, as compared to 75% in adult pigs, notwithstanding a similar plasma protein concentration[41].

Apart from concentrations of binding proteins such as albumin, other factors are also able to influence the binding of drugs in the newborn, such as the presence of foetal albumin, substances of maternal origin, high concentration of free fatty acids and bilirubin. Data describing the influence of these factors on binding are, however, mostly restricted to humans[15].

RENAL EXCRETION

In mammalian species, drugs or their metabolites are excreted by glomerular filtration or by a combination of glomerular filtration and active tubular secretion, while passive tubular reabsorption can also occur. Renal function of newborn mammals is not fully developed at birth. This can result in a reduced excretion of drugs. Species differences in the maturity of renal function at birth have been reported. Newborn ruminants, for example, possess a much more mature renal function than other mammals[8]. One should also keep in mind that the rate of postnatal development of renal function can vary considerably from one species to another.

Glomerular filtration

From Table 16.3, it is clear that the development of glomerular filtration takes only a few days in newborn ruminants and in man and pig as well this development takes place in the first week of life. A somewhat slower postnatal development of glomerular filtration occurs in dogs and rodents. As a result, one can expect that the clearance of drugs which are mainly eliminated by glomerular filtration, are already high in the early stages of life in most mammalian species. For gentamicin, an antibiotic almost entirely eliminated by glomerular filtration, a high clearance value was found in newborn calves[4] and man[1].

Table 16.3 Rate of postnatal development of renal function in different species; time required to reach adult
values

	Glomerular filtration	Tubular secretion
Cattle	very fast (1-3 days)	very fast (1-3 days)
Goat	very fast (1-3 days)	fast (1-2 weeks)
Sheep	very fast (1-3 days)	fast (1-2 weeks)
Dog	intermediate (2-3 weeks)	slow (4-8 weeks)
Rodent	intermediate (2-3 weeks)	slow (4-8 weeks)
Pig	fast (1-2 weeks)	slow (4-8 weeks)
Man	fast (1-2 weeks)	very slow (> 20 weeks)

Tubular function

Maturational changes in tubular function can also
influence the elimination of some drugs. From Table 16.3,
it is obvious that the species differences in postnatal
development of tubular function are more pronounced than
those of glomerular filtration. In the newborn calf renal
tubular function is already fully developed a few days
after birth. A somewhat slower development was found in
goats and sheep. In the dog, rodent and pig, several
weeks are required before tubular secretion reaches full
maturity. In human neonates, tubular secretion develops
very slowly, over months. These important species
differences in development of tubular secretion can lead
to large variations between different species in the
clearance of drugs excreted by tubular secretion in the
newborn. It has, for example, been shown that the
evolution in the elimination of benzylpenicillin, a drug
almost entirely excreted by tubular secretion, is faster
in the calf than in the pig[21].

BIOTRANSFORMATION

In neonates, drug metabolizing activity is in general low.
Intraspecies differences in maturity at birth and in the

Table 16.4 Postnatal development of biotransformation :
time required to reach adult values.

Horse	1-2 weeks
Rodent	1-3 weeks
Ruminant	3-5 weeks
Dog	3-5 weeks
Pig	4-6 weeks
Humans	4-12 weeks

---

rate of postnatal development have been reported. A sim-
plified representation of the development of drug metabo-
lising capacity in man and other mammals is given in Table
16.4. In the human neonate and in piglets, several weeks
are needed for development of the enzyme system,
associated with drug biotransformation[13,22]. From the few
studies dealing with the pharmacokinetics of antibiotics
in equine species, it can be inferred that the major
metabolic pathways develop very rapidly after birth in
foals[3].

Postnatal development of drug metabolism is, however,
more complex as indicated in Table 16.4. The rate at
which biotransformation achieves adult levels of activity
varies considerably according to the drug and the
metabolic pathway studied. In general, at the moment of
birth, the cytochrome P_{450}-dependent mixed function
oxidase system and the glucuronide conjugating system are
deficient in mammals. Other metabolizing steps such as
acetylation, sulphate and glycine conjugation have been
reported to be already well developed in neonates[2]. The
postnatal development of the sulphonamide biotransformation in different domestic animal species reflects
these findings. Low hydroxylation and low glucuronidation
have been demonstrated during the first days of life for
sulphadimidine[25] and sulphadiazine[9] in pigs, for sulphadimidine in calves[18,19], for sulphadoxine in goats[17] and
for sulphamerazine in sheep (unpublished results);

acetylation of sulphonamides is not deficient in these animal species. For some pathways, such as dealkylation, it has been reported that the activity can exceed several times the adult value at some stages of the evolution of the young mammals[14].

CONCLUSIONS

At the time of birth large intraspecies variations in maturity exist, and the rates of postnatal development are likewise different from species to species. Therefore, important differences in the pharmacokinetics of a foreign compound can be expected between neonates of different species, although only few studies in this field have been performed.

References
1. Assael, B.M. (1982). Pharmacokinetics and drug distribution during postnatal development. Pharmacol.
   Ther. 18:159-197.
2. Baggot, J.D. (1977). Principles of Drug Disposition
   in Domestic Animals. Philadelphia: W.B. Saunders.
3. Baggot, J.D. and Short, C.R. (1984). Drug disposition
   in the neonatal animal, with particular reference to
   the foal. Equine Vet. J. 16(4):364-367.
4. Clarke, C.R., Short, C.R., Hsu, R. and Baggot, J.D.
   (1985). Pharmacokinetics of gentamicin in the calf :
   developmental changes. Am. J. Vet. Res. 46:2461-2466.
5. De Backer, P. and Bogaert, M.G. (1983). Drug bioavailability in the developing ruminant. In: Ruckebush, Y., Toutain, P.L. and Koritz, G.D. (eds). Veterinary Pharmacology and Toxicology, pp.133-140.
   Lancaster: MTP Press L.
6. De Backer, P., Debackere, M., De Corte-Baeten, K.
   (1978). Plasma levels of chloramphenicol after oral
   administration in calves during the first weeks of
   life. J. Vet. Pharmacol. Ther. 1:135-140.
7. De Backer, P., Belpaire, F.M., Bogaert, M.G. and
   Debackere, M. (1982). Pharmacokinetics of sulfamera-
   zine and antipyrine in neonatal and young lambs. Am.
   J. Vet. Res. 43:1744-1751.
8. Friis, C. (1983). Postnatal development of renal
   function in goats. In: Ruckebush, Y., Toutain, P.L.
   and Koritz, G.D. (eds). Veterinary Pharmacology and
   Toxicology, pp.57-62. Lancaster: MTP Press L.
9. Friis, C., Gyrd-Hansen, N., Nielsen, P., Olsen, C.E.
   and Rasmussen, F. (1984). Pharmacokinetics and
   metabolism of sulphadiazine in neonatal and young
   pigs. Acta Pharmacol. Toxicol. 54:821-826.
10. Groothuis, D.G. (1983). De farmacokinetiek bij vlees-

kalveren en de activiteit van antibacteriële middelen
met betrekking tot salmonella dublin infecties.
Doctoraal proefschrift, Utrecht.

11. Gyrd-Hansen, H., Friis, C., Nielsen, P. and Rasmussen,
F. (1984). Metabolism of trimethoprim in neonatal and
young pigs : comparative in vivo and in vitro studies.
Acta Pharmacol. Toxicol. 55:402-409.

12. Hill, K.J. (1968). Abomasal function. In: Handbook
of Physiology. Alimentary Canal, vol. V, pp.2747-2759.
Baltimore: Williams and Wilkins.

13. Leat, W.M.F. (1970). Carbohydrate and lipid metabolism in the ruminant during postnatal development.
In: Phillipson, A.T. (ed.). Physiology of Digestion
and Metabolism in the Ruminant, pp.211-222.
Newcastle-upon-Tyne: Oriel Press.

14. Mannering, G.J. (1985). Drug metabolism in the newborn. Fed. Proc. 44:2302-2308.

15. Morselli, P.L., Franco-Morselli, R. and Bossi, L.
(1980). Clinical pharmacokinetics in newborn and
infants. Age related differences and therapeutic
implications. Clin. Pharmacokinet. 5:485-527.

16. Nielsen, P. and Rasmussen, F. (1976). Influence of
age on trimethoprim and sulfadoxone in goats. Acta
Pharmacol. Toxicol. 38:113-119.

17. Nielsen, P., Romvary, A. and Rasmussen, F. (1978).
Sulfadoxine and trimethoprim in goats and cows :
absorption fraction, half-lives and the degrading
effect of the ruminal flora. J. Vet. Pharmacol. Ther.
1:37-46.

18. Nouws, J.F.M., Vree, T.B., Baakman, M. and Tijhuis, M.
(1983). Effect of age on the acetylation and
deacetylation reactions of sulphadimidine and
N^4-acetylsulphadimidine in calves. J. Vet. Pharmacol.
Ther. 6:13-22.

19. Nouws, J.F.M., Vree, T.B., Baakman, M., Driessens, F.,
Breukink, H.J. and Meviu, D. (1986). Age and dosage
dependency in the plasma disposition and the renal
clearance of sulfadimidine and its N_4-acetyl and
hydroxy metabolites in calves and cows. Am. J. Vet.
Res. 47:642-649.

20. Ruckebush, Y. (1983). Perinatal pharmacology in rumi-
nant models. In: Ruckebush, Y., Toutain, P.L. and
Koritz, G.D. (eds). Veterinary Pharmacology and
Toxicology, pp.3-22. Lancaster: MTP Press L.

21. Short, C.R. (1983). Developmental patterns of penicillin G excretion. In: Ruckebush, Y., Toutain, P.L.
and Koritz, G.D. (eds). Veterinary Pharmacology and
Toxicology, pp.63-72. Lancaster: MTP Press L.

22. Short, C.R. (1984). Drug disposition in neonatal
animals. J. Am. Vet. Med. Assoc. 184:1161-1162.

23. Short, C.R. and Clarke, C.R. (1984). Calculation of
dosage regimens of antimicrobial drugs for the neonatal patient. J. Am. Vet. Med. Assoc. 185(10):
1088-1093.

24. Silverio, J. and Poole, J.W. (1973). Serum concentrations of ampicillin in newborn infants after oral

administration.   Pediatrics 51:578-580.
25. Svendsen, O. (1976).   Pharmacokinetics of hexabarbi-
    tal, sulphadimidine and   chloramphenicol   in   neonatal
    and young pigs.   Acta Vet. Scand. 17:1-14.

17
Comparative pharmacokinetic studies of sulphonamides

T. B. VREE, J. F. M. NOUWS AND Y. A. HEKSTER

ABSTRACT

In species-dependent pharmacokinetics there are three main
variables : the structure of the drug, the mechanism and
route of metabolism, and renal excretion. When the drug
is administered orally, the structure and characteristics
of the gastrointestinal tract are an additional factor
which may dominate the overall pharmacokinetic behaviour.
Sulphonamides are metabolized by acetylation-deacetylation
reactions and by hydroxylation. Hydroxylation is possible
at different positions in the N_1-substituent group. The
ratio between acetylation and hydroxylation depends on the
structure of the sulphonamide and the species. Renal
function, as expressed by inulin or creatinine clearance,
is almost independent of the species and related to the
body weight. The renal excretion mechanisms of
sulphonamides and their metabolites are governed by the
molecular structure and kidney architecture, but not by
animal species.

There are three main variables governing the
pharmacokinetics of sulphonamides in animals. These are
(1) the molecular structure of the sulphonamide; (2) the
variation in metabolic pathways and variations in the
enzyme concentration in each species; and (3) renal

excretion. By selecting one sulphonamide for a comparative study it is possible to study both species-dependent metabolism and renal clearance.

METABOLISM
Acetylation
Acetylation as a metabolic pathway for sulphonamides is well known and most studied in man. Acetylation is carried out by N-acetylases and acetylcoenzyme-A. There exists a "fast-slow" acetylation phenotype. Fast acetylators have an additional enzyme available, which is missing in slow acetylators. The N-acetylase composition differs in each species. Fast-slow acetylation has been demonstrated in man, monkeys and rabbits, and seems to be absent in ruminants. The structure of the sulphonamide also has an influence on "fast-slow" acetylation. A clear phenotype in man is established only for the 2-sulphanilamide-pyridine and -pyrimidine derivatives as exemplified by sulphadimidine (Figure 17.1). There are three phenotypes in man characterized by homozygotic and heterozygotic fast acetylation and heterozygotic slow acetylation. The homozygotic slow acetylation must also exist but has not as yet been demonstrated. This acetylation probably exists in ruminants.

Acetylation is part of an acetylation-deacetylation equilibrium, the position of which depends on the molecular structure of the sulphonamide and the species[14,15]. Dogs (and dog-related species) show an extremely high rate of deacetylation, so that no acetylation appears to take place[13,15]. Pigeon and sheep show equal rates of deacetylation and acetylation.

Acetylation is one of the basal conjugation reactions in life: it is present in old species such as turtles and snails[11,12] and is present at the time of birth[5,7].

Hydroxylation
The hydroxylation pathway of sulphonamides, known since 1944[8], has been investigated less than the acetylation

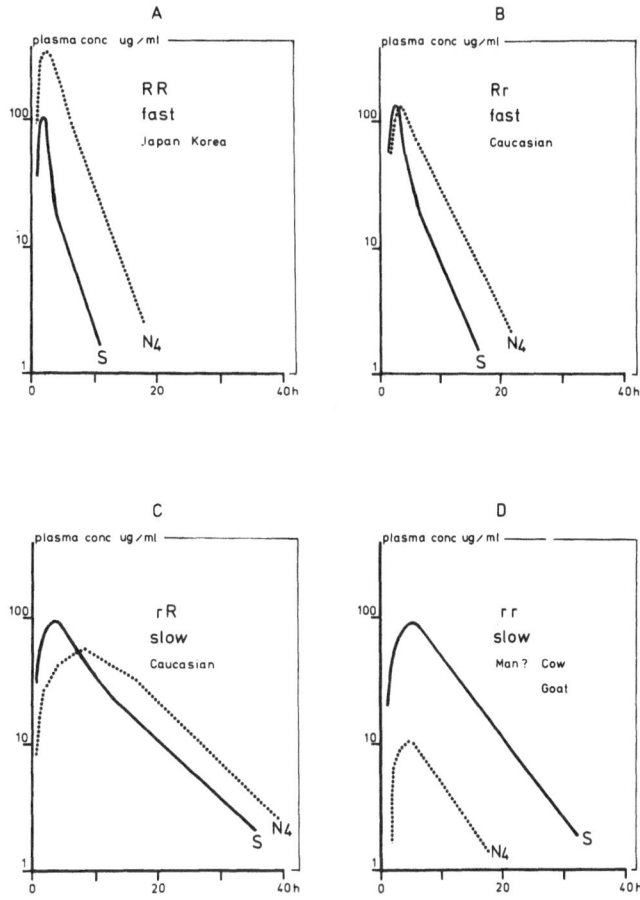

Figure 17.1   Plasma concentration-time curves of sulphadimidine in four different acetylator phenotypes. Three
phenotypes – A, B, and C – have been detected in man; possibility D occurs only in animals.

pathway. The reasons for not studying this pathway are,
firstly, that the Bratton and Marshall reaction cannot
discriminate   between   parent   drug   and N_4-hydroxy-
metabolites; and secondly, that the synthesis of these
hydroxymetabolites presents difficulties.   The synthesis
of   5-hydroxysulphapyridine is reported by Scudi and
Childress[9]. Hydroxylation of sulphonamides in man is
reported for sulphapyridine[3,10], and recently in man for

sulphamethoxazole, sulphadiazine, sulphatroxazole and sulphadimidine[4,14,16]. In the veterinary literature the metabolites are identified in urine extracts by thin layer chromatography and mass spectrometry. Biosynthesis of N_1-hydroxysulphonamides is possible, using the dog as the hydroxylating animal due to its lack of acetylation activity. No metabolites that interfere in the isolation and identification procedures are produced by this species[13,14]. Synthesis of these hydroxymetabolites in the dog is species-dependent. The hydroxymetabolites can be excreted by active tubular secretion, or they can be first glucuronidated before they are excreted.

Renal excretion

Sulphonamides are excreted by means of both passive and active processes depending on their molecular structure[16]. Active proximal tubular secretion is the excretion mechanism for sulphamethiazole, sulphathiazole and sulphisomidine, while all other sulphonamides are excreted by passive processes. All N_4-acetylsulphonamides and hydroxyglucuronide metabolites are also excreted by active tubular secretion. Passive excretion comprises glomerular filtration and passive tubular reabsorption, characterized by the variables urine flow and urine pH. Man shows variations in urine pH, between pH 5 and 7, while ruminants have a highly alkaline pH (8-9) and in the dog pH ranges from 6 to 9. Urine flow rate is species-dependent and varies between individual animals. In man there is an average flow of 1 ml/min, while cows have a flow of 10-30 ml/min, goats 0.5 ml/min and snails 0.01 ml/min. A high urine flow and alkaline urine pH minimize the passive tubular reabsorption of sulphonamides. The glomerular filtration rate, as monitored by creatinine clearance, depends on the species and is related to body weight. It varies from 2 ml/min in the mouse, to 120 ml/min in man and to 500-700 ml/min in cows.

Edwards[2] has shown that the renal glomerular function, as indicated by inulin clearance, seems to be independent of the species. It is related to body weight and basal metabolic rate: it removes the waste products of food (energy) constituents, the quantity of the daily food intake and waste produced being related to the body size.

Once excreted by the kidney glomerulus and tubule, the drug can be reabsorbed according to its pKa value and lipid solubility from both the renal tubule and the bladder[17]. A high rate of urine flow and frequent micturition decrease the rate of reabsorption and increase the overall renal clearance. With the selection of a specific sulphonamide as test substrate, two kinetic variables, structure and renal clearance, are constant for most species. Species-related differences in pharmaco-kinetics of the sulphonamide can therefore be ascribed to differences in metabolism (pathways and rates).

The percentage of the dose excreted in the urine as each metabolite reflects the yield of the metabolic pathways for each species when the renal clearance of the metabolite is considered species-independent. When the latter assumption is correct, then the plasma concentration of parent drug and metabolites will in addition reveal the relative importance of each metabolic pathway.

MATERIALS AND METHODS
Drugs
Sulphonamides were obtained from De Onderlinge Pharma-ceutische Groothandel OPG (Utrecht, the Netherlands). N_4-acetylsulphonamides (N_4), and hydroxysulphonamides (SOH) were synthetized and isolated according to Vree et al.[13,14].

Animals
Animals were obtained from the Central Animal Laboratory, University of Nijmegen, Dotulabs (Nijmegen) and the Institute of Veterinary Pharmacology (University of Utrecht, the Netherlands).

HPLC analysis

Deglucuronidation, sample preparation and HPLC analysis were performed as described elsewhere[6],[7].

RESULTS

Sulphamethoxazole

Sulphamethoxazole is predominantly acetylated in man and animals such as the pigeon, penguin, cat, and sheep. There is a small percentage of hydroxylation (10-20% of the dose). Deacetylation is substantial in cat and sheep, minimal in man and maximal in the dog[15]. Cats are slow acetylators due to a substantial rate of deacetylation as illustrated in Figures 17.2 and 17.3. Fish and water turtles acetylate about 5% of the dose of sulphamethoxazole.

Sulphatroxazole

Sulphatroxazole, a 4-methyl substituted analogue of sulphamethoxazole, is predominantly eliminated by hydroxylation in man and the dog (70%), but it is mainly acetylated in cows. Sulphamethoxazole and sulphatroxazole are both hydroxylated at the 5-methyl group. The hydroxymetabolite of sulphatroxazole is excreted renally by active tubular secretion in man and is not glucuronidated. Although in man hydroxylation is the main metabolic pathway (70%), it is a relatively slow process, resulting in a half-life of 25 h[14]. Hydroxylation of sulphatroxazole is species-dependent and in calves acetylation dominates the metabolic process, which is opposite to the finding in man.

Sulphapyridine

Sulphapyridine is hydroxylated and acetylated to a great extent in man. That hydroxylation is a major process is indicated by the fact that 70% of the dose of the metabolite N_4-acetylsulphapyridine is hydroxylated. It is not certain whether 5-hydroxysulphapyridine becomes acetylated. Sulphapyridine shows a clear "fast-slow"

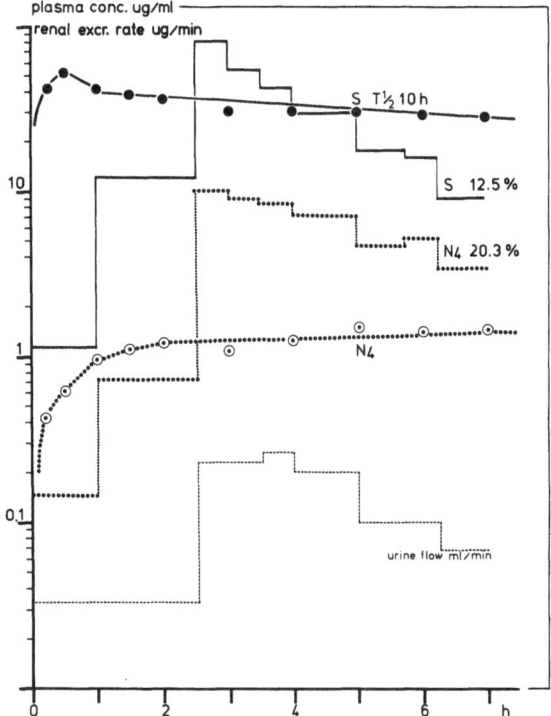

Figure 17.2   Plasma concentration-time curves and renal excretion rate-time profiles of sulphapyridine (S) and its metabolite N_4-acetylsulphapyridine (N_4) in a cat after a rapid intravenous infusion of 78 mg of sulphapyridine.

acetylation phenotype, which is reflected in the half-lives of elimination of the two groups. This behaviour indicates that acetylation governs the overall metabolic elimination in man. The hydroxylation of N_4-acetylsulphapyridine in man is an unusual phenomenon, because a drug conjugate is further metabolized (Figure 17.4). Dogs, goats and cats are unable to hydroxylate the N_4-acetylsulphapyridine; they deacetylate this compound first and then hydroxylate it.

Sulphamerazine
Sulphamerazine is predominantly acetylated in man by a

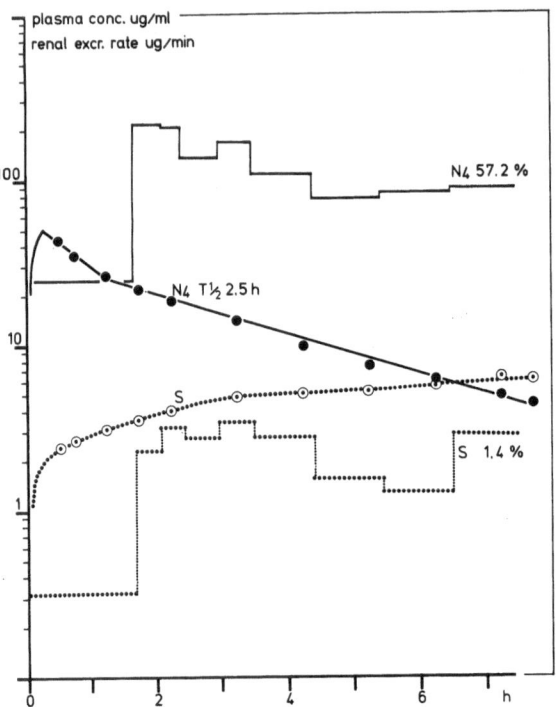

Figure 17.3   Plasma concentration-time curves and renal excretion rate-time profiles of N₄-acetylsulphamethoxazole (N₄) and its metabolite sulphamethoxazole (S) in a cat after an intravenous dose of 79 mg of N₄-acetyl-sulphamethoxazole.

"fast-slow" acetylation-deacetylation phenotype. Deacetylation is measurable in man. Hydroxylation in man accounts for maximally 10-20% of the administered dose. The dog hydroxylates sulphamerazine predominantly at the 4-position, while the sheep, goat, and cow hydroxylate mainly the 6-methyl group[1,13,14].

Sulphadimidine
Sulphadimidine is acetylated according to the "fast-slow" acetylation phenotype in man, while the percentage of hydroxylation in the two groups remains low and constant (10%). In ruminants, hydroxylation is the

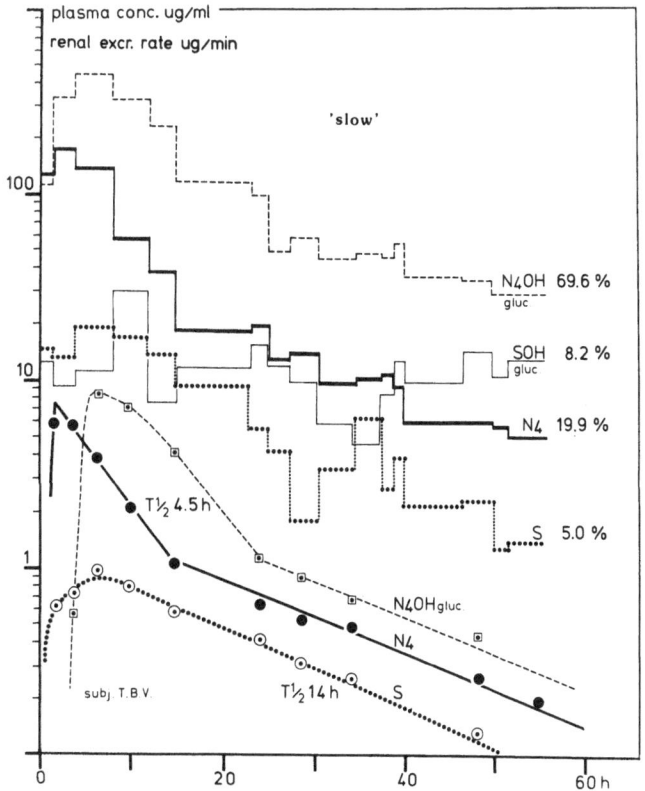

Figure 17.4   Plasma concentration-time curves and renal
excretion rate-time   profiles   of N_4-acetylsulphapyridine
(N_4)   and its hydroxymetabolites in man after an oral dose
of 593 mg of N_4-acetylsulphapyridine. Here a conjugate is
hydroxylated   into N_4-acetyl-5-hydroxysulphapyridine
(glucuronide)   (N_4OH).   The   parent   drug   is   also
deacetylated   into   sulphapyridine (S) and subsequently
hydroxylated   into 5-hydroxysulphapyridine (glucuronide)
(SOH). The hydroxylation of the N_4-acetyl derivative does
not occur in dog, cat or goat.

predominant metabolic pathway.   Hydroxylation   at   the
6-methyl position is dominant over the hydroxylation at
the 5 position in the cow, sheep, and goat, while   in   the
horse   the   position   is   reversed.   At a dose of 100-200
mg/kg, the 6-methyl hydroxyl derivative is capacity-

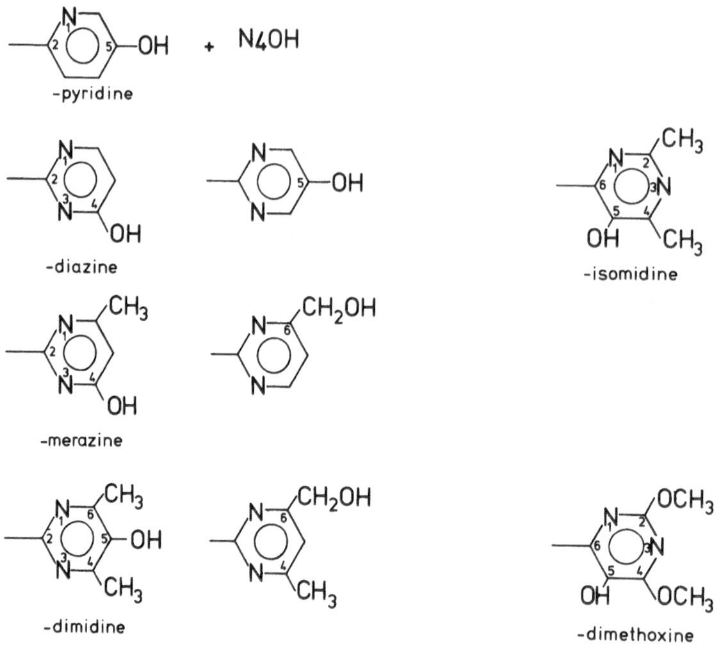

Figure 17.5 Structural formulae of the hydroxymetabolites of sulpha-2-(6)-pyrimidines.

limited in the cow, but not in the horse. 6-Hydroxyme-thylsulphadimidine is excreted renally by passive processes only, while 5-hydroxysulphadimidine is rapidly glucuronidated and excreted by active secretory processes. For this reason the plasma concentration of 5-hydroxysul-phadimidine in cows is much lower than that of 6-hydroxy-methylsulphadimidine. Pigs are unable to hydroxylate sulphadimidine. Fish, turtles and snails acetylate and hydroxylate sulphadimidine very slowly. Birds must possess additional metabolic pathways as so much of the dose remains unaccounted for.

Half-life of elimination
There are striking differences between man and other mammals in the elimination half-life of sulphonamides. In man the half-life ranges from 1 h for sulphamethiazole to 100 h for sulphadoxine, while in other animals the range

is much smaller (2-10 h). This variation is obtained with
high doses of 100-200 mg/kg, resulting in capacity-limited
elimination and wide variation in reported half-life. The
short half-life of sulphonamides in animals is predominantly caused by the high rate of hydroxylation and not by
acetylation. In man acetylation (never hydroxylation) is
the rate-governing step in the elimination half-life.

DISCUSSION

Metabolism is not equivalent to elimination from the body.
The parent drug is removed but another compound, which may
or may not be pharmacodynamically active replaces it.
Metabolism converts the parent drug into a suitable form
so that it can be conjugated and actively excreted. If
the parent drug or a metabolite is excreted by active
tubular secretion, then clearly no conjugation is needed
nor does it occur. All hydroxymetabolites and N_4-acetyl-
metabolites formed from sulphonamides show plasma
concentration-time curves running parallel to that of the
parent drug. This means that the intrinsic elimination of
the metabolites is higher than that of the parent drug.
The hydroxymetabolites are eliminated by glucuronidation
and renal excretion, the glucuronides and N_4-acetyl
conjugates by active renal excretion.

When renal function and the mechanism of excretion are
constant for a sulphonamide in each species, then the
different yields in metabolites in the urine or blood
reflect the different metabolic rates and pathways. In
this series of mammals, the number of metabolic pathways
is constant; there are two hydroxylation reactions and one
acetylation-deacetylation equilibrium. The rate constants
of each metabolic pathway differ among the species: they
are species/gene/enzyme related. Figure 17.5 summarizes
the hydroxymetabolites of some sulphapyrimidines.

References
1. De Backer, P. (1986). Comparative neonatal pharmacokinetics. In: Van Miert, A.S.J.P.A.M., Bogaert, M.G.
   and Debackere, M. (eds). Comparative Veterinary

Pharmacology, Toxicology and Therapy. Proc. 3rd EAVPT Congress. Part II, Invited Lectures. Lancaster : MTP Press.

2. Edwards, N.A. (1975). Scaling of renal functions in mammals. Comp. Biochem. Physiol. 52A:63-66.

3. Hansson, K.-A. and Sandberg, M. (1973). Determination of sulphapyridine and its metabolites in biological materials after administration of salicylsulphapyridine. Acta Pharm. Suecica 10:87-92.

4. Hekster, Y.A. and Vree, T.B. (1982). Clinical pharmacokinetics of sulphonamides and their N$_4$-acetyl derivatives. Antibiot. Chemother. 31:22-118.

5. Nouws, J.F.M., Vree, T.B., Tijhuis, M.W. and Baakman, M. (1983). Effect of age on the acetylation and deacetylation reactions of sulfadimidine and N$_4$-acetylsulfadimidine in calves. J. Vet. Pharmacol. Ther. 6:13-22.

6. Nouws, J.F.M., Vree, T.B., Breukink, H.J., Baakman, M., Driessens, F. and Smulders, A. (1985). Dose dependent disposition of sulfadimidine, its N$_4$-acetyl-, and its hydroxy metabolites in plasma and milk of dairy cows. Vet. Q. 7:177-186.

7. Nouws, J.F.M., Vree, T.B., Baakman, M., Driessens, F., Breukink, H.J. and Mevius, D. (1986). Age and dosage dependency in the plasma disposition and the renal clearance of sulfadimidine and its N$_4$-acetyl and hydroxy metabolites in calves and cows. Am. J. Vet. Res. 47:642-649.

8. Scudi, J.V. (1944). Excretion of metabolic products of sulfapyridine in the dog. Proc. Soc. Exp. Biol. Med. 55:197-199.

9. Scudi, J.V. and Childress, S.J. (1956). Constitution of the hydroxysulfapyridine isolated from dog urine. J. Biol. Chem. 218:587-593.

10. Schröder, H. and Schröder, B. (1973). Isolation and excretion of a hydroxylated metabolite of sulphapyridine from human urine. Acta Pharm. Suecica 10:263-268.

11. Vree, T.B. and Vree, J.B. (1983). Acetylation of sulphamethoxazole by fresh water turtles Pseudemys scripta elegans. J. Vet. Pharmacol. Ther. 6:237-240.

12. Vree, T.B. and Vree, M.L. (1984). Acetylation of sulphamethoxazole by the snail Cepaea hortensis. J. Vet. Pharmacol. Ther. 7:239-241.

13. Vree, T.B., Tijhuis, M.W., Nouws, J.F.M. and Hekster, Y.A. (1984). Isolation and identification of 4-hydroxysulfamerazine and preliminary studies on its pharmacokinetics in dogs. Pharm. Weekbl. Sci. Ed. 6:80-87.

14. Vree, T.B., Hekster, Y.A. and Tijhuis, M.W. (1985). Metabolism of sulfonamides. Antibiot. Chemother. 34:5-65.

15. Vree, T.B., Hekster, Y.A., Nouws, J.F.M. and Dorresteijn, G.M. (1985). Pharmacokinetics of sulfonamides in animals. Antibiot. Chemother. 34:130-170.

16. Vree, T.B. and Hekster, Y.A. (1985). Renal excretion

of sulfonamides. Antibiot. Chemother. 34:66-121.
17. Wood, J.H. and Leonard, T.W. (1983). Kinetic implica-
    tions of drug resorption from the bladder. Drug Metab.
    Rev. 14:407-423.

18
Species differences in protein binding

F. BELPAIRE

ABSTRACT

Protein binding influences the disposition of a drug, and knowledge of the protein binding in different species can sometimes help to explain differences in pharmacokinetics and pharmacodynamics which occur. Comparison of protein binding of drugs in different species is only of value if a systematic and careful comparison of binding in different animal species has been performed since percentage binding depends on a number of factors such as methodology used, the concentration of drug tested and intra-individual and interindividual differences in binding. Species variations in the degree of binding of those drugs mainly bound to albumin have been noted. They are in general more extensively bound in humans than in other mammalian species. For most drugs the extent of binding is usually within a range which permits a classification of high, moderate and low, whatever the species. For other drugs such as salicylates and valproate, pronounced interspecies differences in binding were found. Species differences in binding of drugs mainly bound to alpha$_1$-acid glycoprotein are more pronounced than for drugs mainly bound to albumin. These differences are mainly due to differences in affinity and capacity. This is illustrated for oxprenolol, propranolol and disopyramide.

INTRODUCTION
Many drugs are to some degree bound to blood constituents such as albumin, alpha$_1$-acid glycoprotein (alpha$_1$-AGP), lipoproteins and erythrocytes. While most drugs are mainly bound to plasma albumin, many basic drugs such as beta-adrenoceptor blockers, antiarrhythmics or tricyclic antidepressants are primarily bound to alpha$_1$-AGP, an acute phase reactant.

   Protein binding influences the disposition of a drug, and knowledge of the protein binding in different species can sometimes help in explaining the differences in pharmacokinetics occurring between these species. Protein binding also affects the intensity of the pharmacological effect : free, unbound drug is pharmacologically active, whereas bound drug is inactive, serving as a depot from which the concentration of free drug in body water is maintained.

   A systematic comparison of protein binding in several animal species has been performed for relatively few drugs. In most cases however, interspecies differences can be inferred from data obtained by different investigators. However, conclusions which are not based on a systematic study can be misleading. Indeed, the percentage binding obtained in a study depends on a number of factors.

FACTORS INFLUENCING BINDING
Methodology
Several methods have been developed to measure protein binding of drugs in plasma or serum. Most commonly, equilibrium dialysis and ultrafiltration are used, each having both advantages and disadvantages. Rarely are the various methods systematically compared and in the few instances when this has been done, different values were often obtained. Even when the same method, such as equilibrium dialysis, is used, there can be interlabo-

ratory variations due to differences in buffer composition, pH, temperature (25 °C or 37 °C) and other factors. These problems must be considered when comparing protein binding data from different laboratories.

Drug concentration

For many drugs, percentage binding is constant within the therapeutic range, because these concentrations are usually much lower than those required for saturation of the binding sites. However, for drugs such as the sulphonamides, salicylates and phenylbutazone, the therapeutic levels approach saturation concentrations, and the percentage binding decreases with increasing drug concentration. Saturation of the protein binding sites and concentration-dependency within the therapeutic range will occur at lower concentration for drugs which bind to alpha$_1$-AGP than for drugs which bind to albumin, because of the lower alpha$_1$-AGP levels in plasma. Comparison of binding percentage between species is useful only when the concentration at which binding is measured is known.

Interindividual and intra-individual differences

Considerable intersubject variability frequently exists in serum binding of a particular ligand; in terms of free fraction a 4 to 5-fold range is not uncommon even in healthy animals or humans. Intersubject variation seems to be more important for drugs mainly bound to alpha$_1$-AGP than for drugs bound to albumin, as illustrated in Figure 18.1. The intersubject variation in serum binding of three drugs mainly bound to alpha$_1$-AGP (lidocaine, oxprenolol and propranolol), and of three drugs mainly bound to albumin (digitoxin, phenytoin and diazepam), was measured by equilibrium dialysis in 21 healthy dogs[4]. The percentage free lidocaine, propranolol and oxprenolol varies considerably, whereas the percentage free digitoxin, phenytoin and diazepam varies to a much lesser extent. The causes of such variations are many, but are clearly related to variations in protein concentration and in binding affinity.

Age, sex, pregnancy and disease states (renal failure, liver disease, inflammatory diseases) also influence the variability. This is also illustrated in Figure 18.1. In 21 dogs with inflammatory diseases, the free percentages of lidocaine, oxprenolol and propranolol are lower than in control dogs, but interindividual variation is also important. For digitoxin, the percentage free drug is higher than in control dogs; for phenytoin there is no difference, and for diazepam the mean percentage free drug is higher. Interindividual variations in binding of digitoxin, phenytoin and diazepam are more important in inflammatory disease than in healthy dogs. These results demonstrate that there is a large interindividual variation in binding of drugs which are mainly bound to alpha$_1$-AGP, whereas this variation is much lower for drugs mainly bound to albumin. Inflammation increases binding of drugs bound to alpha$_1$-AGP, but does not change much binding of drugs mainly bound to albumin.

Finally, genetic factors are probably also important, but this is largely an unexplored area.

SPECIES DIFFERENCES IN BINDING OF DRUGS MAINLY BOUND TO ALBUMIN

Species variations in the degree of binding to serum proteins have been found for digitoxin, furosemide, sulphonamides, phenylbutazone[3]. Drugs which are mainly bound to albumin are in general more extensively bound in human beings than in other mammalian species. Nevertheless, the extent of binding of most drugs is usually within a range which permits the binding of drugs to be classified as high, moderate or low, regardless of species[3]

In one study digitoxin binding was high, whereas for digoxin it was low in several mammalian species, but interspecies differences were present for each drug. The fraction of digitoxin bound ranged from 92% in man to 81% in the pony, and for digoxin values between 17 and 40% in

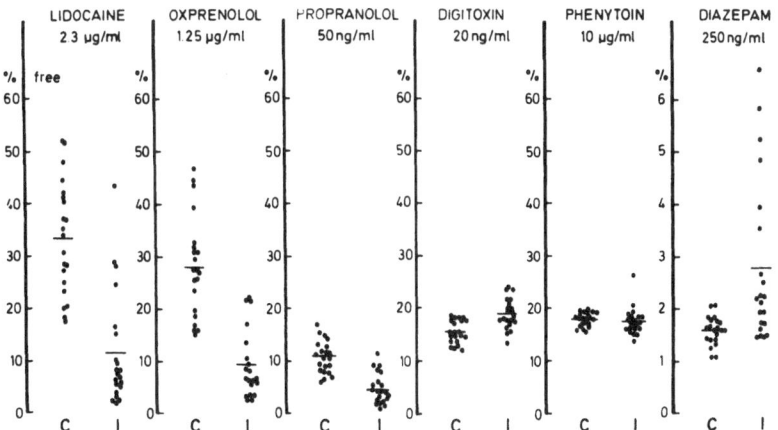

Figure 18.1 Percentage free lidocaine, oxprenolol, propranolol, digitoxin, phenytoin and diazepam in the serum
of 21 healthy dogs (C) and of 21 dogs with inflammatory
disease (I). The initial concentrations used for the in
vitro equilibrium dialysis are mentioned for each drug.

the different species were reported[1].

The binding of morphine, studied in 13 mammalian
species, was low and ranged from 11% in swine to 24% in
cattle[2].

The binding of furosemide was high in all species and
varied from 95% in man to 83% in the cat[10]. For
digitoxin, digoxin, morphine and furosemide species
differences were relatively small.

For salicylates, more pronounced interspecies
differences in binding were found by Sturman and Smith[11]
who reported that species could be separated into two
groups. In baboons, horses, dogs, rats, mice, turkeys and
toads, there was a low protein binding capacity for
salicylate (less than 15% bound at a salicylate
concentration of 5 µg/ml). In the second group (rhesus
monkey, rabbit, guinea-pig and man) there was a much
larger affinity (more than 70% bound at a salicylate
concentration of 5 µg/ml).

More recently, Löscher[9] demonstrated for valproate, a

drug mainly bound to albumin, striking differences in the degree of binding between man (95%), dog (79%), rat (63%) and mouse (12%).

The differences in the extent of binding among species may reflect different affinities for binding to albumin, as well as differences in albumin concentration. Variation in the chemical structure of albumin from different species probably accounts for both quantitative and qualitative differences in binding of a given compound[7,12].

SPECIES DIFFERENCES IN BINDING OF DRUGS MAINLY BOUND TO ALPHA₁-AGP

For drugs mainly bound to $alpha_1$-AGP, such as oxprenolol, propranolol and disopyramide, the differences in extent of binding between species are more pronounced than for drugs mainly bound to albumin. Data in the literature are sparse. Figure 18.2 shows the binding of oxprenolol (1.25 µg/ml) and propranolol (10 ng/ml) to serum and to albumin (4 g%) in man, dog, rat and rabbit, and to human $alpha_1$-AGP (70 mg%)[5]. In the four species, albumin binding is lower than serum binding and is quite similar in all species, indicating that in each species except the rabbit, other binding proteins are involved, probably $alpha_1$-AGP. Indeed, as shown for man, binding to $alpha_1$-AGP was more pronounced than to albumin. The importance of $alpha_1$-AGP binding for the species differences is also suggested by the fact that serum binding in the rabbit, which is low and little higher than the binding to albumin, increases markedly after induction of arthritis. Inflammatory diseases enhance the concentration of $alpha_1$-AGP in man, dog and rat. In healthy rabbits the concentration of $alpha_1$-AGP is probably very low or the protein has a low affinity for the drugs studied. Species differences in capacity constant were demonstrated for both drugs; species differences in affinity constant were present only for propranolol. These results suggest that in man, dogs and rats but

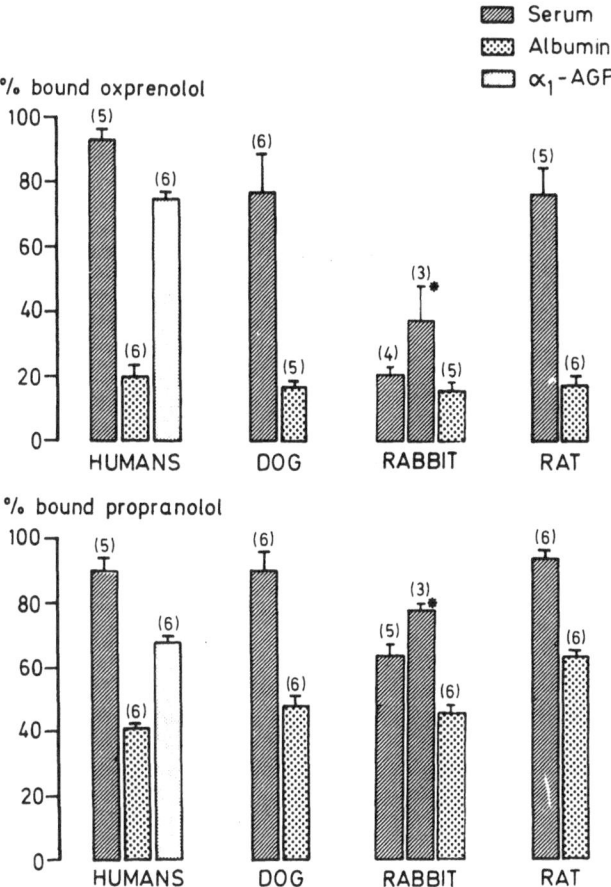

Figure 18.2   Percentage binding of oxprenolol (1.25 µg/ml)
and propranolol (10 ng/ml) to serum and to albumin (4 g%)
of different species and to human alpha$_1$-AGP (70 mg%).
Means (+SEM) are given: the number of experiments is given
between brackets. *Serum of arthritic rabbits. (From reference[5], with permission).

much less in rabbits, oxprenolol and propranolol bind to
alpha$_1$-AGP and that species differences in binding are due
to differences in concentration of alpha$_1$-AGP and affinity
constants.

     Similar results were found for disopyramide, another
drug mainly bound to alpha$_1$-AGP in man[8]. Interspecies

variations in binding of disopyramide to serum in most
animal species (rabbit 5%, man 85%, horse 90%) were due to
differences in affinity for binding to $alpha_1$-AGP. There
was no relationship between disopyramide binding and the
capacity constants.

CONCLUSIONS

Protein binding markedly influences the disposition of
drugs, and some of the differences in the pharmacokinetics
among species can partly be explained by differences in
protein binding. This is illustrated for diazepam.
Klotz[6] found a significant correlation between the free
fraction of diazepam and the slow disposition constant ß,
which characterizes elimination processes. This might
indicate that plasma protein binding determines the
hepatic elimination of this drug.

References
  1. Baggot, J.D. and Davis, L.E. (1973). Plasma protein
     binding of digitoxin and digoxin in several mammalian
     species. Res. Vet. Sci. 15:81-87.
  2. Baggot, J.D. and Davis, L.E. (1973). Species diffe-
     rences in plasma protein binding of morphine and
     codeine. Am. J. Vet. Res. 34:511-514.
  3. Baggot, J.D. (1977). Principles of drug disposition
     in domestic animals. Philadelphia: W.B. Saunders.
  4. Belpaire, F.M., Bogaert, M.G. and De Rick, A. (1984).
     Variability of serum binding of drugs in healthy dogs
     and in dogs with inflammatory disease. London: IUPHAR
     9th International Congress of Pharmacology. Abstracts:
     88P. London: Macmillan press.
  5. Belpaire, F.M., Braeckman, R.A. and Bogaert, M.G.
     (1984). Binding of oxprenolol and propranolol to
     serum, albumin and alpha_1-acid glycoprotein in man and
     other species. Biochem. Pharmacol. 33:2065-2069.
  6. Klotz, U., Antonin, K.H. and Bieck, R. (1976). Pharma-
     kinetics and plasma binding of diazepam in man, dog,
     rabbit, guinea pig and rat. J. Pharmacol. Exp. Ther.
     199:67-73.
  7. Kragh-Hansen, U. (1981). Molecular aspects of ligand
     binding to serum albumin. Pharmacol. Rev. 33:17-53.
  8. Lima, J.J. and Haughey, D.B. (1981). Disopyramide
     binding to serum protein in man and animals. Drug
     Metab. Dispos. 9:582-583.
  9. Löscher, W. (1979). A comparative study of the pro-
     tein binding of anticonvulsant drugs in serum of dog
     and man. J. Pharmacol. Exp. Ther. 208:429-435.
 10. Neff-Davis, C.A. and Davis, L.E. (1982). Serum pro-

tein binding of furosemide in several species. J. Vet. Pharmacol. Ther. 5:293-294.

11. Sturman, J.A. and Smith, M.J.H. (1967). The binding of salicylate to plasma proteins in different species. J. Pharm. Pharmacol. 19:621-623.

12. Thorp, J.M. (1972). Inter- and intra-species diffe-rences in the binding of anionic compounds to albumin. In: De C. Baker, S.B. and Neuhaus, G.A. (eds). Toxi-cological problems of drug combinations. Proc. of the Meeting of the Eur. Society for the Study of Drug Toxicity, Berlin 1971, vol. 13, pp.98-109. Den Haag: De By.

Drug Residue Toxicology

19
The target animal species in drug toxicity studies: an evaluation of its usefulness and limitations

T. A. J. M. DE ROIJ

ABSTRACT

In the safety evaluation of animal drugs both the target animal species and man have to be considered. In the case of feed additives the environment is a third factor. The value of the target animal species in safety evaluation can be increased considerably if more advantage is taken of information obtained either directly or indirectly from target animal studies. In particular, this applies to studies of drug pharmacokinetics and metabolism and to toxic effects in the target animal. The ultimate goals have to be to obtain more relevant data for a well-balanced risk assessment and concomitantly aim at a reduction of the total testing programme.

INTRODUCTION

Drug development has evolved from a somewhat "haphazard" activity, having many aspects in common with medieval alchemy, to an enterprise requiring a multidiscipli- nary approach in a well-structured and equipped setting. Use is made of the ever-increasing insight into the pa- thogenesis of diseases, knowledge of chemical struc- ture-activity relations and new technological methodo- logies.

The expansion of the scientific and technological

possibilities for developing better and safer drugs has been accompanied by and is to some extent interrelated with a considerable increase in the regulatory requirements that have to be fulfilled before the use of a drug is approved. Consequently, development time and cost for a completely new drug are long and high, respectively. A recent survey conducted by the US Animal Health Institute Market Research Committee showed that to develop a new anthelmintic for use in cattle takes approximately 8 years and costs $16 million.

A substantial part of that sum is spent on safety testing. The cost of a full battery of toxicity tests for a pharmaceutical product is estimated to be approximately $4 million. In the case of drugs for animal usage, the cost of residue-related safety studies has to be added. This means that between 30 and 40% of the development cost of a new animal drug is spent on safety testing.

The wording "full battery of toxicity tests" implies that testing is usually carried out following rigidly fixed protocols. Animal species used, number of animals per group, dosing regimen, parameters studied etc. are standardized as much as possible to ensure that the test results are acceptable to regulatory authorities. This situation is unsatisfactory.

Both the academic world and industry put much effort in the design and development of testing methods that are an alternative to presently used methods. To be a useful alternative, new testing methods should enable a more reliable prediction to be given of the health hazards of a drug to man, by providing information on the basic mechanisms underlying the toxic effects[1,10]; they should minimize the number of animals used and they should be less expensive and time-consuming. Furthermore, the availability of a series of tests from which a choice can be made depending on the requirements in a particular case, leads to more flexible testing procedures. Finally, they should not be additional to presently used testing programmes, but replace parts of it.

In this chapter an overview is presented on how the target animal species can be used more efficiently in the safety evaluation of animal drugs, thus possibly leading to a reduction of the total testing programme.

TARGET ANIMAL VERSUS LABORATORY ANIMAL

In the safety evaluation of animal drugs both the target animal species and man have to be considered. In the case of drugs that are administered repeatedly on a large scale, the environment is the third entity to be taken into account. The safety for man relates to the actual contact with drugs during manufacture and handling as well as to the consumption of edible tissues and products from drug-treated food-producing animal species.

If a particular drug was initially developed for human application, the results from a number of toxicity studies in laboratory animal species are usually already available. These relate only to the drug itself, not to metabolites occurring as residues in edible animal products. However, a separate veterinary drug development is not uncommon as with growth promoters, coccidiostats, antibiotic feed additives and anthelmintics.

Data on efficacy, target animal tolerance and drug residues can only be obtained in studies with the target species. These studies can by themselves provide a great part of the information necessary for a risk assessment relating to man.

PHARMACOKINETICS AND METABOLISM STUDIES

Studies on the pharmacokinetics and metabolism of animal drugs in the target animal are a first example of how target animal studies can provide much more information relevant to safety evaluation and not merely information on one aspect, namely the occurrence of residues in edible tissues.

The pharmacokinetics and metabolism of a drug can vary widely from one species to another. Therefore, studies pertaining to these aspects with animal drugs have to be carried out in the target animal species itself. The methodology used is usually that of administering a certain quantity of radiolabelled drug at one or more appropriate sites in the molecule, together with the non-labelled drug. The radiolabel should preferably be C14, the appropriate sites are those in which the radiolabel is not easily lost by metabolic degradation.

Information obtained in these studies relates to

(1) total residue level as a function of withdrawal time;
(2) extraction and concentration procedures;
(3) percentages of extractable and non-extractable residues.

The extractable residue fraction consists of compounds (parent drug and metabolites) that are free, that is, unbound, or relatively easily released from their binding sites by the extraction procedures used. The non-extractable fraction is much less easily dealt with, in view of the analytical difficulties encountered in its identification. It consists of fragments of the original drug molecule formed by extensive biodegradation and incorporated into endogenous tissue structures, residues that are covalently bound to DNA and other macromolecules and residues that are not covalently bound, but yet cannot be extracted with available procedures.

Covalently bound metabolites are a subject of special concern, since covalent binding of reactive metabolites to macromolecules such as DNA is considered a first step in carcinogenesis and teratogenesis. The actual toxicological significance of bound residues for the consumer is far from clear, however, but this subject will not be discussed in this chapter.

Aspects that can be investigated in conjunction with pharmacokinetics and metabolism studies are : the bioavailability of the residues, the mutagenic activity of the extractable residues and the environmental fate of excreted residues.

Bioavailability

The total residue usually is a complex mixture of parent drug and bound or free metabolites. Consequently, the bioavailability of the residues is not uniform and is certainly not identical to that of the parent drug or known metabolites incorporated as pure chemicals in the diet, if only because the residues are embedded in the tissue matrix.

However, if the residue complex contains toxic components, their effect in man (the consumer) can only be expressed in terms of bioavailability. An indication on residue bioavailability is obtained by feeding the target animal tissues originating from metabolism studies and containing radiolabelled residue complex to one or more laboratory animal species (model consumers). By determining faecal and urinary excretion of radioactivity, the fraction of the total residue that is absorbed after oral administration is assessed. Additional analyses may include level of radioactivity in several tissues of the model consumers. Further refinements of this procedure are possible by determining absorption before and after extraction of the free residue fraction from the target animal tissues. In this way the bioavailability of the extractable residue fraction can be distinguished from that of the non-extractable fraction. (For a more general overview of this relay bioavailability methodology see[3]).

Examples of an application of the above principles include trenbolone[5] and ronidazole[8,9]. In the case of trenbolone no difference was observed between excretory patterns of radioactivity in rats before and after extraction of the residue-containing tissues with ethyl acetate. With ronidazole the residue bioavailability studies have been of considerable support in confirming the hypothesis that a substantial fraction of the persistent residues in swine muscle tissue is due to endogenous substances (drug-derived fragments incorporated into endogenous structures).

Mutagenic activity

An important element in the safety assessment of animal drug residues is the provision of data to establish that residues are not carcinogenic, whatever the underlying mechanism of carcinogenicity may be. Before a decision is taken on the need to commence carcinogenicity testing all available information on chemical structure of the parent compound and level and composition of the residue complex in the edible tissues should be taken into consideration. In a number of situations the value of this prescreening assessment can considerably be increased by evaluating the mutagenicity of the extractable residue complex. In previous parts of the testing programme extraction and concentration procedures have been established. These can be applied to tissues from target animals to which non-labelled drug has been administered. The concentrated extract is subsequently subjected to a limited series of mutagenicity tests.

An extension of this testing method, which mimics the processes occurring in the gastrointestinal tract of man, consists of administering the residue-containing tissue to laboratory animals and investigating whether the mutagenic activity of the extractable residues is altered by gastrointestinal metabolic processes.

Requirements that have to be fulfilled for the above procedure to be successful are :

(1) extraction and concentration methods must be suitable to provide an extract that can be used in several tests;
(2) the residue components must be sufficiently stable to withstand extraction and concentration;
(3) the amount of residue must be sufficiently high.

Johnston and Hopke[4] have made an estimate of the probability of detecting a mutagen with the Ames assay for any weight of compound assayed. The estimate was based upon data from 157 chemicals that gave a positive response

in the Ames test. Their results are of great help for the
design and analysis of experiments to detect mutagens,
especially mutagens present in complex, chemically
unidentified mixtures such as food, effluents, drug
residues, drinking water etc.

As far as the present author is aware the literature
gives no example of the application of the above procedure
to drug residue complexes.

Environmental fate

If a drug for use in animals is applied as a feed
additive, which implies large-scale use, an assessment
should be made of its environmental impact. A substantial
portion of the drug is excreted in urine and faeces, which
are subsequently used for soil fertilization. The
residues of the drug present in manure could be persistent
and have an adverse effect on manure degradation and soil
organisms and processes. The fate of the residues in the
environment can be investigated by using the excreta of
target animals, with which metabolism studies were
conducted. De Vries and de Roij have conducted some
experiments (unpublished results) following this procedure
regarding sulphadimidine.

A representative sample of urine and faeces from pigs,
that were administered an oral dose of ^{14}C-sulphadimidine
together with a non-labelled sulphadimidine containing
ration, was applied to soil columns. The columns were
eluted daily during 2 months (equivalent of 9 mm
rain/day). After 2 months the soil columns were dissected
and analysed for extractable sulphadimidine and its major
metabolite N_4-acetylsulphadimidine, extractable radioactivity and non-extractable radioactivity. No radioactivity could be detected in the leaching water.

From the upper 8 cm of the column, 15% of the applied
sulphadimidine and 40% of the applied N_4-acetylsulpha-
dimidine were recovered by extraction. The greatest part
was retained in the upper 4 cm. Approximately 6% of the
total radioactivity applied was extractable from the upper

8 cm, whereas 50% appeared to be non-extractable. Around 40% was lost, probably by the formation of volatile radiolabelled compounds.

From these and other experiments it was concluded that both sulphadimidine and its major metabolite are rather strongly adsorbed to soil particles. A substantial part of these compounds may be transformed to volatile degradation products.

TOXICITY STUDIES IN THE TARGET ANIMAL

At practical use levels, an animal drug must not be toxic for the target species. Its safety margin has to be as wide as possible. Animal drugs can be tested directly in the target species using doses sufficiently high to establish a safety margin. Parameters studied include growth rate, feed and water intake, and also biochemical and haematological values, histology, immunology and reproduction. It may seem unnecessary to include the latter aspects in target animal toxicity tests. However, it must be realized that studying the toxic effects of animal drugs in the target animals not only yields information on the potential toxicity of the parent drug, but also of the metabolites, to which man can be exposed by consuming edible animal products. In fact, it is the best example of the auto-exposure concept that is being propagated in US drug regulations[2,7]. Data on functional, biochemical and structural changes, resulting from exposure of the target animal to a drug, can therefore be very useful for an extrapolation to man.

One limitation might be that, in comparison with the commonly used laboratory animal species, the target animal is less uniform from a genetic point of view and that less baseline data are available on biochemistry, haematology, histology etc.[6]. This will partly be compensated for by the increasing knowledge of basic mechanisms of toxic actions of chemicals. Furthermore, an extrapolation from target species to man will in principle be as good or as bad as an extrapolation from laboratory species to man.

CONCLUSION

The safety evaluation of new drugs, whether for human or animal use, has become a long and arduous process. Much time and money are spent to guarantee as far as possible, that, under the conditions of use, drugs are safe, or that the risk of the occurrence of unwanted effects is acceptable.

For animal drugs, this not only relates to the target species, but also to man who may be exposed to drug residues in the edible products of treated animals. In the last 10-15 years there has been a growing tendency to put more emphasis on the latter aspect. Although the wholesomeness of our food is an extremely important issue, one should strive for a well-balanced approach in this respect. It is not realistic to try to assess the carcinogenicity of the last drug-derived molecule in edible tissues. Moreover, requirements of this nature will greatly hinder the further development of new drugs.

It has been shown in this chapter that in the process of safety evaluation there are a number of opportunities to obtain relevant information that, when used properly, could result in an increase in testing efficiency and a decrease in testing requirements.

References
1. Aldridge, W.N. (1981). Mechanism of toxicity. New concepts are required in toxicology. TIPS 2:228-231.
2. Farber, T.M. (1980). Problems in the safety evaluation of tissue residues. J. Environ. Pathol. Toxicol. 3:73-79.
3. Huber, W.G., Becker, S.R. and Archer, B.P. (1980). Bioavailability of residues : current status. J. Environ. Pathol. Toxicol. 3:45-63.
4. Johnston, J.B. and Hopke, P.K. (1980). Estimation of the weight-dependent probability of detecting a mutagen with the Ames assay. Environ. Mutag. 2:419-424.
5. Ross, D.B. (1981). Toxicology and residues of trenbolone acetate as a model. In : Jasiorowski, H. (ed.). Steroids in Animal Production, pp.227-235. Warsaw : ARS Polona-Ruch.
6. Stevenson, D.E. (1979). Current problems in the choice of animals for toxicity testing. J. Toxicol. Environ. Hlth 5:9-15.
7. Weber, N.E. (1983). Metabolism and kinetics in the

regulation of animal drugs. J. Anim. Sci. 56:244-251.
8. Wolf, F.J., Bayliss, F.P., Smith, G.E., Rosenblum, C.,
    Meriwether, H.T., Alvaro, R.F., Wolf, D.E., Koniuszy,
    F.R. and Jacob, T.A. (1983). Disposition of
    ronidazole in swine. 1. Radiocarbon content of
    tissues. J. Agric. Food Chem. 31:559-564.
9. Wolf, F.J., Alvaro, R., Steffens, J.J., Wolf, D.E.,
    Koniuszy, F.R., Green, M.L. and Jacob, T.A. (1984).
    Tissue residues due to ronidazole : bioavailability of
    residues in swine muscle on ingestion by the rat.   J.
    Agric. Food Chem. 32:711-714.
10. Zbinden, G. (1978). Application of basic concepts to
    research in toxicology. Pharmacol. Rev. 30:605-616.

20
The use of pharmacokinetics in chronic toxicity testing

H. G. VERSCHUUREN AND R. H. REITZ

ABSTRACT

The usefulness of a unified pharmacokinetic model for the chronic testing of drug residues is described. The model was very suitable for the disposition and metabolism rate of methylchloroform (MC) in humans, rats and mice, at various exposure levels and with two different routes of administration. The physiological parameters fed into the model take account of old and young animals. The model could provide more reliable estimations of health hazards for the chemicals in our environment.

INTRODUCTION

Chronic toxicity studies are indispensable for the evalua-tion of risks to humans, resulting from the exposure to drugs, food additives, residues of pesticides or feed additives, and to many industrial chemicals. The design of the studies, including the choice of the dose levels requires forward projection of available knowledge. Nevertheless, sometimes results are obtained at high dose levels, qualitatively different from those obtained at intermediate and low dose levels[3,7,14].

This phenomenon has stimulated research into the fate of chemicals in the body of animals at different dose levels. Changes in absorption, distribution and metabolism in a dose-dependent manner have, with hindsight, provided the key for the explanation of the findings obtained in many experiments. More scientists are now prepared to make use of pharmacokinetic data, in setting dose levels for chronic toxicity and carcinogenicity studies. The underlying principle is that data obtained under unusual conditions, such as extremely high dose levels, cannot be used directly to predict the fate of the chemical and the effects it will have on the animal at lower dose levels.

The development of mathematical models has advanced our ability to predict the events. A unified pharmacokinetic model was developed, suitable for predicting the disposition of methylchloroform in young and old animals, in several species, including man, and by two routes of administration.

Methylchloroform (1,1,1-trichloroethane, or MC) had been investigated in man as well as in animals[9,12] in separate experiments. However, a comprehensive unified model capable of describing the pharmacokinetics of methylchloroform in several species after administration by different routes has not been reported before. This model was developed, based on physiological parameters to simulate methylchloroform disposition in mice, rats and humans, following inhalation exposure. The simulation was compared with actual data generated for these three species. In addition, by changing the physiological parameters, the predicted disposition in elderly rats and mice was compared with data obtained by Schumann et al.[13]. Furthermore, the model was used to predict the disposition of methylchloroform given in drinking water and these findings were compared with actual data obtained by Reitz et al.[11]. Methylchloroform was used to develop this model, because of the multitude of actual data points available. The significance of the model for other chemicals including veterinary drugs is discussed below.

METHODS

Four-compartment model

A four-compartment physiological model, similar to that developed by Ramsey and Andersen[10] was used (Figure 20.1).

Physiological parameters

Body weights were as follows : humans : 83 kg; young rats: 215-250 g depending on the average actual weight in a particular study; elderly rats : 468 g; young mouse : 29 g; elderly mouse : 37.5 g.

Volumes of individual tissue

The volumes of individual tissue compartments (in litres) were calculated by multiplying the total body weight by the relative percentage for each tissue, assuming unit density (1 g/ml) for all tissues. The relative percentages of individual tissue compartments in humans were taken from Davis and Mapleson[5], who obtained much of their data from the report of the Task Group on reference man[6], and these are summarized in Table 20.1. Relative percentages of the tissue compartments in young rats were taken from reference[4]. Relative percentages of the tissue compartments in elderly rats were assumed to be identical to those of young rats, except that the relative fat content was increased to 28.3%, with a corresponding decrease in the relative percentage of the slowly perfused compartment from 63.5 to 61.3% (see Table 20.1). Volumes of the tissue compartments in young mice were assumed to be identical to those of young rats except that the percentage of body fat was set at 2% of total body weight. The relative percentages of the tissue compartments in elderly mice were equal to those of young mice except that the fat compartment was increased from 2% to 16% of body weight (see Table 20.1). The values used for relative fat content of the older animals were chosen by the computer to give the best possible simulation of the experimental data.

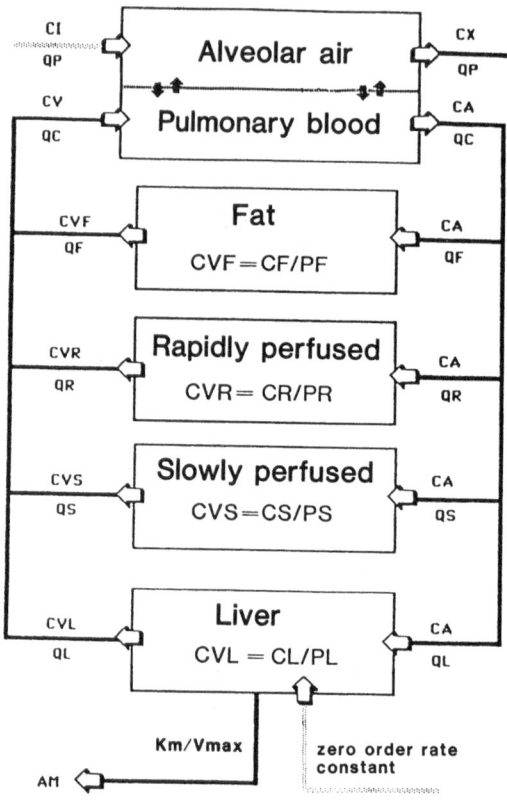

Figure 20.1 Physiological model used to describe the pharmacokinetics of methylchloroform in rats, mice and humans during inhalation and drinking water exposures to methylchloroform. C = concentration; CI : concentration in inhaled air; CX = concentration in expired air; CV = concentration in venous blood; CA = concentration in arterial blood; CVF = concentration in venous blood draining adipose tissue; CR = concentration in rapidly perfused compartment; CS = concentration in slowly perfused compartment; CL = concentration in liver; Q = flow in litre/h; QP = alveolar ventilation rate; QC = cardiac output; QF = flow through fat compartment; QR = flow through rapidly perfused compartment; QS = flow through slowly perfused compartment; QL = flow through liver compartment; PB = blood/air partition coefficient (pc); PF = blood/fat partition coefficient; PL = liver/

blood partition coefficient; PR = rapidly perfused/blood partition coefficient; PS = slowly perfused/blood partition coefficient; Km = Michaelis constant; Vmax = maximum velocity of metabolism.

Cardiac output and alveolar ventilation

Cardiac output and alveolar ventilation for humans were taken from Davis and Mapleson[5]. Cardiac output and alveolar ventilation for the other species were scaled to the 0.7 power of body weight, as outlined by Ramsey and Andersen[10]. All values are tabulated in Table 20.1.

Flows to individual tissue groups

Flows to the individual tissue groups were calculated by multiplying the relative percentage of flow to each tissue by the appropriate cardiac output. It was assumed that the same percentage of cardiac output would perfuse the tissue groups in all three species, and the percentages were taken from Davis and Mapleson[5]. All values are tabulated in Table 20.1.

Partition coefficients

Tissue/air partition coefficients were determined for rat blood, liver, fat and muscle using the vial equilibration technique of Andersen et al.[2]. Tissue/blood partition coefficients for rat fat, muscle, and liver were than calculated by dividing the measured tissue/air partition coefficient by the blood/air coefficient for rat blood. To estimate the blood/tissue partition coefficients for the rapidly and slowly perfused compartments, the partition coefficients for liver/blood and muscle/blood were doubled (see Table 20.1). This gave a good fit with experimental data, and was rationalized by considering that other components of these heterogeneous compartments such as brain and skin contain more lipid than liver and muscle, respectively. Blood/air partition coefficients for human and mouse blood were determined by the method of M.L. Gargas and M.E. Andersen (personal communication).

Table 20.1 Parameters used in the physiologically based pharmacokinetics model for methylchloroform. The abbreviations are : Rat 1, young rats (2-4 months); Rat 2, old rats (18.5 months); Mouse 1, young mice; Mouse 2, elderly mice. Parameters used for drinking water simulation in rats are very close to Rat 1 and are not shown.

	Human	Rat 1	Rat 2	Mouse 1	Mouse 2
Weights in kg					
Body weight	83.0	0.215	0.468	0.029	0.038
Liver*	2.6	4.1	4.1	4.1	4.1
Rapidly perfused*	3.1	6.2	6.2	6.2	6.2
Slowly perfused*	52.4	63.5	61.3	63.5	63.5
Fat*	19.5	7.1	28.3	2.0	16.0
Flows in litres/h					
Alveolar ventilation	300.0	4.64	7.98	1.14	1.37
Cardiac output	388.8	6.01	10.4	1.48	1.77
Liver**	24	24	24	24	24
Rapidly perfused**	53	53	53	53	53
Slowly perfused**	18	18	18	18	18
Fat**	5	5	5	5	5
Partition coefficients					
Blood/air	2.5	6.2	6.2	10.8	10.8
Liver/air	12.5	12.5	12.5	12.5	12.5
Rapidly perfused/air	25.0	25.0	25.0	25.0	25.0
Slowly perfused/air	14.5	14.5	14.5	14.5	14.5
Fat/air	280.0	280.0	280.0	280.0	280.0
Metabolic constants					
Vmax (mg/h)	3.91	0.0604	0.104	0.0149	0.0178
Km (mg/litre)	3.5	3.5	3.5	3.5	3.5

* Percentage of body weight
** Percentage of cardiac output

Tissue/blood coefficients for human and mouse tissues were calculated by dividing the measured or estimated tissue/air partition coefficient for the corresponding rat tissue by the blood/air coefficient for the other species. Partition coefficients used in these simulations are listed in Table 20.1.

Values of Vm and Km

The values of Vm and Km were manually adjusted to fit the data gathered by Schumann et al.[12] describing the metabolism of inhaled methylchloroform in young rats. The value of Vm was then scaled to the 0.7 power of body weight for the other species (see Table 20.1). Km was held constant at 3.5 mg/l methylchloroform for all three species.

Computer programs

Simultaneous differential equations describing the fate of methylchloroform were formulated as a computer program as outlined by Ramsey and Andersen[10]. Simulations were conducted with a software package developed by Agin and Blau[1] and were run on an IBM 3033N computer.

RESULTS

In models such as those shown in Figure 20.1, tissues have been grouped together according to relative blood flow rates and tissue/blood partition. In this particular example, we have five groupings : (1) the lung, where gas exchange occurs; (2) the fat bed, with relatively high affinity for methylchloroform; (3) the rapidly perfused tissues (such as kidney); (4) the slowly perfused tissues like muscle; and (5) the metabolizing tissues (which comprise the liver in this particular case).

Methylchloroform may enter this system either through the inhaled air (inhalation exposure) or the gastrointestinal tract. Uptake from the gastrointestinal tract was assumed to occur rapidly, and was simulated by assuming input directly into the liver for drinking water

exposures.   Metabolism of methylchloroform is assumed to
occur according to saturable Michaelis-Menten kinetics.

Simultaneous differential equations to describe the
movement of methylchloroform in each of these compartments
can be formulated if we know the flows and partition
coefficients associated with each step. The first set of
predictions related to the concentration-time course in
venous blood in rats. Figure 20.2 shows a solid line for
the prediction, open circles for the low (150 ppm) and
triangles for the high exposure level (1500 ppm)[12]. A
good fit was obtained quickly without the necessity of
extensive adjustments with model parameters.

In addition to predicting the time course of methylchloroform in venous blood, the physiological model is
capable of describing a variety of other properties which
may be verified experimentally. For each of the
parameters the ratio of the model prediction to the actual
data is calculated for exposure to 150 and 1500 ppm. For
concentrations in the blood at the end of the 6 hour
exposure this ratio was 1.66 at 150 ppm and 1.9 at 1500
ppm. Equally so the ratio for the body burden (total
amount present in the body) at the end of the 6 hour
exposure was 1.11 and 1.36 respectively; for the amount
metabolized : 1.07 and 0.92; for the concentration in fat
1.95 and 1.69; for the concentration in the liver 1.05 and
1.44. The ratio of predicted to actual data varied
between 0.92 and 1.98, with a mean ratio of 1.51 in rats.
The fitting of five additional parameters, keeping the
ratio within a factor of 2, is really remarkable.

The rat model was then used as a basis for
extrapolation to the B6C3F1 mouse. This entailed scaling
the flows and metabolic rates and incorporating a new (experimentally determined) partition coefficient.

The time profile of methylchloroform in venous blood is
shown in Figure 20.3 for 150 and 1500 ppm exposures during
6 h. Methylchloroform reached higher peak blood levels in
mice (about 4-fold) but was eliminated five to ten times
more rapidly after termination of exposure. The

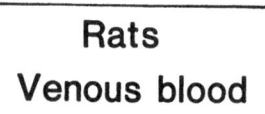

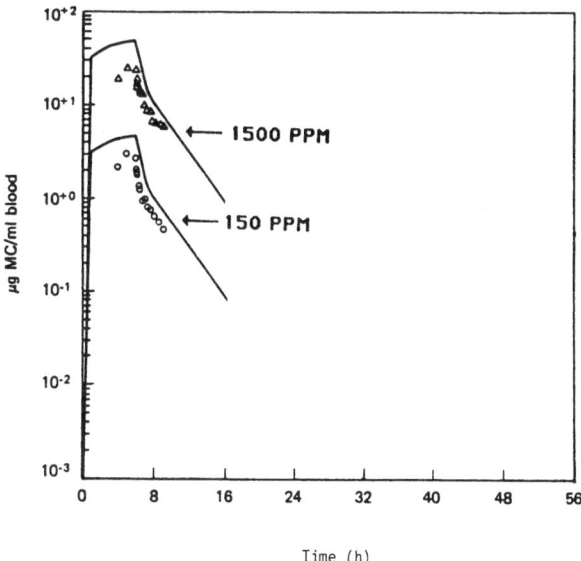

Figure 20.2 Concentrations of methylchloroform in venous
blood of rats resulting from a 6 h exposure to 150 or 1500
ppm of methylchloroform.

physiological model accurately predicted both these facts
without any adjustments to model parameters.

In addition to the venous blood levels of methylchloroform in mice, the model was used to describe several other
properties of this agent. Again, an excellent agreement
was obtained between the model predictions and the actual
data. The ratio of predicted to actual data for the 150
and 1500 ppm exposure levels was as follows : for
concentrations in the blood at the end of the 6 hour
exposure the ratio was 0.93 and 0.78 for 150 and 1500 ppm
respectively; for the body burden after 6 hour exposure
0.69 and 0.77; for the amount metabolized 0.78 and 0.69;
for the concentration in the fat 1.29 and 1.07 and for the
concentration in the liver 1.00 and 1.22 respectively.

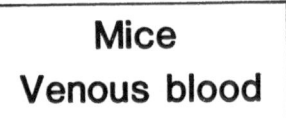

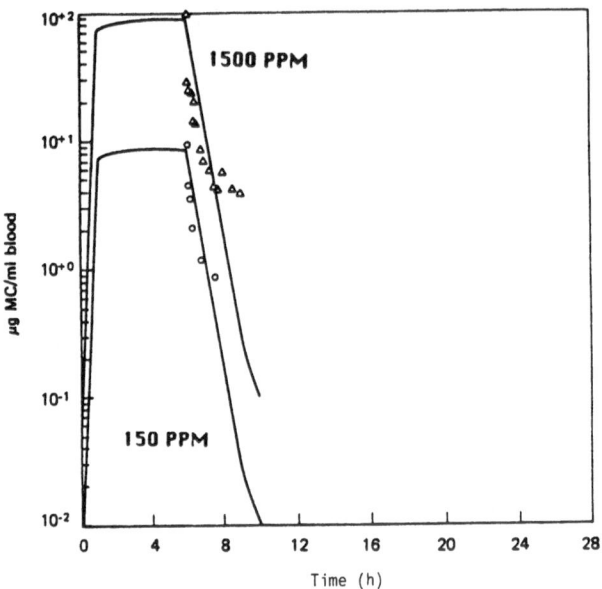

Figure 20.3 Concentrations of methylchloroform in venous blood of mice resulting from a 6 h exposure to 150 or 1500 ppm of methylchloroform.

With slight modifications, it proved possible to use this model to describe the disposition of methylchloroform in rats after consumption of drinking water containing 4.4 mg/ml of ^{14}C methylchloroform. Rats were given free access to treated water for 8 h, resulting in a mean dose of 143 mg/kg. During and following exposure, the rats were housed in glass metabolism cages, and the radio-activity in expired air was collected with activated charcoal traps. The concentration of methylchloroform in expired air predicted by the model as well as the concentration actually obtained are shown in Figure 20.4. Methylchloroform elimination was well described for the first 30 h. After this period, the model predicted less

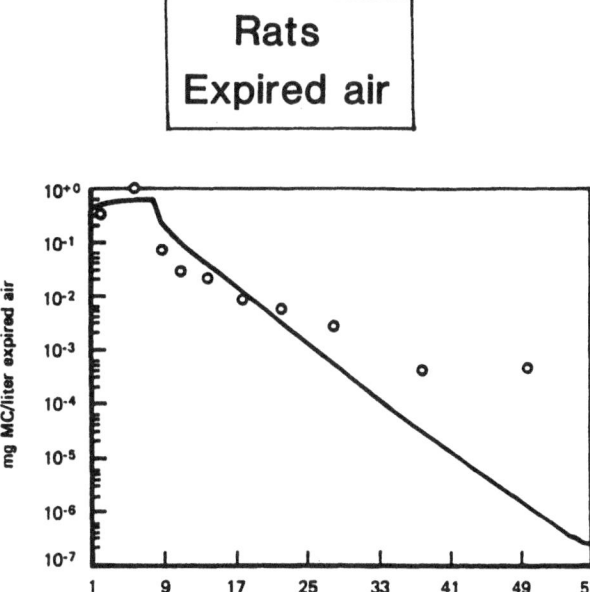

Figure 20.4   Concentrations of methylchloroform in expired
air collected from rats during and following exposure to
saturated solutions (4.4 mg/ml) of methylchloroform in water for 8 h.

radioactivity in expired air than was actually observed.
However, at this point, 99.9% of the administered radioactivity had been recovered, so the last few radioactive
counts may represent a slowly eliminated volatile metabolite of methylchloroform, such as trichloroethanol. The
model predicted 5.3 μmol of methylchloroform would be
metabolized, and 8.0 μmol were actually recovered, giving
a prediction ratio of 0.66.
     The ultimate test of any extrapolation procedure is how
well it can predict human data from animal experiments.
In this case, we already had the human data available, but
we proceeded as if we had only animal data to check the
usefulness of this procedure. The model was used,
unchanged, to predict the disposition of methylchloroform
after either 35 or 350 ppm inhalation exposures in humans.

Data gathered by Nolan et al.[9] for periods up to 10 days post-exposure are shown in Figure 20.5. Blood levels of methylchloroform during exposure were slightly lower than model predictions, but the degree of agreement was excellent.

Similarly, the concentrations of methylchloroform in expired air obtained by Nolan et al.[9] were compared with the model predictions. The expired air concentrations during exposure were perfectly predicted. There were slight discrepancies in the 20–40 h post-exposure period. The methylchloroform metabolites recovered by Nolan were 68% and 62%, respectively, of the values predicted by the model for 350 and 35 ppm.

Finally, the model was used to describe a hypothetical human exposure to methylchloroform in drinking water. For this simulation it was assumed that humans consume two litres of water/day, and that this water contains 0.31 ppm methylchloroform. This value was chosen as a "worst case", because this is the highest concentration reported in drinking water supplies by the United States EPA. For mathematical convenience, it was assumed that people consume small amounts of water periodically throughout the day, therefore the input of methylchloroform was simulated as a zero order process equal to the average rate of uptake. The stimulation was then run for periods varying from 1 to 100 days.

It was apparent from these simulations that steady state is approached within just a few days. Furthermore, the body burden of methylchloroform after 100 days of water consumption was only 2.7 times higher than that present after a single day of drinking such water.

The model also made it possible to calculate the average body burden of methylchloroform in humans under these conditions. We compared this value to the average body burden of methylchloroform present in animals at the "no observed effect level" in chronic studies conducted at Dow. The "no observed effect levels" we observed were 875 ppm for rats and 1500 ppm for mice. The body burdens of

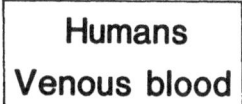

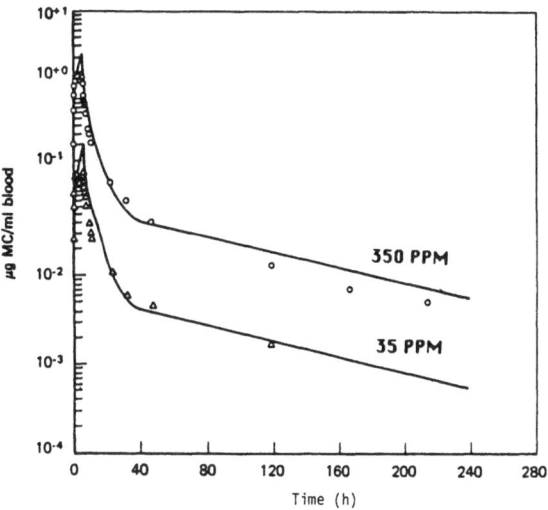

Figure 20.5 Concentrations of methylchloroform in venous blood collected from humans during and following exposure to 35 ppm (open triangles) or 350 ppm (open circles) of methylchloroform for 6 h.

methylchloroform failing to produce toxicity in these animals were five to six orders of magnitude higher than those predicted to occur in humans consuming such water.

DISCUSSION

From the results obtained, the conclusion may be drawn that for methylchloroform a unified pharmacokinetic model can be successfully applied. The model was fed with the relevant physiological data, and a limited number of experimental determinations of partition coefficients and metabolism, and disposition studies.

   The same model was able to describe a wide variety of data in humans, rats and mice over a broad range of inhalation exposures. This was so even when the exposure levels were high enough to cause saturation of metabolism.

Another feature of this model was its ability to describe the disposition of methylchloroform given to rats by different routes, inhalation or drinking water.

With all the close fits between actual data and model predictions, one could confidently move to the next step : prediction into an area where no confirmatory data are available. Reitz[11] used the model for the risk evaluation relevant to an assumed drinking water contamination with methylchloroform. The body burden for humans is predicted, to be five to six orders of magnitude below the "no observed effect levels" in experimental animals.

The use of this model could mean a significant step forward in calculating the potential health hazards of chemicals in our environment. It is obvious that this promising model should be further tested with other chemicals, including veterinary drugs. Those chemicals with data available on partition coefficients and metabolism/disposition in more species should be selected for this purpose. The results obtained in the application of this model should stimulate investigations to obtain the appropriate pharmacokinetic data available before starting a long term study. Knowing the fate of the chemical in the body at several dose levels can be an enormous help in estimating the toxicological impact involved.

References
1. Agin, G.L. and Blau, G.E. (1982). Application of DACSL (Dow Advanced Continuous Simulation Language) to the design and application of chemical reactor systems. Amer. Inst. Chem. Eng. Symp. Ser. No.214, 78:108-118.
2. Andersen, M.E., Gargas, M.L. and Ramsey, J.C. (1984). Inhalation pharmacokinetics : evaluating systemic extraction, total in vivo metabolism, and the time course of enzyme induction for inhaled styrene in rats based on arterial blood : inhaled air concentration ratios 1. Toxicol. Appl. Pharmacol. 73:175-187.
3. Anderson, M.W., Hoel, D.G. and Kaplan, N.L. (1980). A general scheme for the incorporation of pharmacokinetics in low-dose risk estimation for chemical carcinogenesis : Example - Vinyl Chloride. Toxicol. Appl. Pharmacol. 55:154.
4. Caster, W.O., Poncelet, J., Simon, A.B. and Armstrong, W.D. (1956). Tissue weights of the rat. I. Normal

values determined by dissection and chemical methods. Proc. Soc. Exp. Biol. Med. 91:122-126.

5. Davis, N.R. and Mapleson, W.W. (1981). Structure and quantification of a physiological model of the distribution of injected agents and inhaled anaesthetics. Br. Journal Anaesth. 53:399-405.

6. Gehring, P.J. (1968). Hepatotoxic potency of various chlorinated hydrocarbon vapors relative to their narcotic and lethal potencies in mice. Toxicol. Appl. Pharmacol. 13:287-298.

7. Gehring, P.J. and Blau, G.E. (1977). Mechanisms of carcinogenesis dose response. J. Env. Path. Toxicol. 1:163-179.

8. International Commission on Radiation Protection (1975). Report of the task group on reference man. W.S. Snyder et al. (eds). ICRP Publication 23. New York : Pergamon Press.

9. Nolan, R.J., Freshour, N.L., Rick, D.L., McCarty, L.P. and Saunders, J.H. (1984). Kinetics and metabolism of inhaled methyl chloroform (1,1,1-trichloroethane) in male volunteers. Fund. Appl. Toxicol. 4:654-662.

10. Ramsey, J.C. and Andersen, M.E. (1984). A physiologically based description of the inhalation pharmacokinetics of styrene in rats and humans. Toxicol. Appl. Pharmacol. 73:159-175.

11. Reitz, R.H., Schumann, A.M., Osborne, D.W. and Nolan, R.J. Pharmacokinetics of 1,1,1-trichloroethane (MC) in humans, rats and mice after inhalation or drinking water administration. The Toxicologist 5:110.

12. Schumann, A.M., Fox, T.R. and Watanabe, P.G. (1982). [14C]methyl chloroform (1,1,1-trichloroethane) : Pharmacokinetics in rats and mice following inhalation exposure. Toxicol. Appl. Pharmacol. 62:390-401.

13. Schumann, A.M., Fox, T.R. and Watanabe, P.G. (1982). A comparison of the fate of inhaled methyl chloroform (1,1,1-trichloroethane) following single or repeated exposure in rats and mice. Fundam. Appl. Toxicol. 2:27-32.

14. Watanabe, P.G., Zemple, J.A., Pegg, D.Y. and Gehring, P.J. (1978). Hepatic macromolecular binding following exposure to vinyl chloride. Toxicol. Appl. Pharmacol. 44:571-579.

21
The Food Animal Residue Avoidance Databank (FARAD): a computer databank of the pharmacokinetics of drugs, pesticides and environmental chemicals in food animals

A. L. CRAIGMILL, S. F. SUNDLOF AND J. E. RIVIERE

ABSTRACT

The Food Animal Residue Avoidance Databank (FARAD) is a computer databank of information on chemicals considered to be actual or potential residue problems in the United States. FARAD has been developed under the auspices of the United States Department of Agriculture Extension Service, Residue Avoidance Program (RAP). FARAD includes a listing of all drugs approved by the Food and Drug Administration for use in food animals, all the tissue, egg and milk tolerances for 119 chemicals, and information on the chemical properties of these chemicals. The major focus of FARAD has been to collect all published information on the pharmacokinetics of these chemicals in food and non-food animal species. FARAD currently contains information on 938 proprietary drug preparations approved by FDA, 253 residue tolerances, and over 3000 pharmacokinetic entries linked to over 700 bibliographic citations. After completion of data extraction and entry into FARAD, this information will be used for making detailed analysis of interspecies differences in pharmacokinetics, to study disease-induced changes in pharmacokinetics, and to study the relationship of serum pharmacokinetics to tissue residues.

INTRODUCTION

The Food Animal Residue Avoidance Databank (FARAD) is being developed as an integral part of the United States Department of Agriculture Extension Service, Residue Avoidance Program (RAP). The RAP project was started to implement educational and field research programs that would help to decrease the incidence of food animal residue violations in the United States. The FARAD is a cooperative pilot project between five states : California, Florida, Idaho, Illinois and North Carolina. The role of FARAD in the Residue Avoidance Program is the acquisition, consolidation and dissemination of residue avoidance information.

MATERIALS AND METHODS

FARAD was first developed using a commercially available relational database management program called dBASE II, and Osborne I microcomputers with 20 megabyte hard disk storage systems. The data file structure and dBASE II program files for FARAD operation were developed at North Carolina State University. The data files and user program files have been successfully transferred to IBM personal computers equipped with hard disk storage devices and to a DEC 11/730 minicomputer. dBASE III, the dBASE II upgrade program for the IBM personal computer, is the software program currently used for data storage and retrieval.

The FARAD is made up of six separate data files that are linked on the generic chemical name. The first of these files is the Tradename file which contains a listing of all the drugs currently approved by the FDA for use in food animals, the manufacturer name, the species for which they are approved, the dosage, route of administration, indications for use, and withdrawal times. The second file is the Generic chemical file which contains information on the chemical formula, pKa, log P (partition coefficient), solubility and analytical methods for 119 different chemicals. The third file is the Tissue

Tolerance file which contains the tolerance levels established for the 119 chemicals in food animal products and the Federal Register reference for each. The fourth is the RAP Project Material file which contains a description of all the educational and research materials developed by all participants in the RAP program, the type of material, the source, and the address of a contact person. The fifth is the Bibliographic Citation file which contains a complete citation of every article from which pharmacokinetic data were extracted. The sixth, and most extensive, file is the Pharmacokinetic file. The information that may be entered into each pharmacokinetic record is shown in Table 21.1. Each record is referenced to a bibliographic citation, and each citation may give rise to multiple pharmacokinetic records.

Data extraction
The Food Safety and Inspection Service gave FARAD a list of 119 chemicals that were considered to have the potential to cause residues in food animal products. In this list there were 42 antibiotics, 26 pesticides, 13 environmental contaminants, 11 anthelmintics, 8 hormones and 14 mycotoxins. This list formed the nucleus of chemicals included in FARAD. Information on the chemical properties of these compounds was obtained from Toxicology Data Bank searches and primary sources. Tissue tolerances were obtained from the Food and Drug Administration and by searching the Federal Register. Literature sources of kinetic information were found by doing computerized searches using AGRICOLA, TOXLINE and MEDLINE and then by searching the bibliographies of each relevant paper for additional citations. Copies of each paper that contained relevant kinetic or residue information were obtained from local libraries or from the National Agricultural Library which provided free document delivery as their contribution to FARAD. All data extraction is carried out at both the University of California and the University of Florida.

Table 21.1 Structure of the pharmacokinetic data file

Field	Field name	Width	Description
1	CIT_NUM	9	Citation number (Bibliographic File)
2	CON_CODE	1	Confidence code
3	GENERIC	61	Generic chemical name
4	DRGCLASS	20	Drug class
5	SPECIES	10	Species code
6	HEALTH	45	Health status
7	DOSE	16	Dose (mg/kg)
8	INTERVAL	8	Dosage interval
9	DOSE_NUM	11	Number of doses given
10	ROUTE	63	Route of administration
11	EXCR	27	Excretion route(s) and percentages
12	VD	32	Volumes of distribution (B, ss, area)
13	CLR	12	Clearance(s)
14	SPB	5	Serum protein binding
15	HLIFE	27	Half-lives (1,2,3)
16	CP	39	Maximum and minimum plasma levels
17	METABOL	65	Measured metabolites
18	OTH_DAT	130	Other useful data
19	LU_DATE	8	Last update to record
20	MATRIX	10	Matrix (serum, liver, kidney, etc.)
21	INTERC	27	Intercepts (A,B,C)
22	RATE	12	Glomerular filtration rate
23	NUM_ANIM	4	Number of animals studied
24	SPECIES2	20	Breed, age, weight

Over 2000 articles have been screened for residue or kinetic data, and over 700 citations have been found that contain useful data. Most articles do not contain all of the parameters listed in Table 21.1, however any useful information found is entered. If the authors have done a pharmacokinetic analysis of the data, their results are entered into FARAD directly. The only changes made are conversions to standard units. There are many papers that contain tissue residue or plasma level data that were not analysed for pharmacokinetic parameters by the authors. These data are extracted and sent to North Carolina State University, which is the site at which data are analysed and entered into FARAD.

Data analysis and entry into FARAD
Data taken from articles that contain residue or plasma level information that has not been analysed for kinetics, are processed through an automated curve stripping program (CSTRIP) for initial parameter estimates and then are analysed using a non-linear regression program (SAS-NLIN) which calculates relevant model-independent curve-fit parameters (slopes, areas, heights, moments). These estimates are then passed to a Fortran program which automatically selects the proper number of exponentials and weighting schemes using parametric and non-parametric statistical tests, and calculates the desired pharmacokinetic parameters. Tissue residue depletion data are analysed using a first-order log-linear regression analysis to determine the half-life of the residue in tissues. These data generated by FARAD are keyed both to the original citation from which the data were extracted, and to FARAD. Copies of all the FARAD-generated data are filed with the original article and data extraction sheets.

There are currently more than 3000 individual pharmacokinetic entries in FARAD that have been taken from over 700 articles. The pharmacokinetic file is projected to contain at least 10,000 records when complete and thus is approximately 30% finished. Completion of data entry is expected by January 1986. New records from recently published articles will be added as they appear in order

to keep FARAD current. The percentage of articles in
FARAD by species is shown in Table 21.2. The make-up of
the kinetic file mirrors the amount of published research
that has been done on the kinetics of chemicals in each
species. Pharmacokinetic data from non-food animals are
included in FARAD because, in many cases, kinetic studies
have not been done in food animals. Limited human kinetic
data are available in FARAD, but not all human data found
are entered.

Table 21.2   Pharmacokinetic file breakdown by species

Species	Per cent
Rodent	22.55
Bovine	20.73
Human	8.86
Canine	8.43
Avian	8.23
Ovine	3.64
Equine	3.45
Porcine	3.02
Caprine	0.91
Feline	0.38
Other	19.82

Data dissemination

The dissemination of residue avoidance information is a
major aspect of FARAD and is carried out at three sites,
the Universities of California, Illinois and Florida.
FARAD is not available "online", but is currently an
expert mediated system. Each call for information is
screened by a toxicologist and the appropriate data are
delivered to the caller. Information contained in any
file except the pharmacokinetic file can be sent without
review by the toxicologist. Due to the complexity of the
pharmacokinetic data, the expert is essential for the

appropriate application of kinetic information to   residue problems.

CONCLUSIONS

The FARAD is a multifaceted computer databank of residue avoidance information. One of its most important elements is a data file of pharmacokinetic information on the fate of chemicals in food animals. FARAD contains   heretofore unpublished   information   generated   from   the analysis of data taken from published articles that   did   not   perform kinetic analysis.   It is a valuable resource for examining interspecies   differences   in   kinetics,   disease-induced differences   in   kinetics,   and   the relationship of serum kinetics to tissue kinetics.

Acknowledgements

This project was funded by the United States Department of Agriculture   Extension   Service   with pass-through funding from the Food Safety and Inspection Service.   Postdoctoral fellow   support was provided for in part by NIEHS training grant ES07046.   This support is gratefully acknowledged.

Inflammation and Anti-Inflammatory Drugs Immunomodulation

22
Modulation of autonomic receptor function by Haemophilus influenzae in the respiratory system

F. P. NIJKAMP, F. ENGELS AND G. FOLKERTS

ABSTRACT

Pretreatment of guinea-pigs with the respiratory pathogen Haemophilus influenzae induces a deterioration of the pulmonary beta-adrenergic receptor system and hyperreactivity of the pulmonary cholinergic receptor system in vitro. This dysfunction of the autonomic nervous system is accompanied by a bronchial hyperreactivity to histamine in vivo, mediated by direct and reflex effects of histamine in the larger airways.

   Guinea-pig pulmonary macrophages stimulated with serum from H. influenzae pretreated animals mimic the deteriorating influence on the beta-adrenergic system in the larger airways in vitro. A role for oxygen-centred radicals is suggested.

INTRODUCTION

Increased bronchial irritability, or hyperreactivity, to a wide variety of different physical and chemical stimuli is a characteristic feature of patients with chronic obstructive lung disease. Airway hyperresponsiveness has often been associated with bronchial inflammation[3]. In healthy subjects respiratory airway infection results in an increased bronchospasm to inhaled methacholine and histamine. The mechanisms responsible for bronchial hyperreactivity are largely unknown, but the experimental evidence suggests that the disorder may stem from disturbances in mechanisms regulating airway smooth muscle tone rather than abnormality in the muscle itself (for reviews see[6,7]). In particular, an imbalance between the bronchoconstrictor parasympathetic cholinergic receptor system and the bronchodilator sympathetic beta-adrenergic system of the autonomic nervous system may predispose to bronchoconstriction[6,7]. Release of acetylcholine at the parasympathetic nerve endings leads to stimulation of cholinergic receptors with a resulting excessive bronchoconstriction response, oedema due to leakage from small vessels and increased mucus secretion. In contrast, stimulation of the beta-adrenoceptors of the sympathetic system by the endogenous hormone adrenaline or the neurotransmitter noradrenaline has opposite effects, that is, dilatation of the airways, vasodilatation, a decrease in the oedema, increased clearance of mucus and furthermore prevention of asthmatic mediator release.

The autonomic receptor system is dynamic and constantly changing. Stimulation decreases the number of receptors, while the absence of stimulation due to decreased concentrations of the specific hormones increases the number of receptors specific for that hormone. An altered function of the beta-adrenoceptors of the effector organs in asthma has been postulated by Szentivanyi[14]. He regards partial beta-adrenergic blockade as the fundamental factor of atopic abnormalities in general and bronchial asthma in particular. This hypothesis was based on an analogy of the symptoms of patients with bronchial asthma to those which could be induced by vaccination with Bordetella pertussis, such as hypersensitivity to pharmacological mediators, immunological reaction to antigen, and a decreased response to beta-sympatho-mimetics. However, B. pertussis lacks an obvious relationship with infections in asthmatic bronchitis, while the taxonomically closely related bacterium Haemophilus influenzae, usually found in the upper respiratory airways, often can be isolated from the deeper airways of patients with asthmatic bronchitis.

Previously we showed that H. influenzae induces a deterioration of the pulmonary beta-adrenergic system and a hyperreactivity of the cholinergic system in experimental animals (for review see[12]). The number of radioligand detectable beta-adrenoceptor binding sites in peripheral lung tissue was significantly reduced 4 days following administration of H. influenzae[10]. Furthermore the tracheal spirals from treated animals showed significantly less relaxation to the beta-sympathomimetic isoprenaline, regardless of whether the trachea was maximally contracted with carbachol or studied with normal intrinsic tone[9].

Besides H. influenzae, other bacterial suspensions also induced significant decreases in the beta-adrenoceptor number, that is, Streptococcus pneumoniae, Bordetella pertussis and Escherichia coli $O_{111}B_4$. S. pneumoniae has entirely different structural components in its cell wall and is not taxonomically related to H. influenzae, suggesting a rather aspecific effect. On the other hand, Staphylococcus aureus, an influenza A virus and Escherichia coli J_5 did not have similar properties. Because both of the other effective species were gram-negative, we tested whether the lipopolysaccharide (LPS) in the cell outer membrane was the responsible structure. The LPS of the effective ($O_{111}B_4$) and ineffective (J_5) E. coli strains were isolated by phenol-water extraction and tested in our experimental model. These LPS preparations showed similar properties to the killed suspensions of complete bacteria. The E. coli $O_{111}B_4$-LPS induced a decrease in beta-adrenoceptor number of approximately 20%, 4 days following vaccination, while the E. coli J_5-LPS was not effective[11].

There is an extensive cross-reaction between polysaccharides of pneumococci and H. influenzae. The difference between E. coli $O_{111}B_4$ and its UDP-gal-epi-merase-deficient mutant J_5 (with lipopolysaccharide that contains only core glycolipid) is mainly located in the repetitive sugar components of the O-antigenic side-chain of the LPS. Thus, probably the common factor of the gram-negative bacilli and the gram-positive cocci (S. pneumoniae) is situated in this immunogenic polysaccharide part of the LPS. Since all previous reports were obtained using isolated bronchial tissue we investigated, in the present experiment, the influence of H. influenzae on in vivo lung function parameters and additionally analysed the role of pulmonary macrophages.

EFFECTS ON LUNG FUNCTION PARAMETERS IN VIVO

The animals used were male guinea-pigs weighing 350-400 g (CPB-TNO, Zeist, The Netherlands). Treatment with H. influenzae was performed 4 days prior to the experiments. The animals were injected intraperitoneally (i.p.) with 5 x 10^8 killed cells (colony forming units)/100 g body weight. Guinea-pigs were anaesthetized with urethane (2 g/kg i.p.) and allowed to breathe spontaneously. The right jugular vein was cannulated for the injection of histamine hydrochloride and atropine sulphate.

Pulmonary resistance and dynamic lung compliance were determined breath by breath by a modified method of Amdur and Mead[1] using a computerized respiratory analyser. In each animal, two dose response curves were performed, one before and one after the administration of atropine, which was administered 15 min before the start of the second dose-response curve. Histamine injections were given with time intervals of at least 10 min. Histamine (0.5-8.0 ug/100 g body weight i.v.), administered as a bolus injection (0.1 ml) caused a dose-dependent increase in pulmonary resistance and a dose-dependent decrease in dynamic lung compliance. Basal values for saline and H. influenzae-treated guinea-pigs for pulmonary resistance were, respectively, 0.080 $\pm$ 0.025 and 0.073 $\pm$ 0.013 $cmH_2O/ml.s^{-1}$ and for dynamic lung compliance 0.431 $\pm$ 0.031 and 0.539 $\pm$ 0.055 ml/cmH_2O, respectively.

In H. influenzae-pretreated animals the increase in

pulmonary resistance was significantly potentiated by 1.0-8.0 µg histamine/100 g body weight i.v. Decreases in dynamic compliance did not differ. Maximal potentiation of the histamine response was observed at 1.0 and 8.0 µg histamine/100 g body weight. Data for increases in pulmonary resistance after histamine expressed as maximal value/basal value were 4.9 ± 0.9 for controls and 16.5 ± 3.8 ($p < 0.01$) for H. influenzae at 1.0 µg histamine and 19.0 ± 3.9 and 51.8 ± 10.6 ($p < 0.01$), respectively, at 8.0 µg histamine. The parasympathetic blocking drug atropine (100 µg/kg body weight i.v.), administered 15 min before the second dose-response curve of histamine, antagonized the potentiating effect at low doses of histamine (1.0-2.0 µg/100 g body weight i.v.) but not at high doses (4.0-8.0 µg/100 g body weight i.v.). At 1 µg histamine data for controls and treated animals were 5.6 ± 2.2 and 7.7 ± 2.0 and at 8 µg 19.0 ± 5.5 and 47.3 ± 9.7 ($p < 0.01$), respectively.

The results show that following pretreatment with H. influenzae there is an increased reactivity to histamine as measured by the potentiated increase in pulmonary resistance. Since the decreases in dynamic lung compliance were not different between the two groups, these data point to hyperreactivity of the larger respiratory airways. Histamine induces airway constriction in guinea-pigs mainly by activation of H_1-receptors. Besides direct stimulation of H_1-receptors of respiratory smooth muscle, bronchoconstriction by histamine in vivo is caused by stimulation of sensory "irritant" receptors which are localized in the major conducting airways. This reflex-bronchoconstriction is mediated through afferent and efferent pathways in the vagus nerve. Since in H. influenzae-treated guinea-pigs atropine antagonizes the potentiating effect at low doses of histamine, hyperreactivity is at least partly mediated by this reflex-arc.

At higher doses of histamine the hyperreactivity is probably due to direct stimulation of histamine receptors on the smooth muscles because atropine does not influence this increased sensitivity. The hyperreactivity at low doses of histamine may be due to increased sensitivity of the muscarinic receptor system since it was shown in in vitro experiments that carbachol induces in H. influenzae pretreated animals an increased contractile response of isolated guinea-pig tracheal spirals[9]. Douglas et al.[5] showed by experiments with beta-adrenergic blocking drugs that an increased histamine sensitivity may also be a function of a beta-adrenergic hyporesponsiveness. In previous work we showed that vaccination with H. influenzae results in impaired beta-adrenergic functioning accompanied by loss in radioligand detectable number of beta-adrenoceptor binding sites in guinea-pig respiratory airways[9,10]. A reasonable suggestion for the hyperreactivity at low and high doses histamine in vivo therefore may also be a beta-adrenoceptor hyporesponsiveness, which needs to be further substantiated.

ROLE OF PULMONARY MACROPHAGES

Pulmonary macrophages constitute the major cellular defence in the lung against bacterial invasion. In order to investigate the possible involvement of pulmonary macrophages in H. influenzae-induced deterioration of lung beta-adrenergic function, we additionally studied the influence of specifically stimulated pulmonary macrophages on the relaxation of isolated guinea-pig tracheal spirals to the beta-adrenoceptor stimulant isoprenaline. Killed, non-capsulated H. influenzae bacteria (10^8 colony-forming units/100 g body weight) were administered by intraperitoneal injection 4 days prior to the experiment. Pulmonary macrophages were isolated from non-treated animals by lung lavage via a tracheal cannula with 4 x 20 ml saline washes, containing 2.6 mM EDTA. The lavage fluid was centrifuged (10 min, 800 g) and the cells were resuspended in warm Krebs-bicarbonate solution. More than 90% of the cells collected were macrophages, the remaining cells being lymphocytes. From a non-treated guinea-pig the trachea was isolated and cut in a spiral fashion[9]. The tracheal preparation was incubated in 2 ml warm Krebs-bicarbonate solution, continually gassed with 95% O_2/5% CO_2, together with the cells obtained in the lung lavage (10^6 cells/ml, 60 min at 37 °C). This resulted in adherence of about 80% of the added macrophages to the tracheal preparation. Subsequently, the tracheal preparation was suspended in an organ bath, containing warm Krebs-bicarbonate solution, and connected to an isotonic smooth muscle transducer (Harvard Bioscience). Specific stimulation of the macrophages was carried out by a 1 h incubation of the tracheal preparation with serum (2% v/v) from an animal pretreated with H. influenzae. Beta-adrenoceptor function of the isolated tracheal spirals was determined by initial contraction with 10^{-6}M of the cholinergic agonist carbachol, after which a cumulative dose-response curve to isoprenaline was constructed. Maximal isoprenaline-induced relaxation was calculated relative to the precontraction to 10^{-6}M carbachol.

Adherence of the macrophages per se did not influence beta-adrenergic function in the trachea. Maximal isoprenaline-induced relaxation was 104 ± 9%, as compared to tracheal spiral relaxation in the absence of macrophages. Stimulation of the pulmonary macrophages with serum from an animal that had been pretreated with H. influenzae, resulted in a highly significant reduction of isoprenaline-induced relaxation (69 ± 5% as compared to non-stimulated pulmonary macrophages). Addition of control serum also led to a decrease of tracheal relaxation, but this effect was not significant. The contractile responses to carbachol did not differ between these experimental groups.

Our data indicate that in guinea-pigs intraperitoneal administration of H. influenzae results in the accumulation of a factor in the serum, which can alter pulmonary macrophage activity. Thus activated, these macrophages may be responsible for the negative effects of H. influenzae on pulmonary beta-adrenergic receptor function and the induction of bronchial hyperreactivity in vivo[9,10,11,12]. The as yet unidentified serum activity may very well represent an important factor in the induction of immune activity in the lungs, and maybe elsewhere.

In an attempt to reveal the mechanism whereby pulmonary macrophages influence tracheal beta-adrenergic receptor function, we studied the role of reactive oxygen species therein. The microbicidal and cytotoxic capabilities of macrophages are determined by their ability to release various lysosomal enzymes and reactive oxygen species like superoxide anion, hydrogen peroxide, and hydroxyl radicals, subsequent to phagocytosis[2]. At the scene of bacterial killing, these oxygen metabolites inevitably leak into the surrounding tissue and may inflict considerable damage.

To assess whether this phenomenon is also responsible for the changes in tracheal beta-adrenergic function, we studied the influence of several enzymes and inhibitors, which interfere with the formation and activity of oxygen metabolites, on the effects of pulmonary macrophages on tracheal spiral relaxation. Carbachol-induced precontraction of the tracheal spirals was not significantly different between the various experimental groups. Addition of thiourea (25 mM) 30 min prior to stimulation of the pulmonary macrophages with serum from a H. influenzae-treated animal, resulted in complete inhibition of macrophage-induced reduction of tracheal relaxation (111 $\pm$ 21% as compared to non-stimulated pulmonary macrophages). Since thiourea is a potent scavenger of the highly reactive hydroxyl radical this points to this oxygen species being responsible for the deterioration of tracheal beta-adrenoceptor function. Catalase (5000 U/ml), an enzyme which catalyses the reduction of hydrogen peroxide to water, was equally effective (102 $\pm$ 9%). The latter may be explained by a diminished availability of hydrogen peroxide for the formation of hydroxyl radicals. Superoxide anion does not seem to be directly involved in the effects of pulmonary macrophages on tracheal relaxation, since superoxide dismutase (300 U/ml), catalysing the conversion of superoxide to hydrogen peroxide, did not affect the decrease in tracheal relaxation (71 $\pm$ 4%).

From the present results we conclude that pulmonary macrophages may be responsible for the negative effects of H. influenzae on tracheal beta-adrenergic receptor function through the release of oxygen radical species, in particular the highly reactive hydroxyl radicals. It has been shown that oxygen radicals can directly damage endothelial cells[8,13]. It is conceivable that low concentrations of radical species could specifically affect the beta-adrenergic receptor moiety. In situations where the integrity of the pulmonary lining material has been affected, such as in chronic obstructive lung diseases (COLD), the negative effects on beta-adreno-ceptors could be even more significant, because of the diminished protective capacity which the lining material normally displays towards radical species[4]. A disturbance of the pulmonary beta-adrenergic system may result in a relative preponderance of the bronchoconstrictive mechanisms and, as a result, may contribute to the reduction of the airflow as is observed in chronic obstructive lung diseases. Therefore, the above-mentioned mechanisms may also apply for patients with chronic asthmatic bronchitis, in other words, they might contribute to exacerbations of bronchial asthma, and to bronchial hyperreactivity in general.

Acknowledgements
This work was subsidized by the Dutch Asthma Foundation.

References
1. Amdur, M.O. and Mead, J. (1958). Mechanics of respiration in unanaesthetized guinea pigs. Am. J.
   Physiol. 192:364-368.
2. Beaman, L. and Beaman, B.L. (1984). The role of oxygen and its derivatives in microbial pathogenesis and

host defense. Ann. Rev. Microbiol. 38:27-48.

3. Boushey, H.A., Holzman, M.J., Sheller, J.R. and Nadel, J.A. (1980). Bronchial hyperreactivity. Am. Rev. Resp. Dis. 121:389-413.

4. Cross, C.E., Halliwell, B. and Allen, A. (1984). Antioxidant protection : a function of tracheo-bronchial and gastrointestinal mucus. Lancet i: 1328-1330.

5. Douglas, J.S., Dennis, M.W., Ridgway, P. and Bouw-huys, A. (1973). Airway constriction in guinea pigs : interaction of histamine and autonomic drugs. J. Pharmacol. Exp. Ther. 184:169-179.

6. Nijkamp, F.P. and Schreurs, A.J.M. (1984). Infection and ß-adrenoceptor function. In: Morley, J. (ed.). Perspectives in Asthma. 1: Beta-adrenoceptors in Asthma, pp.129-139. London: Academic Press.

7. Nijkamp, F.P. (1985). Hyperreactivity, inflammation and the ß-adrenoceptor. In: Bonta, I.L., Bray, M.A. and Parnham, M.J. (eds). Handbook of Inflammation, pp. 335-354. Amsterdam : Elsevier Science Publishers BV.

8. Sacks, T., Moldow, C.F., Craddock, P.R. and Bowers, T.K. (1978). Oxygen radicals mediate endothelial cell damage by complement-stimulated granulocytes. J. Clin. Invest. 61:1161-1167.

9. Schreurs, A.J.M., Terpstra, G.K., Raaijmakers, J.A.M. and Nijkamp, F.P. (1980). Effects of vaccination with Haemophilus influenzae on adrenoceptor function of tracheal and parenchymal strips. J. Pharmacol. Exp. Ther. 215:691-696.

10. Schreurs, A.J.M. and Nijkamp, F.P. (1982). Haemophilus influenzae-induced loss of lung beta-adrenoceptor binding sites and modulation by changes in peripheral catecholaminergic input. Eur. J. Pharmacol. 77:95-102.

11. Schreurs, A.J.M., Verhoef, J. and Nijkamp, F.P. (1983). Bacterial cell-wall components decrease the number of guinea pig lung beta-adrenoceptors. Eur. J. Pharmacol. 87:127-132.

12. Schreurs, A.J.M. and Nijkamp, F.P. (1984). Haemophilus influenzae and the beta-adrenergic system : a review. Vet. Res. Commun. 8:1-14.

13. Shasby, D.M., Vanbenthuysen, K.M., Tate, R.M., Shasby, S.S., McMurtry, I. and Repine, J.E. (1982). Granulocytes mediate acute edematous lung injury in rabbits and in isolated rabbit lungs perfused with phorbol myristate acetate : role of oxygen radicals. Am. Rev. Resp. Dis. 125:443-447.

14. Szentivanyi, A. (1968). The beta-adrenergic theory of the atopic abnormality in bronchial asthma. J. Allergy 42:203-232.

23
Impairment of pulmonary homeostatic and antimicrobial defence mechanisms by infectious bovine rhinotracheitis and parainfluenza-3 virus infections

P. O. OGUNBIYI, P. D. CONLON AND P. EYRE

ABSTRACT

In calves, infectious bovine rhinotracheitis and para-influenza-3 viruses caused significant inhibition of the macrophage chemiluminescence reaction. Similar effects were observed due to parainfluenza-3 virus in guinea-pigs. Beta-adrenergic receptors in both macro- phages and airway smooth muscle were disrupted by virus infection. The viruses caused marked hyperreactivity in airway smooth mus-cle and in mast cell histamine release. Hyperreactivity may be a factor in bovine virus infection and may predis-pose to opportunistic secondary bacterial colonization. Levamisole and verapamil prevent some of the virus-induced responses. These drugs may be useful in the management of secondary bacteria pneumonia.

INTRODUCTION

Respiratory tract infections, particularly influenza virus, rhinovirus and Haemophilus influenzae in man, are known to induce or exacerbate obstructive pulmonary disease and to increase airway reactivity to bronchocon-strictors (such as histamine, acetylcholine). Szentivanyi and others have proposed that impaired beta-adrenoceptor activity might predispose to bronchoconstriction in asthma[5,6,8]. Busse[1] reported a decreased granulocyte

245

response to isoprenaline in asthma during respiratory virus infection.

The bovine "shipping fever" complex (bovine pasteurellosis) is an economically important disease of poorly understood multiple aetiologies. Infectious bovine rhinotracheitis (IBR) virus and parainfluenza-3 virus (PI-3) have been implicated as predisposing to pulmonary pasteurellosis[10]. Viral impairment of pulmonary homeostasis may contribute to secondary bacterial infection.

MATERIALS AND METHODS

Experiments were conducted in calves and guinea-pigs. Jersey (male) calves were purchased locally at birth. They ranged from 2 to 5 months of age at the time of experiment. All animals were examined clinically every day. Immediately prior to virus infection, nasopharyngeal swabs/cultures were carried out for common viral and bacterial pathogens. Also, standard immunological tests for virus antibodies were conducted. Calves were divided randomly into treatment groups. One group acted as controls to provide uninfected tissue samples. A second group of calves was infected with IBR virus and a third group was infected with PI-3 virus. The second group received a field isolate of IBR virus at a dose of 2.5×10^5 TCID$_{50}$ in saline, aerosolized for 10 min. The third group was aerosolized for 15 min with a field strain of PI-3 virus at the rate of 5×10^6 TCID$_{50}$ in saline. All groups underwent bronchoalveolar lavage (BAL) after 4 days and were euthanized on day 6 post-infection. Lavage fluid was centrifuged and the cell suspension differentially counted. Viability of more than 95% was determined by trypan blue exclusion. Alveolar macrophages (AM) were challenged with opsonized zymosan and release of superoxide radicals and H_2O_2 was measured as chemiluminescence following reaction with luminol. The effects of virus infection on luminescence were estimated as well as the effects of added drugs. Following euthanasia a bronchus (3 mm diameter) was taken from each calf, cut spirally and

mounted in O_2-Krebs-Henseleit solution at 37 °C at a
resting tension of 2 g. Cumulative dose-response curves
to bronchoconstrictor and bronchodilator drugs[3] were
established in both control and virus-infected animals.
In one group of calves, lung mast cell histamine was released using the calcium ionophore : A23187. Histamine
concentration was measured spectrophotofluorimetrically
before and after PI-3 virus infection.

In a further experiment, adult guinea-pigs were aerosolized with PI-3 virus (1×10^5 $TCID_{50}$/15 min). Alveolar
macrophages were harvested at day 4 and animals were
euthanized at day 6 for mast cell histamine release and
airway smooth muscle studies.

Two groups of guinea-pigs were treated daily, for 3
days, with verapamil, 5 mg/kg, intramuscularly, or levamisole, 2.2 mg/kg, subcutaneously, during PI-3 virus infection. Bronchoalveolar lavage (BAL) was performed 4 days
post-viral exposure (PVE) and the animals were sacrificed
on day 6 PVE. Alveolar macrophage activity, pulmonary
smooth muscle responses and mast cell mediator release
were then examined.

RESULTS
In control calves, isoprenaline and dobutamine significantly inhibited alveolar macrophage chemiluminescence,
dose-dependently, and their effects were blocked by
propranolol (a non-selective beta-antagonist) and atenolol
($beta_1$-antagonist), respectively. Salbutamol and terbutaline ($beta_2$-selective agonists) were of low potency and
inconsistent in effect. PGE_2 also modulated alveolar
macrophage function. Both IBR and PI-3 virus infections
significantly inhibited the alveolar macrophage chemiluminescence in calves, and the same observation was made
following PI-3 virus infection in guinea-pigs. $Beta_1$-
adrenoceptor agonist effect was negated by PI-3 and IBR
viruses in calves and PI-3 virus in guinea-pigs. The
virus effect on $beta_2$-adrenoceptor activity was inconsistent (Figure 23.1). The modulating action of PGE_2 was

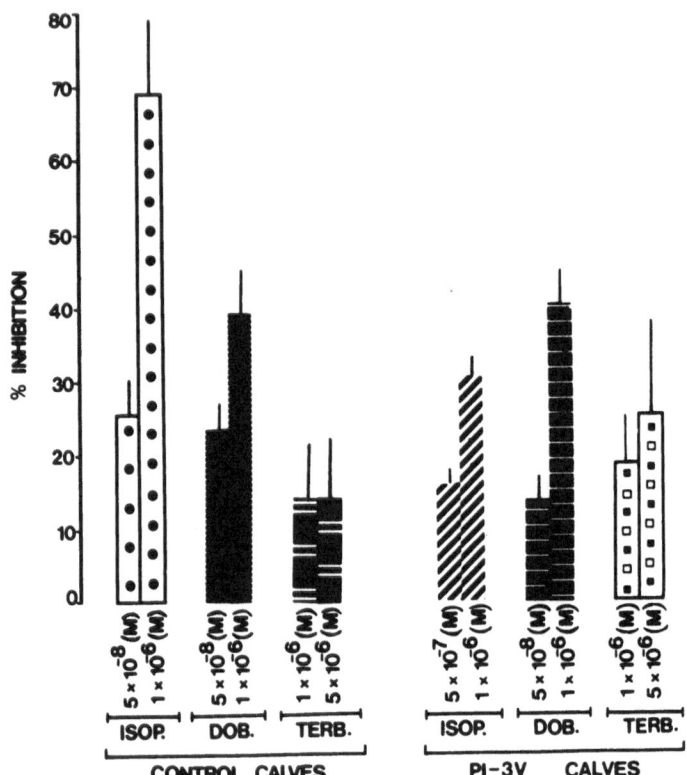

Figure 23.1   Inhibition of the chemiluminescence of alveolar macrophages by different concentrations   of   isoprenaline   (ISOP),   dobutamine   (DOB)   and   terbutaline   (TERB)   in
control and parainfluenza-3 virus-infected calves; n =   5.
Vertical bars are SEM.

not   affected   by PI-3 virus.   IBR virus was not tested in
this case.

Pulmonary virus infection induced   significant   impairment   of   bronchodilator   responses   and   tracheal   relaxation
to beta$_2$-sympathomimetics,   histamine   H$_2$-agonists,   adenosine   diphosphate   (ADP)   and adenosine triphosphate (ATP)
(purinergic agonists)   in calves and guinea-pigs, respectively (Figure 23.2).   At the same time, the potency and efficacy of carbachol and histamine H$_1$-agonists, as broncho-
constrictors, was enhanced.

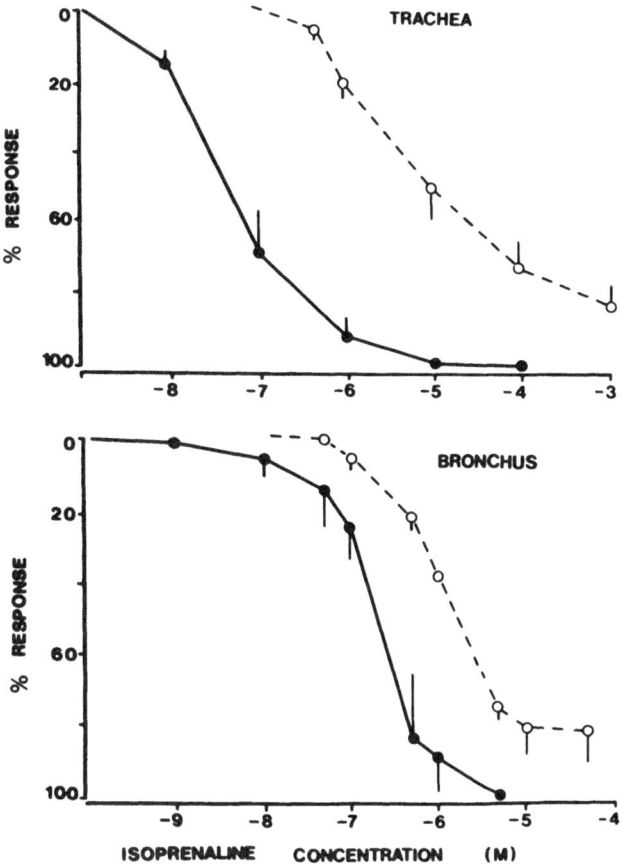

Figure 23.2   Log concentration-response curves for isoprenaline in the trachea (upper panel) and bronchus (lower
panel) of control (●——●) and infectious bovine rinotra-
cheitis (IBR) virus-infected (o--o) calves; n = 5. Drug
doses are final molar bath concentrations. Values are
means ± SEM.

Infection with PI-3 virus in calves and guinea-pigs resulted in a 10-fold increase in calcium ionophore A23187-
induced histamine release by the pulmonary mast cells. IBR
virus was not examined in this case. The spontaneous
histamine release from the mast cell was also significantly increased in the infected animals.
Both verapamil and levamisole significantly reversed or

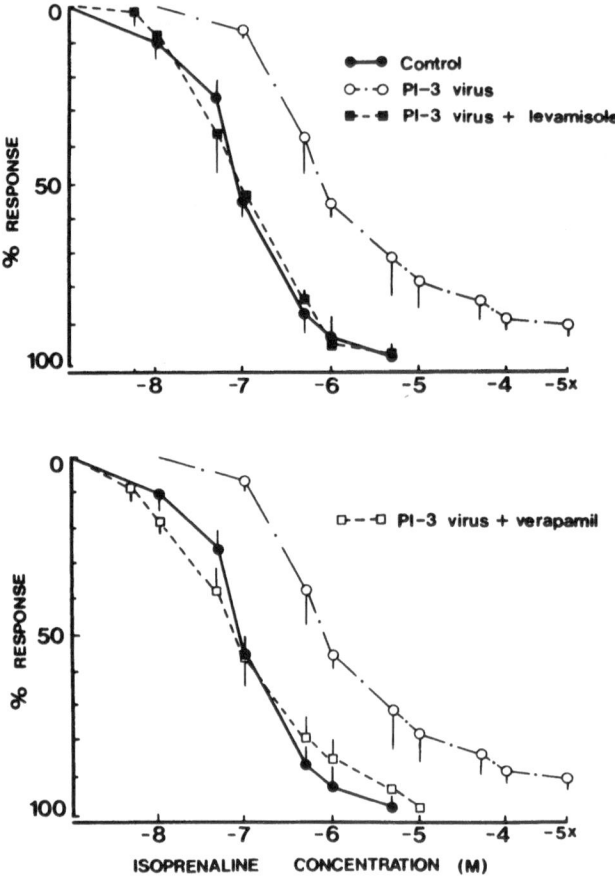

Figure 23.3 Log concentration-response curves for isoprenaline in the trachea of control and parainfluenza-3
(PI-3) virus-infected guinea-pigs and of (PI-3) virus-
infected guinea-pigs pretreated with levamisole (upper
panel) and verapamil (lower panel); n = 9. Drug doses are
final molar bath concentrations. Values are means ± SEM.

prevented smooth muscle hyperreactivity induced by the
virus (Figure 23.3).   These drugs also reversed the
virus-induced   suppression of the alveolar macrophage
activity and the beta-adrenoceptor effects on alveolar
macrophages were partly restored.   Levamisole was more
effective than verapamil at the dosages studied, and
neither drug had any effect in uninfected animals. In the

mast cell, levamisole did not influence Ca^{2+} A23187-indu-
ced mediator release, whereas verapamil attenuated the
enhanced histamine release.

DISCUSSION

The present results indicate a virus-induced airway smooth
muscle hyperreactivity, which is presumably due, partly,
to blunting of the pharmacological inhibitory mechanisms.
Also occurring are lung mast cell hyperreactivity and
alveolar macrophage hyporeactivity. The mechanisms by
which a variety of stimuli induce smooth muscle
hyperreactivity are poorly understood although a number of
factors have been suggested[7]. There are indications that
alveolar macrophages may contribute to the observed impairment in pulmonary beta-adrenoceptor-mediated effects[2].

These studies demonstrated the presence of beta-adrenergic receptors on the alveolar macrophages. Catecholamines are known to modulate the functions of immunocompetent cells and this may also be applicable to alveolar
macrophages. The expression of immunological receptors on
macrophages are altered during inflammatory responses in
the lung[9]. It is, therefore, highly probable that
alveolar macrophage pharmacological receptors are similarly altered. Since alveolar macrophages are the first
line of defence against pulmonary insults, such alterations may be important in the pathogenesis and pathophysiology of pulmonary diseases.

We propose that the down-regulation of the pulmonary
inhibitory homeostatic system and the enhanced excitatory
mechanisms (for example, the "leaky" mast cell phenomenon)
with the resulting homeostatic disturbances, will lead to
increased tissue damage. All of these changes, together
with virus-induced tissue damage, increased mucus
production and alveolar exudate will create a favourable
microenvironment for opportunistic bacterial infection.

Levamisole and verapamil reversed the virus-induced
responses in macrophages and smooth muscle. The mechanisms involved in these actions are not known. However,

the Ca²⁺ antagonizing action of verapamil and the effect
of levamisole on intracellular cyclic nucleotides⁴ may be
involved. These drugs are worthy of clinical evaluation
in pulmonary disease, although we recognize the limitation
imposed by the cardiovascular actions of calcium antagonists.

References
1. Busse, W.W. (1977). Decreased granulocyte response to
   isoproterenol in asthma during upper respiratory
   infections. Am. Rev. Resp. Dis. 115:783-790.
2. Engels, F., Oosting, R.S. and Nijkamp, F.P. (1985).
   Pulmonary macrophages induce deterioration of guinea-
   pig tracheal beta-adrenergic function through release
   of oxygen radicals. Eur. J. Pharmacol. 111:143-144.
3. Eyre, P. (1971). Pharmacology of bovine pulmonary
   vein anaphylaxis in vitro. Br. J. Pharmacol. 43:
   302-311.
4. Mikulikova, D. and Trnavsky, K. (1980). Effect of
   levamisole on lysosomal enzyme release from polymorphonuclear leukocytes and intracellular levels of cAMP
   and cGMP after phagocytosis of monosodium urate
   crystals. Agents Actions 10:374-377.
5. Nijkamp, F.P. and Schreurs, A.J.M. (1984). Infection
   and ß-adrenoceptor function. In : Morley, J. (ed.).
   Beta Adrenoceptor in Asthma, pp.129-146. London: Academic Press.
6. Norris, A.A. and Eyre, P. (1982). Pharmacological
   abnormality in bronchial asthma and the role of
   respiratory pathogens. Med. Hypotheses 8:199-205.
7. Stempel, D. and Boucher, R.C. (1981). Respiratory
   infection and airway reactivity. Med. Clin. N. Am.
   65:1045-1053.
8. Szentivanyi, A. (1968). The beta-adrenergic theory of
   the atopic abnormality in bronchial asthma. J.
   Allergy 42:203-232.
9. Warr, G.A., Jakab, G.J. and Hearst, J.E. (1979). Alterations in lung macrophage immune receptor(s) activity associated with viral pneumonia. J. Reticulo-
   endothel. Soc. 26:357-366.
10. Yates, W.D.G. (1982). A review of infectious bovine
    rhinotracheitis, shipping fever pneumonia and viral-
    bacterial synergism in respiratory disease of cattle.
    Can. J. Comp. Med. 46:225-263.

24
The potential of biological response modifiers in the treatment of malignancies in animals and man

E. J. RUITENBERG, W. H. DE JONG, P. A. STEERENBERG, W. R. KLEIN AND
V. P. M. G. RUTTEN

ABSTRACT

Bacillus Calmette-Guérin (BCG) was able to induce regression of established tumours in an experimental guinea-pig tumour system, and in two spontaneously occurring tumours of farm animals. In the guinea-pig tumour system a tumour line-specific immunity remained, indicating that antigen presentation occurred during BCG-induced tumour regression. In bovine ocular squamous cell carcinoma (BOSCC) and sarcoid tumours of the skin in the horse a substantial number of animals showed tumour regression (approximately 70%). Local BCG immunotherapy seems promising especially for equine sarcoid tumours of the skin. These findings are discussed in relation to the results obtained with BCG immunotherapy in clinical trials in man.

INTRODUCTION

Immunotherapy for cancer has been intensively studied[2,9]. The results in clinical trials have generally been disappointing, and it is now clear that immunotherapy is not a panacea for cancer treatment. However, the interest in cancer immunotherapy has intensified studies of the immune reactions of the host against its tumour. More knowledge on tumour immunology is therefore now available than in the early days of cancer immunotherapy. It has now become apparent that there are many agents and products that can interact with the immune system. These agents have recently been designated biological response modifiers (BRMs)[11]. Interpreted most widely these BRMs modify or change the relationship between tumour and host with resultant therapeutic effects, and BRMs include the classical immunostimulants like Bacillus Calmette-Guérin (BCG) and Corynebacterium parvum. BCG is the most widely studied immunostimulating agent and some tumours in man, such as squamous cell carcinomas of the head and neck region[3] and bladder carcinomas[14], respond favourably to local BCG immunotherapy. Based on results in an experimental guinea-pig tumour system (the line ten hepatocellular carcinoma), experiments were performed in spontaneously occurring tumours of farm animals (bovine ocular squamous cell carcinoma [BOSCC] and equine sarcoid tumours of the skin).

MATERIALS AND METHODS

Line ten tumour system

The line ten hepatocellular carcinoma was originally induced by orally feeding diethylnitrosamine to strain 2 guinea-pigs. The tumour has been converted to ascites form and is maintained by intraperitoneal passages. One x 10^6 viable line ten tumour cells were inoculated on the flank. BCG (one x 10^7 culturable particles) was administered intralesionally. Tumour growth was measured twice weekly with vernier callipers. This line ten tumour is non-immunogenic; after conventional immunization procedures with irradiated tumour cells or amputation of a growing tumour, no tumour immunity is induced[17]. After BCG administration (either admixed with tumour cells or intratumorally) the surviving animals are immune against the line ten tumour. For immunological studies, spleen cells of line ten immune animals were obtained and used in both in vitro and in vivo experiments.

Spontaneously occurring tumours

In addition to the guinea-pig tumour system local (intralesional) immunotherapy with BCG was performed on two spontaneously occurring tumours of farm animals – bovine ocular squamous cell carcinoma and fibroepithelial sarcoid tumours of the skin of horses. For both tumours a randomized clinical trial was performed using extensive surgery as treatment for the control group.

RESULTS

Line ten tumour system

Intralesional treatment of an established intradermally growing line ten tumour resulted, within 4-5 weeks, in complete tumour regression (Figure 24.1). The BCG-induced inflammation resulted in a granulomatous reaction in which cells of the macrophage lineage were predominantly present. The animals became immune against the line ten tumour, as a second tumour cell challenge of these BCG-cured animals was rejected (Figure 24.1). The line ten tumour is by itself non-immunogenic[17], the resulting tumour immunity remaining after addition of BCG to a line ten tumour challenge or after intralesional BCG treatment. It is therefore concluded that, during the BCG-induced tumour rejection, antigen presentation must have occurred resulting ultimately in specific immune T cells.

Some aspects of this immunity were further investigated using spleen cells from line ten immune guinea-pigs (data not shown). Line ten immune guinea-pigs were obtained after a primary immunization with a mixture of BCG and line ten tumour cells. The results of these investigations[4,5,15] can be summarized as follows : the tumour immunity, induced after BCG treatment (either intratumorally or BCG admixed with line ten tumour cells), could be transferred to naive non-immune strain 2 guinea-pigs using spleen cells of line ten immune animals. These line ten immune spleen cells showed a specific tumour rejection capacity; the line ten tumour was rejected and an antigenically distinct line one tumour was

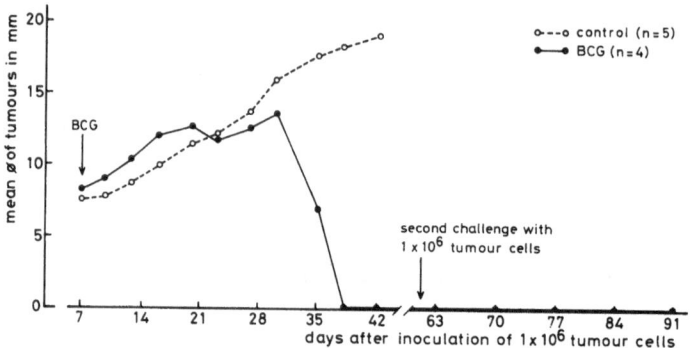

Figure 24.1 Effect of BCG-RIVM (1 x 10⁷ culturable particles intralesionally) at day 7 after tumour cell inoculation) on growth of the line ten hepatocellular carcinoma
in strain 2 guinea-pigs.

not. The transferred immunity was long-lasting; at 160
days after adoptive transfer tumour cells were still
rejected. For this rejection in vivo proliferation seemed
necessary.   In vitro the line ten immune spleen cells
showed a non-specific cytotoxic activity, whereas in a
lymphocyte stimulation assay line ten tumour antigen was
specifically recognized. In addition, these immune spleen
cells showed in vivo a specific migration to the line ten
challenge site.
    In this non-immunogenic tumour system it is concluded
that BCG treatment resulted in the induction of a
tumour-specific, long-lasting solid immunity against the
line ten tumour. This immunity is carried by cells with a
helper and/or amplifier function.

Spontaneously occurring tumours
In bovine ocular squamous cell carcinoma (BOSCC),
intralesional BCG treatment (either as live BCG or a
non-living BCG cell wall preparation) resulted in almost
complete tumour regression in 60-70% of the treated
animals. In approximately 50% of these BCG-cured animals
tumour recurrence occurred (Table 24.1).   No serious
side-effects of the BCG treatment were observed.   In

Table 24.1 Intralesional BCG treatment of bovine ocular squamous cell carcinoma (BOSCC)[a] : I = Regression of pri-mary tumour; II = Local recurrence; III = Intercurrently killed; IV = Metastases at necropsy[b]

Treatment	n[a]	I	II	III	IV
No treatment	10	2/10[c]	0/2	7/10	5/10
Surgery[d]	10	-	0/10	1/10	1/10
BCG lot 048	10	5/10	0/5	4/10	3/10
BCG lot 060	10	7/10	4/7	1/10	2/10
BCG cell walls	10	7/10	4/7	5/10	3/10

[a] BOSCC tumour size ranging from 1 x 1 to 4 x 4 cm.

[b] Regional lymph node (lymphonodulus subparotidealis) and/ or lung.

[c] Number of animals with regression versus number of ani-mals treated.

[d] Surgery : total block resection including primary tumour, eye, lymphonodulus subparotidealis, lymphonodulus retro-pharyngealis, parotid salivary gland and part of the mandibular salivary gland.

sarcoid skin tumours of the horse, 70-90% of the BCG-treated tumours showed complete and long-lasting regression (Table 24.2). Some animals now have a follow-up period of more than 2-3 years. No recurrences were observed.

In BOSCC no evidence for the induction of tumour immunity was found, the appearance of recurrences generally at the same localization of the regressed primary tumour suggesting that the cured animals were not immune. The BOSCC-bearing cows could be divided into three groups : animals not responding to therapy (±33%); animals showing long-lasting regression (±33%); and ani-mals showing regression followed by recurrences (±33%). Whether this also reflects a difference in immune reactivity remains to be established. In comparison with

Table 24.2 Intralesional BCG treatment of fibroepithelial (sarcoid) tumours of the skin in horses : I = Complete regression; II = Partial regression; III = No regression

Treatment	n[a]	Mean area (cm^2)	I[b]	II	III
Cryosurgery[c]	26(10)	8.0	26(100%)	–	–
BCG[d]	29(10)	10.8	24(83%)	–	5(17%)
BCG cell walls[e]	16(10)	11.0	11(69%)	4(25%)	1(6%)

[a] Number of tumours with number of animals in brackets.
[b] Number of tumours with percentage in brackets.
[c] Intensive cryosurgery existing of several freeze-thaw cycles (mean number of treatments 3.0).
[d] Mean number of BCG treatments 3.6.
[e] Mean number of BCG cell wall treatments 3.4.

the guinea-pig studies, the group with long-lasting regression is particularly interesting. For sarcoid tumours of the skin of the horse, BCG immunotherapy seems to be indicated; in a prognostically unfavourable group of animals (treated outside the randomized clinical study) complete cure was obtained in eight of eleven animals (data not shown). These animals were not included in the clinical trial because the localization of the tumours (preventing surgery) made them unsuitable for randomization.

DISCUSSION
Bacillus Calmette-Guérin is one of the oldest and best-known biological response modifiers (BRMs). From the late 1960s onwards attempts were made to use BCG for cancer therapy and to date several hundred clinical trials have been performed in man, most of them with disappointing results. What then is the reason that BCG is still used for cancer immunotherapy ? It is well known

that BCG has a profound effect on the immune system and both activation and suppression may occur. Whether the final result of BCG administration is activation (the desired effect) or not, depends on many factors, including the dose of BCG, the route of administration, the immuno-assay in which BCG is studied, the genetic background of the host animal and the BCG vaccine itself (strain of BCG, amount of dead material present, and additives in the vaccine). Only recently has more detailed knowledge become available on the relation between the immune system and cancer, and there remains much still to be learned. Part of the therapeutic failure of BCG in many trials may be attributable to the fact that the agent was used without an understanding of the relationships between the immune system and cancer and its influence on this relation.

In experimental animal tumours such as the line ten hepatocellular carcinoma, and in spontaneously occurring tumours such as BOSCC and equine sarcoid tumours of the skin, the authors and others[8,10] have clearly demonstrated that BCG has the ability to inhibit tumour growth and to induce tumour regression. In the line ten tumour system the tumour size seems a limiting factor for BCG immunotherapy; only tumours of 10 mm diameter or less (which is relatively large in a species as small as the guinea-pig) can be cured, whereas larger tumours (more than 12 mm) cannot[18]. In the study with BOSCC no indications were found that the tumour size was related to the clinical outcome[8]. However, the tumour size in this study was limited, as it ranged from 10 x 10 to maximally 40 x 40 mm. For sarcoid tumours of the skin the total tumour mass was correlated with the clinical result, larger tumours showing less regression (unpublished data from this laboratory). Although BCG has been administered by most routes, there seems to be a general consensus that the best responses are obtained with local application, although the intralesional administration of BCG may have the disadvantage of associated toxicity[13,16]. Those clinical trials in man with BCG which resulted in a beneficial effect are mainly those in which the agent was administered locally[3,6,14]. The benefits of local application of BCG in recurrent bladder carcinoma, in particular, are now well established[14].

In experimental animal tumour systems in syngeneic inbred animals BCG immunotherapy induced immunity against the tumour in several tumour systems (present data and[1,12,18]). In the line ten tumour system this is a remarkable change as the tumour by itself is non-immunogenic[17]. Why BCG causes this change from non-immunogenic into an immunogenic tumour is still unknown. However, that immunotherapy may result in tumour immunity is an important phenomenon as it implies that residual minimal (metastatic) disease and/or recurrences may be cured. In contrast, the data obtained in our study with BOSCC (see Table 24.1) do not indicate that the tumour regression was followed by tumor immunity[8].

In the various animal tumour systems, as in man, differing results were obtained with BCG immunotherapy. Hence, the result of cancer immunotherapy seems to be at least partially dependent on the tumour system itself. At present BCG immunotherapy seems only indicated for transitional bladder carcinoma[14]. For other tumours like carcinoma of the head and neck region, some leukaemia and lymphoma subgroups and gastric cancer, promising preliminary results have been obtained, although there is still doubt whether BCG immunotherapy is indeed effective for these cancers. The use of BCG as adjuvant in autologous tumour cell vaccines may introduce a new area for the clinical use of BCG, since colon cancer patients were recently found to show an immune reaction against their own tumour after vaccination with a mixture of BCG and autologous tumour cells[7].

Acknowledgements
The financial support of the Koningin Wilhelmina Fonds (Netherlands Cancer Foundation) for W.H. de Jong is grate-

fully acknowledged.

References
1. Baldwin, R.W. and Pimm, M.V. (1973). BCG immunotherapy of a rat sarcoma. Br. J. Cancer 28:281-287.
2. Baldwin, R.W. and Pimm, M.V. (1978). BCG in tumor
   immunotherapy. Adv. Cancer Res. 28:91-147.
3. Bier, J., Rapp, H.J., Borsos, T., Zbar, B., Klein-
   schuster, S., Wagner, H. and Rollinghof, M. (1981).
   Randomized clinical study on intratumoral BCG cell
   wall preparation (CWP) therapy in patients with
   squamous cell carcinoma in the head and neck region.
   Cancer Immunol. Immunother. 12:71-79.
4. De Jong, W.H., Van de Plas, M.M.T., Steerenberg, P.A.,
   Kruizinga, W. and Ruitenberg, E.J. (1985). Selective
   localization of tumor immune spleen cells at the tumor
   challenge site after adoptive transfer of line 10
   tumor immunity in strain 2 guinea pigs. J. Immunol.
   134:2032-2040.
5. De Jong, W.H., Steerenberg, P.A., Van de Plas, M.M.T.,
   Kruizinga, W. and Ruitenberg, E.J. (1985). T-cell
   involvement in adoptive transfer of line 10 tumor
   immunity in strain 2 guinea pigs. J. Natl. Cancer
   Inst. 75:483-489.
6. Goodnight, J.E. and Morton, D.L. (1978). Immunotherapy for malignant disease. Ann. Rev. Med.
   29:231-283.
7. Hoover, H.C., Surdijke, M., Dangel, R.B., Peters, L.C.
   and Hanna, M.G. (1984). Delayed cutaneous hypersensitivity to autologous tumor cells in colorectal
   cancer patients immunized with an autologous tumor
   cell : bacillus Calmette-Guérin vaccine. Cancer Res.
   44:1671-1676.
8. Klein, W.R., Ruitenberg, E.J., Steerenberg, P.A., De
   Jong, W.H., Kruizinga, W., Misdorp, W., Bier, J.,
   Tiesjema, R.H., Kreeftenberg, J.G., Teppema, J.S. and
   Rapp, H.J. (1982). Immunotherapy by intralesional
   injection of BCG cell walls or live BCG in bovine
   ocular squamous cell carcinoma : a preliminary study.
   J. Natl. Cancer Inst. 69:1095-1103.
9. Mitchell, M.S. and Murahata, R.I. (1979). Modulation
   of immunity by bacillus Calmette-Guérin (BCG).
   Pharmacol. Ther. 4:329-353.
10. Murphy, J.M., Severin, G.A., Lavach, J.D., Hepler,
    D.I., Lueker, D.C. (1979). Immunotherapy in ocular
    equine sarcoid. J. Am. Vet. Med. Assoc. 174:269-272.
11. Oldham, R.K. (1983). Biological response modifiers.
    J. Natl. Cancer Inst. 70:789-796.
12. Salomon, J.C. and Lynch, N. (1976). Intralesional
    injection of immunostimulants in rat and mouse tumors.
    Cancer Immunol. Immunother. 1:145-151.
13. Schwarzenberg, L., Simmler, M.C. and Pico, J.L.
    (1976). Human toxicology of BCG applied in cancer
    immunotherapy. Cancer Immunol. Immunother. 1:69-76.
14. Shapiro, A., Kadmon, D., Catalona, W.J. and Ratliff,
    T.L. (1982). Immunotherapy of superficial bladder

cancer. J. Urol. 128:891-894.

15. Shu, S., Steerenberg, P.A., Hunter, J.T., Evans, C.H. and Rapp, H.J. (1981). Adoptive immunity to the guinea pig line 10 hepatoma and the nature of in vitro lymphoid tumor cell interactions. Cancer Res. 41:3499-3506.

16. Sparks, F.C. (1976). Hazards and complications of BCG immunotherapy. Med. Clin. N. Am. 60:499-509.

17. Zbar, B., Bernstein, I.D. and Rapp, H.J. (1971). Suppression of tumor growth at the site of infection with living bacillus Calmette-Guérin. J. Natl. Cancer Inst. 46:831-839.

18. Zbar, B., Bernstein, I.D., Bartlett, G.L., Hanna, M.G. and Rapp, H.J. (1972). Immunotherapy of cancer : regression of intradermal tumors and prevention of growth of lymph node metastases after intralesional injection of living Mycobacterium bovis. J. Natl. Cancer Inst. 49:119-130.

25
Immunological defence mechanisms as a target for antibiotics

J. L. GRONDEL AND W. B. VAN MUISWINKEL

ABSTRACT

When the immunological defence mechanisms fail to prevent
the establishment of infections within the host, the
consequence is disease. Particularly under these circumstances, antibiotics have proved to be of remarkable value
for therapeutic treatment of bacterial infections. The
antibiotic generally interferes with the metabolism of the
pathogen, allowing the immune system to eliminate it. In
this way, the antibiotic cooperates with the immune
system. However, the effect of antibiotics on immunological processes is rarely taken into consideration.

In this paper, we selectively review antimicrobial
agents used in veterinary and human medicine with regard
to their effects on non-specific and specific defense
mechanisms.

INTRODUCTION

The barriers, which bacteria have to overcome when
invading a host, are either non-specific or specific. In
both types of resistance, humoral factors and specialized
cells play pivotal roles, forming an elaborate network of
physical, chemical and cellular defence mechanisms,
including the immune system.

The skin with its low pH and bactericidal fatty acids,

and mucous epithelial surfaces containing growth-decreasing factors or phagocytizing cells, are examples of non-specific, external defence. In addition to this barrier, internal non-specific defence is mediated by serum factors (such as transferrin and alternative complement route) and phagocytizing cells (macrophages and granulocytes). Specific defensive responses against invading microorganisms are effected by the immune system.

An immune response is a rather complex interaction between distinct leucocyte populations and humoral factors, and can be characterized by two phenomena : amplification and regulation. Foreign materials (anti-gens) are processed by macrophages and presented to antigen-sensitive lymphocytes in the correct physical configuration. The lymphocytes are required for antibody formation and cellular immune responses. These cells and their products contribute to the rapid elimination of antigen.

When defence mechanisms fail to prevent the establishment of an infective agent in the host, the consequence will be disease. Under these circumstances, antibiotics have proved to be of remarkable value for the therapy of bacterial infections. The antibiotic generally inhibits growth of the pathogen, allowing the immune system to eliminate it. In this way, the antibiotic cooperates with the immune system. However, the effect on the immune status of animal or man is rarely taken into consideration when choosing an antibiotic for therapeutic use.

The importance of antimicrobial agents for the maintenance of animal health is generally accepted in animal husbandry. Besides being used for prevention and control of bacterial diseases, antibiotics are sometimes used because of their growth-promoting effects. However, it is also known that some of these drugs can lead to adverse immunotoxic effects, and that prolonged use will increase the risk for raising drug-resistant bacterial strains.

Several studies have been performed on the interaction between antibiotics and the immune system in mammals, birds and fish. Impairment of the immune system may have serious implications for the outcome of therapy, especially when a relatively long recovery period is required.

Many reports have described either positive, negative or no effect at all on the defence system. However, the picture is based on effects of different antibiotics studied in many animal species. Only a limited number of studies are available concerning the effects of antibiotics upon specific immunological processes such as antigen processing, proliferation and maturation of lymphocytes and the production of immunoregulatory factors.

The effects of a wide range of antimicrobial agents on the mammalian immune response in vivo as well as in vitro have been reviewed by Finch[13] and Hauser and Remington[24]. In this chapter, we selectively review antimicrobial agents used in veterinary and human medicine with regard to their effects on non-specific and specific defence mechanisms.

NON-SPECIFIC DEFENCE MECHANISMS
Chemotaxis and phagocytosis

Chemotaxis and subsequent phagocytosis, important neutrophil and macrophage functions in defence against bacterial infections, are suppressed by several antibiotics in vitro and in vivo. In particular, tetracyclines have been shown to interfere with these leucocyte processes. Both spontaneous and induced migration of human leucocytes in vitro were severely depressed by lymecycline[7], doxycycline[7] and tetracycline[14-16]. On the other hand, the chemotactic response of bovine polymorphonuclear leucocytes (PMN) was not inhibited in the presence of tetracyclines, streptomycin or penicillin at concentrations normally achieved in blood during systematic treatment. In local therapy, as with intramammary injections and topical applications, higher concentrations will be achieved.

Ziv et al.[45] and Dulin et al.[12] examined intramammary injected antibiotic products and corresponding vegetable based vehicles for their effect on phagocytosis by bovine neutrophils. The concentrations used in the phagocytosis assay were similar to those found in milk immediately, and 6 and 12 h after injection. The results indicated that some antibiotics, including penicillins alone or in combinations, chloramphenicol, cephalosporin, tetra-cycline, erythromycin, gentamicin and nitrofurantoin as well as the vehicles in which they are suspended cause a reduction in phagocytic capability of bovine milk PMN.

Phagocytosis and humoral factors
In the initial phase of phagocytosis a phagocyte has to recognize and attach firmly to the foreign particle. These processes are facilitated by a subcomponent of the complement system (C3b) and immunoglobin after binding at the particle surface (opsonization). The phagocytic cells expose receptors for C3b and the Fc portion of certain immunoglobulins at their cell surface.

Athlin et al.[3] showed that doxycycline at therapeutic concentrations (5 µg/ml) did not affect the adherence of yeast cells to human blood monocytes in vitro. However, the median value of engulfed yeast cells by doxycycline-treated monocytes was 30% lower than in control cultures, though statistically not significant.

Augmentation of the effects of cephalosporins on host defences were reported by Lam and co-workers[26]. In their studies, microdiffusion chambers containing either E. coli alone or E. coli plus PMN were implanted intraperitoneally in mice receiving a single dose (3 mg/kg) of cefotaxime, moxalactam or the new product CPW 86-363. It was demonstrated that moxalactam and CPW 86-363 led to a significant reduction in viability of the microorganisms in the chambers containing both leucocytes and bacteria.

Milatovic[28] has shown that pretreatment of Pseudomonas aeruginosa with a third of the minimum inhibitory concentration (MIC) of azlocillin, carbenicillin, cefoperazone or piperacillin changed the opsonic requirements of these bacteria. P. aeruginosa exposed to the beta-lactam antibiotics were opsonized and engulfed by human PMN without participation of the complement system. It was suggested that the filament formation induced by these antibiotics is accompanied by changes of bacterial surface characteristics. Antibiotic-mediated bacterial killing by serum factors has been reported by Lam et al.[26]. The survival of a previously serum resistant E. coli strain was evaluated in media containing fresh human serum and a low concentration (MIC/4) of the cephalosporins moxalactam, cefotaxime or CPW 86-363. Cefotaxime and CPW 86-363 improved the bactericidal activity of serum.

Tetracycline, oxytetracycline, lymecycline and doxy-cycline have been found to suppress the bactericidal effect of serum on E. coli[14]. This effect can be reversed by the addition of Mg^{2+} ions. Lochmann et al.[27] reported a significant deficiency in the values of C3, the key-molecule in the complement system, in rabbits immunized with staphylococcal haemolysin and simultaneously given antibiotics (chloramphenicol or oxytetracycline). Inter-ference with the complement system by sulphonamides and penicillins has been reported by Von Zabern et al.[43].

Human PMN showed enhanced intracellular killing of untreated Pseudomonas aeruginosa after pretreatment (and subsequently washing) of the leucocytes in vitro with nocardin A, a monocyclic beta-lactam antibiotic. These augmenting effects occurred at much lower concentrations than those which exert antibacterial effects without PMN[5].

Studies by Hawkey et al.[23] with three antipseudomonal antibiotics, gentamicin, azlocillin and carbenicillin, did not reveal significant effects on the phagocytic function of human PMN in vitro.

Cannon et al.[9] investigated the in vitro effect of several antibacterial drugs including sulphonamides and trimethoprim on neutrophil function. Human PMN were pretreated with 10 µg/ml of each drug at 37 °C for 60 min.

Sulphamethoxazole, sulphanilamide, trimethoprim, brodimo-
prim and cotrimoxazole significantly increased neutrophil
activity, whereas sulphamerizine, sulphadiazine and
ceftriazone did not change the phagocytic process. Wolff
and Stankova[44] investigated whether sulphamethoxazole and
trimethoprim (1:5) improved alveolar mononuclear phagocyte
oxygen metabolism and intracellular killing of Staphylococcus aureus. Rats were given sulphamethoxazole/trime-
thoprim 10/50 mg/day for 6 weeks. It was shown that
neither the hexose-phosphate shunt activity, nor the
oxygen metabolism or the intracellular killing properties
were affected.

Clindamycin is a well-established drug in the treatment
of serious anaerobic infections. Subinhibitory concentrations of clindamycin interfered with the adhesion of E.
coli to buccal epithelial cells and also promoted
phagocytosis and killing by human PMN[6]. Obviously, the
adherence to phagocytes was not affected. Here too, it
was suggested that alteration of the bacterial cell wall
may inhibit adherence to epithelial cells, necessary for
initiation/establishment of infection, and render the
organism more susceptible to phagocytosis.

SPECIFIC DEFENCE MECHANISMS
Antibody-mediated immune response
When antigen enters the body, it must be processed by
macrophages and presented to T and B lymphocytes capable
of a specific response. Depending on the nature of the
antigen, the B cell receives appropriate stimuli from T
helper cells and macrophages, and it will start to divide.
While the antigen specific B cells expand, some of these
cells will start to differentiate into plasma cells, which
specialize in immunoglobulin synthesis and secretion.

One of the protective effects of antibodies is mediated
by the constant region (Fc) of the antibody molecule.
After combining with antigen, antibody acquires the
ability to activate the complement cascade, to bind to
phagocytes or to provoke degranulation of mast cells and

basophils.   Thong   and   Ferrante[38]   investigated   the   effect
of doxycycline on antibody responses to   sheep   red   blood
cells   (SRBC) in mice.   According to these authors a daily
dose of 100 mg/kg intraperitoneally for   5   days   was   the
usual   therapeutic regime in mice.   Under these experimental conditions, the anti-SRBC response of the   antibiotic-
treated   animals   was   not   significantly   affected.   In a
detailed study in rats by Van   den   Bogert   and   Kroon[39],
oxytetracycline   was   administered   by   continuous,
intravenous infusion (20 mg/kg/day). It   was   shown   that
the   primary   response   to SRBC was severely impaired when
the drug was given for more than 48 h after priming.   The
kinetics of   the IgM response (for example peak day) were
not changed, but the amount   of   antibodies   produced   was
much   lower.   The   anamnestic   response   to   SRBC   was
completely depressed when oxytetracycline was given during
the   first   48   h   of   the   primary   response.   There was
concluded   from   these   experiments   that   oxytetracycline
interferes   with   T   cell   proliferation   and   memory cell
formation.

Gillissen[18] and Gillissen and Pusztai-Markos[19] examined
several cephalosporins and cephamycins in respect of their
effect on humoral immunity. The   response   was   evaluated
with   the   direct plaque-forming cell assay (IgM-producing
spleen cells).   Mice were injected intravenously only once
with   antibiotics   on the same day as being immunized with
SRBC.   The results   showed that three (cefotetan 30 mg/kg,
cefmenoxime 30 mg/kg, and   cefoxitin 20 mg/kg) out   of six
antibiotics reduced the antibody response.   On   the   other
hand,   the   remaining   antibacterial   agents   (cefotaxime,
cefsulodin and cefoperazone) had an enhancing   effect.   A
totally   different   picture   emerged when the effects of 7
day's therapy on the primary humoral reaction to SRBC   was
investigated in mice[33].   Cefotaxime, amikacin, mezlocillin
and piperacillin inhibited the IgM response by 88, 55, 100
and 56%, respectively.   Clindamycin did not interfere with
the response.   The   mezlocillin-induced   suppression   was
long-lasting, being still present 20 days after completion

of the treatment.

It is known that multiple injections of the same drug result in different pharmacokinetics compared to a single dose. This may explain the contradictory results presented by Gillissen and Pusztai-Markos[19] and Roszkowski et al.[33].

Adverse effects of antibiotics on the development of gut-associated lymphoid tissue (GALT) and serum immunoglobulin levels in chickens and turkeys were investigated by Naqi et al.[29] and Cook et al.[11], respectively. The treatment started by dipping eggs in a gentamicin solution (500 mg/l) for 15 min before incubation. The newly hatched birds were each injected with 0.2 mg (chickens) or 1 mg (turkeys) of gentamicin subcutaneously and fed a commercial diet containing chlortetracycline 200 mg/kg for the duration of the study (turkeys : 21 days; chickens : 28 days). In the antibiotic-treated chickens a lowered IgG level was observed at 21 days. By day 28, all serum Ig fractions (IgM, IgG, IgA) were below control values. Also the number of IgM, IgG and IgA-bearing lymphocytes in caecal tonsils and large intestine were reduced as compared to controls. Furthermore, the growth-rate of the bursa of Fabricius was lower than normal.

Feeding antibiotic-containing diets, as well as application of antimicrobial agents with drinking water, may change the enteric microflora. Consequently, the antigenic load and/or composition will be altered.

Oxytetracycline, administered in therapeutic doses for 6 days starting 1 day before immunization, affected the primary and the secondary response to SRBC in chickens (unpublished data). The primary plaque forming spleen cell response was delayed or suppressed in animals which received the antibiotic by intramuscular injection or by oral application (drinking water). Surprisingly, however, the haemagglutination titre was enhanced. The secondary direct plaque-forming cell response was not significantly changed by oxytetracycline, when it was administered orally during the development of the primary response.

However, the peak response of the indirect plaque forming cells was delayed for 1 day. Both the total and 2-mercaptoethanol-resistant haemagglutination titres were enhanced.

Despite the fact that oxytetracycline affected the development of the antibody forming cells in the spleen, the anti-SRBC-titres increased. This indicates that other lymphoid tissues such as bone marrow may also be important sites for antibody synthesis.

It has been shown in fish that oxytetracycline administered as a food additive or by intraperitoneal injection severely reduced the in vivo immune response. It was observed that the plaque-forming cell response against SRBC was depressed by 80-95% after treatment of carp[31,32]. Furthermore, it was demonstrated that oxytetracycline caused a delay in the peak response rather than suppression (unpublished data). Clear immunosuppression was shown in rainbow trout after feeding with pellets containing oxytetracycline[1,40].

Mitogenic stimulation

Mitogens can stimulate cell division. Certain mitogens have the ability to activate T or B cells specifically. The plant lectins phytohaemagglutinin (PHA) and concanavalin A (con A) provoke T cells to proliferate, whereas lipopolysaccharide (LPS), derived from Gram-negative bacteria, can function as B cell mitogen. Lymphocyte mitogenesis can be measured by adding tritiated thymidine to the culture medium. The amount of radioactivity incorporated into newly synthesized DNA is regarded as an estimate of cell proliferation.

The effect of a wide range of antibiotics on human T and B lymphocytes was studied in vitro by Banck and Forsgren[4]. In their study 14 antibiotics (aminobenzylpenicillin, benzylpenicillin, carbenicillin, cefazolin, cephalothin, chloramphenicol, 5-fluorocytosine, gentamicin, kanamycin, lymecycline, nalidixic acid, sulphamethoxazole, tetracycline chloride and trimethoprim) did not inhibit or stimulate the PHA response when 50 µg of each drug/ml was added for 3 days. Inhibitory effects on both T and B cell mitogenic responses were detected for erythromycin, clindamycin and rifampicin at relatively high concentrations. However, doxycycline, nitrofurantoin and fusidic acid significantly depressed both mitogenic responses at low concentrations. These antibiotics had to be present in culture from day 1 or 2 onwards to exhibit a strong suppressive effect. No significant effect was observed after addition of the drugs for the last 24 h combined with tritiated thymidine.

Lymecycline and tetracycline chloride (25 µg/ml) did not influence the thymidine incorporation into PHA-activated cells, whereas minocycline inhibited this process significantly.

Anderson et al.[2] investigated the effect of erythromycin on mitogenic stimulation of human peripheral blood leucocytes. Erythromycin base at concentrations of $1 \times 10^{-6}M - 1 \times 10^{-3}M$ did not affect the PHA-induced proliferation. Only at higher concentrations was a dose-dependent suppression observed. Ingestion of a single dose of 500 mg erythromycin stearate by normal volunteers was not associated with a significant change in mitogenic responsiveness to PHA or con A, measured 90 min and 4 days after drug intake. The authors observed consistently a slight, but statistically insignificant, increase in thymidine incorporation into con A-activated leucocytes.

Sulphonamides and trimethoprim did not modify the mitogenic response of human PBL[9]. However, a highly significant increase in lymphocyte transformation was produced by co-trimoxazole.

In mice, the immunodepressive effect of antibacterial agents was tested in a detailed study by Voiculescu et al.[41]. It was demonstrated that erythromycin, colistin and chloramphenicol strongly inhibited the antigen-dependent B cell blastogenesis in vitro, related to in vivo antibiotic treatment. A T helper-cell deficiency in the colistin- and chloramphenicol-treated animals was suggested by the authors, because the B cell response could be restored by supplementation with autologous T helper-cells.

These careful studies indicate clearly that certain antibiotics selectively interfere with the immune system.

Roszkowski et al.[33] and Borowski et al.[8] showed that the cephalosporin cefotaxime affected the mitogen-induced proliferation of mouse spleen cells in vitro only at high concentrations. Cephradine was inhibitory at therapeutic levels. Furthermore, Borowski demonstrated that mezlocil-lin and piperacillin severely reduced the mitogenic res-ponse to con A and lipopolysaccharide. Amikacin and clin-damycin did not influence the proliferation. When the animals were injected with different concentrations of antibiotics (cefotaxime, amikacin, mezlocillin, pipera-cillin or clindamycin) twice a day for 7 consecutive days, only clindamycin did not affect the lymphocyte stimulation induced by con A or lipopolysaccharide. Cefotaxime and amikacin were effective only in the highest doses tested : 1.2 mg/day and 0.3 mg/day, respectively.

To investigate whether fish leucocytes, obtained from different lymphoid organs, were sensitive to antibiotic treatment in vitro, both phytohaemagglutinin and lipopoly-saccharide mitogenic responses were evaluated in the presence of various concentrations of oxytetracycline in carp[20]. It was demonstrated that this drug significantly inhibited thymidine incorporation. The 50% inhibition level was reached at a concentration of 4-6 µg/ml. Furthermore, oxytetracycline caused a dose-dependent delay in the leucocyte response rather than a true suppressive effect[22]. Obviously, the impairment of cellular functions like DNA synthesis was not due to cytotoxicity as was suggested in previous investigations.

Sulphatroxazole/trimethoprim (5:1), sulphadimethoxine, sulphadimidine, lincomycin/spectinomycin (1:2) and ampi-cillin did not suppress the mitogenic response. On the contrary, at low concentrations an increased thymidine uptake was observed. Gentamicin and furaltadone showed a

dose-dependent inhibition. Chloramphenicol was stimulatory at concentrations below 5 μg/ml, whereas higher quantities became suppressive.

Immunoregulatory factors

Immune responses, both cell-mediated and antibody-mediated, are under strict control, mediated by a number of
different mechanisms. Today, many soluble factors
produced by immunocompetent cells are known to exert a
regulatory effect. In this section we will describe the
effect of several antimicrobial agents on immunoregu-
lation.

In 1974 Serrou[36] published a report on the suppressive
influence of rifampicin on migration inhibition factor
(MIF) secretion by human lymphocytes. Inhibition of
protein and lymphokine synthesis was also observed when
tetracycline was present in human leucocyte cultures[17].

The effects of erythromycin on the release of
prostaglandin E2 (PGE2) by mitogen-stimulated mononuclear
leucocytes were investigated by Anderson et al.[2]. This
drug caused significant inhibition of PGE2 release by
resting and mitogen-activated cells at relatively low
concentrations. According to the literature PGE2 exerts
immunosuppressive activities. Therefore, Anderson et al.[2]
concluded that the observed increase in leucocyte
transformation following erythromycin ingestion, can be
explained by reduced PGE2 production.

The above-mentioned modification of the phytohaemagglutinin response of mouse T cells by erythromycin, colistin
and chloramphenicol, was also observed in experiments with
T helper or T suppressor soluble factors[42]. These data
confirmed the T helper-cell deficiency in antibiotic-
treated animals as well as the T suppressor-cell enhancement in chloramphenicol-treated mice. Furthermore, a significant immunosuppressive activity has been demonstrated
using the migration inhibition assay, following in vivo
treatment with the same antibiotics. On the other hand,
benzylpenicillin, streptomycin, kanamycin and tetracyclin

did not affect the inhibition of macrophage migration.

A T cell-dependent immune response is amplified by the action of both interleukin 1 (IL-1) and interleukin 2 (IL-2). Both factors are proliferation and/or differentiation signals for T and B lymphocytes during the response[30,37]. The amplification process is dependent upon both the level of interleukin synthesis and induction of interleukin receptors. Interleukins have been isolated and characterized in many mammalian species. The existence of interleukin-like factors has also been demonstrated in birds[34,35] and fish[10,21], emphasizing the phylogenetic importance of amplifying/regulatory factors for a standard immune reaction.

In chickens, the early stages of the mitogen-induced T cell proliferation can be inhibited by oxytetracyclin[23]. In this study, supernatants of con A-induced spleen cell cultures were harvested at different time intervals and tested for their growth-promoting activity on T cell blasts, in order to determine the IL-2 production in the presence or absence of oxytetracycline. The antibacterial agent did not seem to have any effect on IL-2 production, whereas the uptake of tritium-labelled thymidine by growth-factor-dependent T cell blasts was severely reduced.

The delayed-type hypersensitivity (DTH) reaction is based upon the interaction between antigen and primed T cells. Several lymphokines are released which account for the typical events during the DTH response. DTH is characterized by the appearance of an induration and erythematous reaction which reaches a maximum at 24-48 h. During this process, macrophages and lymphocytes infiltrate and accumulate at the inflammation site.

Thong and Ferrante[38] have shown that mice treated in vivo with different tetracycline analogues have a reduced capacity to mount DTH responses to SRBC. A significant reduction (30-45%) was observed in experimental groups treated once with doxycycline, rolitetracycline and tetracycline. Oxytetracycline did not evoke a significant effect. The suppressive effect of doxycycline was more pronounced when the drug was administered on the day of challenge than 2 days prior to priming. This suggests an interference with macrophages and/or lymphocytes.

A severely depressed DTH response was observed in rats when oxytetracycline (20 mg/kg/day) was administered continuously, starting just before the moment of priming[39]. Furthermore, it was shown that oxytetracycline, only suppressed the response when the drug was present between 18 and 72 h after priming. According to these authors, this implies that during this particular period the number of T cell divisions is large enough to reduce the mitochondrial ATP-generating capacity in the presence of the drug. Consequently, inhibition of cell proliferation will occur.

In contrast to tetracyclines, several cephalosporins and cephamycins significantly enhanced the DTH response in mice[19]. The antibiotics were given once (30 mg/kg) on the day of immunization or 3, 2 and 1 days before. Pretreatment of the animals with drugs (cefotaxime, cefoxitin, cefsulodin, cefoperazone, cefotetan and cefmenoxime) resulted in a more pronounced effect. However, 7 days of chemotherapy with cefotaxime suppressed the DTH response[33].

CONCLUSIONS
It is clear that some of the commonly used antimicrobial agents can interfere with non-specific and/or specific defence systems. Antibiotics may exert suppressing as well as enhancing immunological side-effects, depending on test models and animal species. Therefore, it is impossible to draw general conclusions on the effects of antibiotics on the immune system as such. We also cannot define the clinical relevance of antibiotic-mediated immunomodulation at the present time. Yet, it is very important to exclude any immunosuppression by certain drugs in either animals or man. This is obvious, because the defence mechanisms have to eliminate the pathogens

finally.

To day, many in vitro and in vivo immunological assays are available and provide us with sensitive tools for monitoring drug effects. However, it is essential to standardize these assays and to incorporate carefully designed studies, which reflect the disease status.

There exists a general relation between the specific growth-rate of bacteria and the nutrient concentration available. In addition, temperature is also an important environmental factor, which determines the rate of all biochemical reactions. For instance, fish pathogens are psychrophilic, which means that their optimal growth-rate is far below 37 °C, in contrast to thermophilic organisms. The immune system of ectothermic animals has to be adapted in such a way that it can mount an adequate response at relatively low temperatures. This biochemical adaptation (for example metabolic rate and membrane lipid composition) may have implications for the pharmacokinetics of the drugs and for the susceptibility of the immunological process to toxic damage. It is clear that antibiotics have been used over a wide range of species. For some species pharmacokinetic data are scarce or even absent. Kinetic data on tissue distribution, plasma disposition and biological half-life time can differ markedly between mammalian species. Moreover, extreme differences may be expected with respect to the pharmacokinetic behaviour of the drug in birds and fish.

The immunoenhancing effects of antibiotics, caused by interference with the bacterial physiology and/or by stimulation of the host immune system are promising. The combined action of immune system and drug will increase the defensive potential. The ultimate goal of antibacterial therapy is to achieve the best action against pathogens with minimal adverse side-effects. It can be seen in Figure 25.1 that many factors determine the clinical efficacy of a selected antibiotic. One of these factors is the binding to plasma proteins, because only free material will pass to the tissues. Another factor is

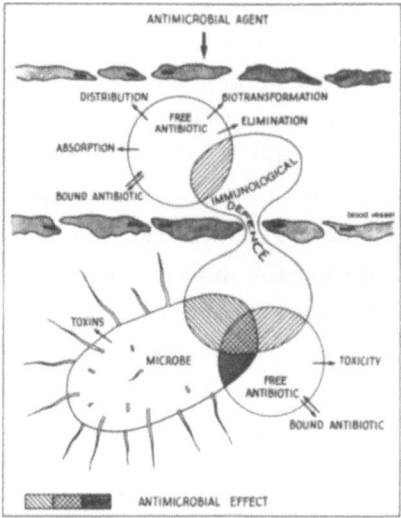

Figure 25.1   Diagram showing the various factors which can influence the outcome of antibiotic therapy.

the amount of unbound drug at the site infection and the degree of interference with local and systemic defence systems.

It is emphasized that a multidisciplinary approach, as is visualized in the diagram, is necessary to tackle the problems efficiently. Immunological, pharmacological and microbiological research has to be extended over a wide range of animal species to support an effective management in animal husbandry and an optimal veterinary practice.

References
 1. Anderson, D.P., Van Muiswinkel, W.B. and Roberson,B.S. (1984). Effects of chemical induces immune modulation on infectious diseases of fish. In : Kende, M., Gainer, J. and Chirigos, M. (eds). Chemical Regulation of Immunity in Veterinary Medicine, pp.187–211.   New York : Alan R. Liss, Inc.
 2. Anderson, R., Fernandes, A.C. and Eftychis, H.E. (1984).   Studies on the effects of ingestion of a single 500 mg oral dose of erythromycin stearate on leucocyte motility and transformatin and on release in vitro of prostaglandin E2 by stimulated leucocytes. J. Antimicrob. Chemother. 14:41–50
 3. Athlin, L., Domellof, L. and Norberg, B. (1984). Adhe- rence and phagocytosis of yeast cells by blood mono-

cytes : effects in vitro of a therapeutic doxycycline
concentration.   Acta   Pathol. Microbiol. Immunol.
Scand. Sect. 92:227-230.
4. Banck, G. and Forsgren, A. (1979). Antibiotics and
suppression   of   lymphocyte   function   in   vitro.
Antimicrob. Agents Chemother. 16:554-560.
5. Banks, R.M. and O'Grady, F. (1983). Therapeutic significance of nocardicin A stimulation of phagocyte
function   in   experimental   Pseudomonas   aeruginosa
infection. Br. J. Exp. Pathol. 64:231-237.
6. Bassaris, H.P., Lianou, P.E. and Papavassiliou, J.T.
(1984).   Interaction of subminimal inhibitory concentrations of clindamycin and Escherichia coli : effects
on adhesion and polymorphonuclear leukocytes function.
J. Antimicrob. Chemother. 13:361-367.
7. Belsheim, J., Gnarpe, H. and Persson, S. (1979).
Tetracyclines and host defense mechanisms : interference with leukocyte chemotaxis. Scand. J. Infect.
Dis. 11:141-145.
8. Borowski, J., Jakoniuk, P. and Talarczyk, J. (1985).
The influence of some cephalosporins on immunological
responses. Drugs Exp. Clin. Res. 11:83-88.
9. Cannon, P., Climax, J., Darragh, A., Lambe, R. and
Lenehan, T.J. (1983).   The action of selected antimicrobial agents on certain functions of human
leucocytes. Br. J. Pharmacol. 80 (Suppl.):596.
10. Caspi, R.R. and Avtalion, R.R. (1984). Evidence for
the   existence of an IL-2 like lymphocyte growth
promoting factor in a bony fish, Cyprinus carpio.
Dev. Comp. Immunol. 8:51-60.
11. Cook, J., Naqi, S.A., Sahin, N. and Wagner, G. (1984).
Distribution of immunoglobulin-bearing cells in the
gut-associated lymphoid tissues of the turkey : Effect
of antibiotics. Am. J. Vet. Res. 45:2189-2192.
12. Dulin, A.M., Paape, M.J. and Ziv, G. (1984). Effect
of   intramammary   injection products on in vitro
phagocytosis. J. Dairy Sci. 67 (Suppl.1):170.
13. Finch, R. (1980). Immunomodulating effects of antimicrobial agents. J. Antimicrob. Chemother. 6:691-699.
14. Forsgren, A. and Gnarpe, H. (1973). Tetracycline
interference with the bactericidal effect of serum.
Nature New Biol. 244:82-83.
15. Forsgren, A. and Schmeling, D. (1977). Effect of
antibiotics   on   chemotaxis   of human leukocytes.
Antimicrob. Agents Chemother. 11:580-584.
16. Forsgren, A., Schmeling, D. and Banck, G. (1978).
Effect of antibiotics on chemotaxis of human
polymorphonuclear leukocytes in vitro. Infection 6
(Suppl.1):S102-S106.
17. Ganguly, R., Pennock, D.G. and Kluge, R.M. (1984).
Inhibition of protein synthesis and lymphokine production by tetracycline. Allerg. Immunol. 30:104-109.
18. Gillissen, G.J. (1982). Antibody production and cellular immunity. In : Eickenberg, U., Hahn, H. and
van Opferkuch, H. (eds). The Influence of Antibiotics
on the Host-Parasite Relationship, pp.5-11. Berlin :

Springer-Verlag.
19. Gillissen, G. and Pusztai-Markos, Z. (1984). Influ-
    ence of antibiotics on immunological parameters : sig-
    nificance in experimental infections. Drugs Exp.
    Clin. Res. 10:813-819.
20. Grondel, J.L. and Boesten, H.J.A.M. (1982). The in-
    fluence of antibiotics on the immune system I. Inhi-
    bition of the mitogenic leukocyte response in vitro by
    oxytetracycline. Dev. Comp. Immunol. (Suppl. 2):
    211-216.
21. Grondel, J.L. and Harmsen, E.G.M. (1984). Phylogeny
    of interleukins : growth factors produced by leukocy-
    cytes of the cyprinid fish, Cyprinus carpio L. Immu-
    nology 52:477-482.
22. Grondel, J.L., Gloudemans, A.G.M. and Van Muiswinkel,
    W.B. (1985). The influence of antibiotics on the
    immune system. II. Modulation of fish leukocytes
    responses in culture. Vet. Immunol. Immunopathol.
    9:251-260.
23. Grondel, J.L., Angenent, G.C. and Egberts, E. (1985).
    The influence of antibiotics on the immune system.
    III. Investigation on the cellular functions of
    chicken leukocytes in vitro. Vet. Immunol. Immunopa-
    thol. 10:307-316.
24. Hauser, W.E. and Remington, J. (1982). Effects of
    antibiotics on the immune response. Am. J. Med.
    72:711-716.
25. Hawkey, P.M., Hawkey, C.A., Richardson, M.D. and War-
    nock, D.W. (1983). In vitro phagocytosis of Candida
    albicans by human polymorphonuclear phagocyte mono-
    layers pretreated with anti-Pseudomonal antibiotics.
    Eur. J. Clin. Microbiol. 2:358-359.
26. Lam, C., Laber, G., Hildebrandt, J., Wenzel, A., Tur-
    nowksy, F. and Schutze, E. (1984). Therapeutic
    relevance of antibiotic-induced augmentation of host
    defences in experimental infections. Drugs Exp. Clin.
    Res. 10:703-711.
27. Lochmann, O., Janovska, D., Vymola, F. and Svandova,E.
    (1979). Effect of antibiotics on the formation of
    specific antibodies. J. Hyg. Epidem. Microbiol.
    Immunol. 23:220-225.
28. Milatovic, D. (1984). Influence of subinhibitory con-
    centrations of antibiotics on opsonization and
    phagocytosis of Pseudomonas aeruginosa by human
    polymorphonuclear leukocytes. Eur. J. Clin. Micro-
    biol. 3:288-293.
29. Naqi, S.A., Sahin, N., Wagner, G. and Williams, J.
    (1984). Adverse effects of antibiotics on the deve-
    lopment of gut-associated lymphoid tissues and
    serum immunoglobulins in chickens. Am. J. Vet. Res.
    45:1425-1429.
30. Oppenheim, J.J. and Gery, I. (1982). Interleukin 1 is
    more than an interleukin. Immunol. Today 3:113-119.
31. Rijkers, G.T., Teunissen, A.G., Van Oosterom, R. and
    Van Muiswinkel, W.B. (1980). The immune system of
    cyprinid fish. The immunosuppressive effect of the

antibiotic oxytetracycline in carp (Cyprinus carpio L.). Aquaculture 19:177-189.

32. Rijkers, G.T., Van Oosterom, R. and Van Muiswinkel, W.B. (1981). The immune system of cyprinid fish. Oxytetracyclin and the regulation of humoral immunity in carp (Cyprinus carpio L.). Vet. Immunol. Immunopathol. 2:281-290.

33. Roszkowski, W., Ko, H.L., Roszkowski, K., Jeljaszewicz, J. and Pulverer, G. (1985). Antibiotics and immunomodulation : effects of cefotaxime, amikacin, mezlocillin, piperacillin and clindamycin. Med. Microbiol. Immunol. 173:279-289.

34. Schauenstein, K., Globerson, A. and Wick, G. (1982). Avian lymphokines, I. Thymic cell growth factor in supernatants of mitogen-stimulated chicken spleen cells. Dev. Comp. Immunol. 6:533-540.

35. Schnetzler, M., Oommen, A., Nowak, J.S. and Franklin, R.M. (1983). Characterization of chicken T cell growth factor. Eur. J. Immunol. 13:560-566.

36. Serrou, B. (1974). Rifampicin and immunosuppression. Lancet ii:172.

37. Smith, K.A., Lachman, L.B., Oppenheim, J.J. and Favata, M.F. (1980). The functional relationship of the interleukins. J. Exp. Med. 151:1551-1556.

38. Thong, Y.H. and Ferrante, A. (1979). Inhibition of mitogen-induced human lymphocyte proliferative responses by tetracycline analogues. Clin. Exp. Immunol. 35:443-446.

39. Van den Bogert, C. and Kroon, A.M. (1982). Effects of oxytetracycline on in vivo proliferation and differentiation of erythroid and lymphoid cells in the rat. Clin. Exp. Immunol. 50:327-335.

40. Van Muiswinkel, W.B., Anderson, D.P., Lamers, C.H.J., Egberts, E., Van Loon, J.J.A. and Ijssel, J.P. (1985). Fish immunology and fish health. In : Manning, M.J. and Tatner, M.F. (eds). Fish Immunology. London : Academic Press.

41. Voiculescu, C., Stanciu, L., Voiculescu, M., Rogoz, S. and Dumitriu, I. (1983). Experimental study of antibiotic-induced immuno-suppression in mice - I. Humoral and cell-mediated immune responsiveness related to in vivo antibiotic treatment. Comp. Immun. Microbiol. Infect. Dis. 6:291-299.

42. Voiculescu, C., Stanciu, L., Voiculescu, M., Rogoz, S., Dumitriu, I. and Nedelcu, C. (1983). Experimental study of antibiotic-induced immunosuppression in mice - II. Th. Ts and NC cell involvement. Comp. Immun. Microbiol. Infect. Dis. 6:301-312.

43. Von Zabern, I., Przyklenk, H., Nolte, R. and Vogt, W. (1983). Effect of sulphonamides and penicillins on the complement system. Immunobiology 165:378-379.

44. Wolff, L.J. and Stankova, L. (1983). Effect of sulfamethoxazole/trimethoprim on alveolar mononuclear phagocyte function. Clin. Res. 31:123.

45. Ziv, G., Paape, M.J. and Dulin, A.M. (1983). Influence of antibiotics and intramammary products on

phagocytosis of Staphylococcus aureus by bovine leukocytes. Am. J. Vet. Res. 44:385-388.

Drug Biotransformation

26
Comparative aspects of drug conjugation in laboratory animals, exotic species and man

J. CALDWELL

ABSTRACT

The great majority of xenobiotics entering the animal body undergo enzymic metabolism in a biphasic sequence of reactions, involving first a reaction of oxidation, reduction or hydrolysis, followed by conjugation of the product with an endogenous moiety. Six major conjugation reactions may be discerned, involving glucuronic acid, sulfate, methyl or acetyl groups, glutathione or one of a number of amino acids. In addition, a number of novel conjugations are known. Although the fundamental pattern of metabolism is common to all species, there occur within the pattern substantial phylogenetic differences, both qualitative and quantitative. These are especially evident with the major conjugation reactions, certain of which exhibit "species defects", for example glucuronidation in the cat and N-acetylation in the dog, while other reactions are restricted in their occurrence to particular groups of species : this is noteworthy with respect to primate species. An understanding of the characteristics of xenobiotic metabolism in particular species may have taxonomic value. It is increasingly appreciated that the conjugation reactions are of considerable pharmacological and toxicological significance, generally by favouring detoxication and excretion. There do exist, however,

circumstances   where   conjugation   results   in   metabolic
activation.   In   either   situation,   the   occurrence   of
substantial   species differences in conjugative metabolism
frequently   underlies   interspecies   differences   in
biological activity of xenobiotics.

When   exogenous   chemicals,   drugs,   agricultural
chemicals, etc. enter the animal body, they undergo one of
four   distinct   fates.   They   may   (a)   be   eliminated
unchanged; (b) undergo   enzymic   metabolism;   (c)   undergo
spontaneous   chemical   transformation;   or   (d) accumulate
unchanged.   Although   examples   of   all   of   these
possibilities   can   be cited, by far the greatest majority
of drugs entering the   body   undergo   enzymic   metabolism.
This is typically a biphasic process (see Figure 26.1), in
which the compound   undergoes   initially   a   phase   I,   or
functionalization   reaction   of   oxidation,   reduction   or
hydrolysis, which serves to introduce within the substrate
a   suitable   functional   group   to act as the site for the
phase II, or conjugation, reactions.

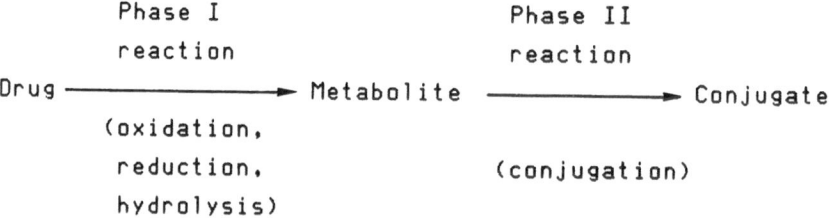

Figure 26.1 The biphasic sequence of drug metabolism

In some cases, a compound may be eliminated as a   phase
I   metabolite,   while   other drugs may undergo conjugation
directly.   The elimination products   of   drugs   will   thus
comprise   some   or   all   of   phase I metabolites, phase II
metabolites, products of the biphasic sequence and,   to   a
greater   or   lesser extent, the unchanged compound.   It is
the   purpose   of   this   chapter   to   review   the   major
conjugation   reactions   of   drug   metabolism   and   their

zoological distribution and to comment upon their significance in pharmacology and toxicology.

The conjugation reactions may be defined as "a group of biosynthetic reactions in which a drug or a metabolite thereof is covalently linked with an endogenous moiety to give a characteristic product known as a conjugate"[3]. The endogenous groupings involved in metabolic conjugation all have well-defined roles in intermediary biochemistry and/or biosynthesis, and these reactions may be viewed as interfaces between drug metabolism and intermediary biochemistry. It is appropriate to consider the conjugation reactions as falling into two groups, a small number of "principal" reactions, whose species distribution, substrate versatility and enzymic mechanism are (reasonably) well understood, and a much larger number of "novel" reactions, which are at present viewed, through the paucity of our knowledge, as restricted in their occurrence to particular combinations of animal species and substrate[3,4]. These novel reactions are outside the scope of the present coverage, but are reviewed at length elsewhere[3,9].

There are six principal metabolic conjugations divided mechanistically into two types[1] : (a) those deriving the required energy from an activated endogenous conjugating agent, generally a nucleotide; and (b) those where the xenobiotic undergoes metabolic activation prior to conjugation. These reactions are shown in Table 26.1.

During the course of evolution, living organisms have developed an immense diversity. The mammalia alone comprise over 4000 species. It is remarkable to note that the biphasic pattern of drug metabolism is found to occur in all mammals (and most other organisms) : however, there occur widespread qualitative and quantitative variations within this fundamental pattern, and these are documented at length in the drug metabolism literature[8,14]. Qualitative differences between species may arise in one of two ways : (a) a species may be (relatively) defective in a reaction of otherwise widespread occurrence; or (b)

Table 26.1   Mechanistic classification of the major conjugation reactions

----

(A) Reactions involving activated conjugating agents
        Glucuronidation (UDPGA)
        Sulphation (PAPS)
        Methylation (S-adenosylmethionine)
        Acetylation (acetyl CoA)
(B) Reactions involving activated xenobiotics
        Glutathione conjugation (epoxides, alkyl and aryl
                                  halides and nitro com-
                                  pounds, etc.)
        Amino acid conjugation   (xenobiotic acyl CoAs)

----

reactions being restricted in their occurrence to
particular species or groups of species. Quantitative
species differences arise from variations in the relative
activities of two or more alternative metabolic options
which a given compound may undergo. It is this last case
which is encountered most frequently.

   A number of so-called "species defects" of metabolic
conjugation have been documented, and a list is presented
in Table 26.2[2,11].

   The best-known of these examples are the defects of
glucuronidation in the cat and related feline species[7] and
of N-acetylation in the dog[5]. It is important to
appreciate that these defects are not absolute, but must
be qualified with reference to the substrate(s) in
question. Thus, the cat is unable to glucuronidate
simple, relatively water-soluble phenols and carboxylic
acids. However, the glucuronidation of more complex,
lipid-soluble substrates proceeds in the cat to the same
extent as in other species. Similarly, dogs are unable to
N-acetylate aromatic amino groups and hydrazides, but do
acetylate the S-substituted cysteines which are the
penultimate intermediates in the conversion of glutathione
conjugates to mercapturic acids. Guinea-pigs, on the

Table 26.2 Some species defects in metabolic conjugation
reactions

Reaction   Affected species

Glucuronidation   Cat and related species
N-Acetylation of   Dog and related species
   aromatic amines
N-Acetylation of   Guinea-pig
   S-substituted cysteines
Sulphation   Pig
Glutamine conjugation   Non-primates
   of arylacetic acids
Glycine conjugation of   Horse
   salicylate (but not
   benzoate)

---

other   hand,   apparently   cannot   N-acetylate   these
substituted cysteines, but do acetylate a variety of other
amines.   The   failure   of   the   guinea-pig   to   excrete
mercapturic   acids   thus   arises   not   from   a   defect   in
conjugation   with   glutathione,   but   rather   from   one   in   the
catabolism of the products of this reaction[2].

For many years, there has been   much   interest   in   the
possibility   that   certain   metabolic   reactions   have   been
restricted by evolutionary pressures to specific groups of
species.   In   particular,   the   close   similarities   between
man and primate species has led   to   numerous   comparative
metabolic   studies   which   have   thus   far   revealed   the
existence of five conjugation reactions which   only   occur
in these species[7,15].   These are :

(1) the glutamine conjugation of arylacetic and aryloxy-
alkyl   acids   (found   in   man,   apes and old and new world
monkeys);
(2) the O-methylation of 4-hydroxy-3,5-diiodobenzoic acid
(man, old and new world monkeys);

(3) the N^1-glucuronidation of certain methoxysulphonamides (all primates);

(4) the quaternary N-glucuronidation of tertiary aliphatic amines (man and apes only);

(5) the C-glucuronidation of pyrazolone rings (man and apes only).

Another example of a metabolic reaction being largely restricted in its occurrence to a group of species is that of taurine conjugation, which occurs at low levels in many species but is particularly well-developed only in carnivores.

Quantitative species differences in the relative extents of competing metabolic options can be seen in the cases of phenols, which may undergo either sulphation or glucuronidation, and carboxylic acids, which are conjugated with amino acids or glucuronic acid. Table 26.3 illustrates this in the case of phenol itself[2].

In other cases, it is found that the physicochemical properties of the drug as well as the animal species in question determine the pattern of conjugation of a particular phenol[12] or carboxylic acid[6].

There are many reasons for the detailed study of

Table 26.3 Species variations due to competing reactions: the conjugation of phenol

Species	Percentage dose conjugated with		Ratio S/G
	sulphate	glucuronide	
Man and old world monkeys	80	12	7
New world monkeys	25	50	0.5
Rat and mouse	45	40	1
Cat	93	1	93
Pig	2	95	<0.1

species differences in drug metabolism, in particular the usefulness of such studies in explaining interspecies variations in pharmacological and toxic effects. Another, less widely appreciated reason is the use of comparative metabolic data in the classification of animals, for which the term "pharmacotaxonomy" has been coined[2]. This is very well illustrated by data from a variety of carnivores examining the species distribution of the glucuronidation defect of the felines and the N-acetylation defect of canines. The data listed in Table 26.4 show that the feline species (cat, lion, lynx, civet) were metabolically completely distinct from the canines (dog and hyena). Although classical taxonomy usually classes the hyena as a feline species rather than a canine, this data suggest that a revision of this view is indicated.

The metabolic conjugation reactions are of great importance for the pharmacological and toxic actions and interactions of drugs and other chemicals, and reasons for this are presented in Table 26.5. By causing substantial changes in the chemical structure and physicochemical properties (the majority of conjugates are more polar and have greater water solubility than their parent compounds) of drugs, the conjugation reactions generally result in the inactivation and facile elimination of drugs from the

Table 26.4 Comparative glucuronidation and acetylation of various substrates amongst carnivores

	Glucuronidation of 1-naphthyl-acetic acid	N-Acetylation of sulphadimethoxine
Cat	0	18
Lion	0	48
Lynx	0	–
Civet	0	66
Hyena	40	0
Dog	20	0

body.   In   a   small number of cases, however, conjugation
may result in metabolic activation, and thus contribute to
the actions of drugs[13].

Species   variations in metabolic conjugation have great
significance as determinants   of   species   differences   in
biological   response.   Thus, cats are far more susceptible
to   the   toxic   effects   of   various   glucuronidogenic
substrates   than   are   rats,   rabbits and other species in
which   this   reaction   is   extant[7].   Similarly,   aromatic
amines produce methaemoglobinaemia far more readily in the
dog than in other species which are   able   to   N-acetylate
these   amines.   The absence of this conjugation in the dog
allows metabolic activation, by N-oxidation, to occur   far
more extensively[3].   Many aromatic amines are carcinogenic,
and the acetylation defect in the dog has a site-directing
influence   upon   their   tumorigenicity[3].   Such amines are
potent bladder carcinogens in the dog, with little   or   no
effect   on other organs, while in the mouse, rat and other
species they produce tumours in a variety of   tissues   but
have   no effect on the urinary bladder.   The relationships
between the oxidation, acetylation, sulphation and   glucuronidation   of   aromatic   amines and their carcinogenicity
are complex[10], but the N-acetylation defect in the dog has
a   major   role   in targetting their carcinogenicity to the
urinary bladder.

The capacity of the   principal   metabolic   conjugations
depends   upon   the   affinities   of the transferase enzymes
involved   both   for   the   xenobiotic   substrate   and   the
endogenous conjugating agent, and upon the availability of
the conjugating agent.   Since these latter have   important
roles   in   intermediary metabolism, their availability for
the conjugation of   xenobiotics   may   be   limited.   This,
together   with   the widespread distribution of conjugation
activity amongst the tissues of the body (notably   in   the
absorptive   and   excretory   organs)   leads   to a number of
pharmacokinetic   consequences   of   conjugation which   are
listed in Table 26.5.   Space does not permit more than the
briefest mention of these, but full descriptions are to be

Table 26.5   Biological   significance   of the conjugation
reactions

Conjugation reactions result in :
(1) Readily excreted end-products of xenobiotic metabolism
(2) Metabolic activation, in certain cases
(3) Detoxication, which may however be defective, due to :
        (a) species defects
        (b) saturation (capacity limitations)
(4) Pharmacokinetic implications, including :
        (a) capacity limitations
        (b) enterohepatic recirculation
        (c) presystemic elimination
        (d) determination of route-of-elimination
        (e) drug-drug interactions
----

found elsewhere[1,4].

In summary, therefore, it will be clear from the above
that the conjugation reactions are of great importance in
the metabolic disposition of drugs and other chemicals in
the animal body, and consequently of pharmacological and
toxicological significance. In the future, our awareness
of metabolic conjugation will develop further in various
ways (a) with enhanced knowledge of both the "principal"
and novel conjugation reactions; (b) the discovery of more
novel conjugations; (c) further recognition of   the
biological consequences of conjugation; and (d) by viewing
the conjugations as interfaces between xenobiotic
metabolism and the biochemistry of endogenous compounds,
with possible pathological sequelae.

References
 1. Caldwell, J. (1980). The conjugation reactions. In :
   Jenner, P. and Testa, B. (eds). Concepts in Drug Metabolism, Part A, pp.211-250. New York :Marcel Dekker.
 2. Caldwell, J. (1980). Comparative aspects of detoxication. In : Jakoby, W.B. (ed.). Enzymatic Basis of
   Detoxication, vol. 1, pp.85-114. New York : Academic
   Press.
 3. Caldwell, J. (1982). Conjugation reactions in foreign

compound metabolism : definition, consequences and species variations. Drug. Metab. Rev. 13:745-778.

4. Caldwell, J. (1982). Conjugation reactions in the metabolism of xenobiotics. In : Arias, I.M., Popper, H., Schachter, D. and Schafritz, D.A. (eds). The Liver : Biology and Pathobiology, pp.281-295. New York : Raven Press.

5. Caldwell, J. (1982). Conjugation reactions of nitrogen centres in xenobiotics. In : Jakoby, W.B., Bend, J.R. and Caldwell, J. (eds). Metabolic Basis of Detoxication, pp.271-290. New York : Academic Press.

6. Caldwell, J. (1982). The conjugation of xenobiotic carboxylic acids. In : Jakoby, W.B., Bend, J.R. and Caldwell, J. (eds). Metabolic Basis of Detoxication, pp.291-306. New York : Academic Press.

7. Caldwell, J. (1985). Glucuronic acid conjugation in the context of the metabolic conjugation of xenobiotics. In : Matern, S., Bock, K.W. and Gerok, W. (eds). Advances in Glucuronide Conjugation, pp.5-18. Lancaster : MTP Press.

8. Caldwell, J. and Paulson, G.D. (1984). Foreign Comound Metabolism. London : Taylor and Francis.

9. Eadsforth, C.V. and Hutson, D.H. (1984). Formation of carbohydrate, sulphate and other xenobiotic conjugates. In : Caldwell, J. and Paulson, G.D. (eds). Foreign Compound Metabolism, pp.171-184. London : Taylor and Francis.

10. Flammang, T.J. and Kadlubar, F.F. (1985). Acetyl CoA-dependent, cytosol-catalysed binding of carcinogenic N-hydroxy-arylamines to DNA. In : Boobis, A.R., Caldwell, J., De Matteis, F. and Elcombe, C.R. (eds). Microsomes and Drug Oxidations, pp.190-197. London : Taylor and Francis.

11. Marsh, M.V., Caldwell, J., Smith, R.L., Horner, M.W., Houghton, E. and Moss, M.S. (1981). The metabolic conjugation of some carboxylic acids in the horse. Xenobiotica 11:655-663.

12. Mulder, G.J. (1982). Conjugation of phenols. In : Jakoby, W.B., Bend, J.R. and Caldwell, J. (eds). Metabolic Basis of Detoxication, pp.247-269. New York : Academic Press.

13. Mulder, G.J. (1984). The role of sulfation and glucuronidation in toxification of xenobiotics. In : Caldwell, J. and Paulson, G.D. (eds). Foreign Compound Metabolism, pp.235-244. London : Taylor and Francis.

14. Parke, D.V. and Smith, R.L. (1977). Drug Metabolism from Microbe to Man. London : Taylor and Francis.

15. Smith, R.L. and Caldwell, J. (1977). Drug metabolism in sub-human primates. In : Parke, D.V. and Smith, R.L. (eds). Drug Metabolism from Microbe to Man, pp.331-356. London : Taylor and Francis.

27
Hepatic microsomes as models for comparative metabolism in vivo

C. H. WALKER

ABSTRACT

Hepatic microsomal systems have been used to study the metabolism of lipophilic xenobiotics. Sometimes these systems give reasonable qualitative and quantitative predictions of metabolism in vivo. In vitro systems such as these can be used to study a much wider range of species than is possible in vivo.

Comparative studies have shown considerable species differences in hepatic microsomal mono-oxygenase activities, which show the general trend mammals>birds>fish. With mammals there is a negative correlation between average mono-oxy-genase activity and log body weight.

With lipophilic xenobiotics particular attention is given to cases where microsomal metabolism is so slow that it may influence rates of excretion and biological half-lives. Here, species differences in enzyme activity may result in corresponding differences in bioaccumulation.

INTRODUCTION

Liposoluble xenobiotics are metabolized by vertebrates, especially in the liver. Although metabolism is usually a detoxifying process, there are important exceptions, where metabolism causes activation (for example, of certain polycyclic aromatic carcinogens and organophosphorous insecticides). Thus, a knowledge of metabolism is an important part of the safety evaluation of drugs, pesticides and other man-made chemicals.

Data are sought on metabolism in vivo in man and in beneficial organisms, but this aim can only be realized to a limited extent. For reasons of cost and because of practical and ethical considerations, only a very limited number of vertebrate species can be studied. This is a serious limitation in the fields of veterinary toxicology and ecotoxicology because there is much evidence of marked species differences in response to toxic agents. For these reasons there is a growing interest in the use of in vitro techniques to predict in vivo metabolism. In vitro techniques are relatively cheap and easy to perform, and can be used to investigate a much wider range of species than is possible by in vivo studies alone.

Many lipophilic xenobiotics undergo their initial biotransformation in the hepatic endoplasmic reticulum. This paper will discuss the use of hepatic microsomes to study metabolism in vitro by different species, and the possibility of using this system to make qualitative and quantitative predictions of metabolism in vivo.

QUALITATIVE COMPARISONS BETWEEN IN VITRO AND IN VIVO METABOLISM

The biodegradable dieldrin analogue HCE (1,2,3,4,9,9-hexa-chloro-1,4,4a,5,6,7,8,8a-octahydro-exo-7,8-epoxy-1,4-metha nonaphthalene) was used as substrate in a comparison between in vivo and in vitro metabolism by the rat, rab-bit, pigeon (Columba livia) and Japanese quail (Coturnix coturnix japonica)[3]. In all species hepatic microsomal metabolism was predominantly by mono-oxygenase attack, with one primary metabolite undergoing further oxidation to two other metabolites as the substrate concentration fell with time. The same metabolic pattern was found in all cases in vivo. Thus, the major in vivo metabolites were correctly predicted by the microsomal model in four contrasting species. In other studies with the rat, hepatic microsomes again provided a good prediction of the major metabolites of phenytoin, griseofulvin, and HEOM (1,2,3,4,9,9-hexachloro-1,4,4a,5,6,7,8,8a-octahydro-6,7-epoxy-1,4-methanonaphthalene; dieldrin analogue)[3].

QUANTITATIVE COMPARISONS BETWEEN IN VITRO AND IN VIVO METABOLISM

Using dieldrin, HCE and HEOM, hepatic microsomal metabolism was compared with in vivo metabolism (biliary excretion) in the male rat. Both microsomal metabolism and biliary excretion were much slower for dieldrin than for the other two compounds[3].

Induction with phenobarbitone caused a 17-fold increase in microsomal mono-oxygenase activity towards HCE in vitro, but there was no significant increase in the rate of biliary excretion of HCE metabolites in vivo. With dieldrin, on the other hand, phenobarbitone induction caused a significant three-fold increase in the maximum rate of excretion, clearly indicating that the enzymic activity was limiting the rate of excretion of metabolites for this compound but not for HCE. A Lineweaver-Burke plot of HCE metabolism by rat microsomes successfully predicted the rate of excretion into bile.

Other workers have successfully used microsomal metabolic data in pharmacokinetic models to predict the rate of loss of lipophilic xenobiotics such as phenytoin, and polychlorinated biphenyl (PCB) isomers[3].

A survey was conducted on the relative mono-oxygenase activities of liver microsomes of different species reported in the literature[2]. Data were collected for 65 vertebrate species, and covered a wide range of assay procedures using different substrates (results are included for ten different substrates). To facilitate comparison between species, activities were calculated relative to those of the male rat. With mammals, there was a good negative correlation between relative activity and body weight (correlation coefficient -0.808). In all cases fish showed lower activities than mammals of the same body size, while most birds had intermediate activities. Cattle, sheep, pigs, cats and dogs fitted into this general pattern, all showing lower relative activities than rats, in keeping with their relatively high body weights[1,2]. The values for dogs, sheep and pigs were close to the regression line. The value for cats fell below the line; the value for cattle was above the line, but the significance of this is uncertain since it was based on only two assay procedures.

DISCUSSION

From the foregoing account, it is clear that microsomal systems can give reasonable qualitative and/or quantitative predictions of the in vivo metabolism of certain lipophilic xenobiotics. However, the examples quoted were for compounds which are metabolized in a relatively simple fashion and which undergo most of their primary biotransformation in the hepatic endoplasmic reticulum. This model would not be appropriate for compounds which are, for example, broken down primarily by blood esterases, or by gut microflora. Anticipation of the likely mechanism and location of biotransformation are needed in the selection of appropriate model systems for in vitro studies. Future progress in this field will depend upon the development, and the successful integration, of a variety of in vitro techniques including the use of perfused organs, cell suspensions and cultures, subcellular fractions and purified enzymes.

Microsomal systems (including induced preparations) may give forewarning of the very slow biotransformation of certain xenobiotics by certain species, with the attendant risk of bioaccumulation. The possibility of using kinetic data to predict bioaccumulation risks was discussed in a recent paper[4]. Where biotransformation rates are very slow, substantial species differences in enzyme activity may be accompanied by corresponding differences in biological half-lives and in susceptibilities to toxic agents.

References
1. Smith, G.S., Watkins, J.B., Thompson, T.N. Rozman, K.
   and Klaassen, C.D. (1984).   Oxidative and conjugative
   metabolism of xenobiotics by livers of cattle, sheep,
   swine and rats.   J. Animal Sci. 58:386-395.
2. Walker, C.H. (1980).   Species variations in some hepatic microsomal enzymes.   Prog. Drug Metab. 5:113-164.
3. Walker, C.H. (1981).   The correlation between in vivo
   and in vitro metabolism of pesticides in vertebrates.
   Prog. Pesticide Biochem. 1:247-285.
4. Walker, C.H. (1985).   Bioaccumulation in marine food
   chains - a kinetic approach.   Marine Env. Res. 17:297-
   300.

28
Pharmacokinetics, hydroxylation and acetylation of sulphadimidine in mammals, birds, fish, reptiles and molluscs

J. F. M. NOUWS, T. B. VREE, H. J. BREUKINK, A.S.J.P.A.M. VAN MIERT AND J. GRONDEL

ABSTRACT

Plasma disposition, plasma protein binding, recovery in urine and renal clearance of sulphadimidine (SDM), its N_4-acetyl (N_4-SDM), its 6-hydroxymethyl (SCH_2OH), its 5-hydroxy (SOH) and its glucuronide (SOH-gluc) metabolites were studied in man, ruminants, horses, pigs, laying-hens and the carp. The elimination half-life depended mainly on the extent of metabolism and the renal excretion rate of the metabolites. N_4-SDM, SCH_2OH and SOH metabolites exhibited higher renal clearance values than SDM. Hydroxylation of SDM predominated over acetylation in horses, ruminants, poultry, turtles and snails. The main metabolite in horses was SOH; in cows, calves, goats, turtles and snails it was SCH_2OH. In ruminants a capacity-limited hydroxylation of SDM to SCH_2OH was observed at dosages of 100-200 mg/kg. Also in laying-hens a capacity-limited elimination-like pattern was obtained following an intravenous SDM dosage of 100 mg/kg. In man and pigs the acetylation pathway was predominant and the elimination half-life in the latter species depended on the position of the acetylation-deacetylation equilibrium. Fish are able to hydroxylate and acetylate SDM.

INTRODUCTION

Sulphadimidine (SDM) is the most widely used sulphonamide for prophylactic and therapeutic purposes in a wide range of species. Between-species differences in elimination half-lives for SDM as well as for other sulphonamides have been reported, and these have been recently reviewed[1]. Most reported pharmacokinetic data have been based on assays performed by the Bratton and Marshall method, which does not distinguish SDM from its hydroxy metabolites[2,5,11]).

Sulphadimidine can be metabolized by hydroxylation at the 5 or 6 position of the pyrimidine ring, and by the acetylation-deacetylation pathway[11-13]. After hydroxylation the metabolites may become glucuronidated (Figure 28.1). The hydroxy metabolites are microbiologically active and they may be potentiated by trimethoprim[6]. Because of its widespread therapeutic use and from the residue point of view, SDM was selected for comparative study of its metabolism, pharmacokinetics and renal clearance of both the parent drug and its metabolites.

MATERIAL AND METHODS

Drugs

Sodium sulphadimidine (33.3%) was obtained from AUV (Cuyk, the Netherlands); N_4-acetylsulphadimidine (N_4-SDM), 6-hydroxymethylsulphadimidine (SCH_2OH) and 5-hydroxysulphadimidine (SOH) were synthesized and isolated according to Vree et al.[11,12].

Experiments

The experiments were performed at different institutes in the Netherlands. SDM was administered intravenously to horses, ruminants, pigs and laying-hens, orally to human volunteers, pigs, turtles and snails, and intraperitoneally to carp. N_4-SDM was administered intramuscularly to carp. From man, horses, ruminants, pigs, laying-hens, and carp heparinized blood samples were taken at regular time intervals, centrifuged, and the plasma was stored at

-20 °C pending HPLC analysis. Urine was collected by either spontaneous voiding, or catheterization, or with special urine collection facilities in man, horses, ruminants and pigs. With respect to carp, turtles, and snails, aquatic water samples were taken at 4-12 h intervals and in the case of carp sampling was followed by refreshment of water.

HPLC analysis

Deglucuronidation, sample preparation and HPLC analysis were performed as described elsewhere[7,8]. SDM, its N_4-SDM and two hydroxy metabolites were determined simultaneously in the samples.

RESULTS

Table 28.1 summarizes the percentages of sulphadimidine and its metabolites in plasma of different species; Table 28.2 presents their plasma protein binding data, Table 28.3 shows the urinary recovery data; and in Table 28.4 the renal clearance values of creatinine and unbound sulphadimidine and its metabolites are summarized.

Man

The main metabolic pathway in man is the acetyl-deacetyl-ation pathway. Hydroxylation only accounts for 10% of the dose. The renal clearance of N_4-SDM is four to five times higher than the creatinine clearance, being lower than in ruminants, but similar to that obtained in pigs, horses and goats. In man, acetylation dominates deacetylation in the acetylation-deacetylation equilibrium, which causes the short elimination half-life. "Slow" and "fast" (Figure 28.2) acetylator phenotypes are distinguishable, exhibiting elimination half-lives ranging between 8.7 and 2 h, respectively (Tables 28.3 and 28.4)[11].

Horses

In the horse, hydroxylation is more important than acetylation, with hydroxylation of the 5 position being

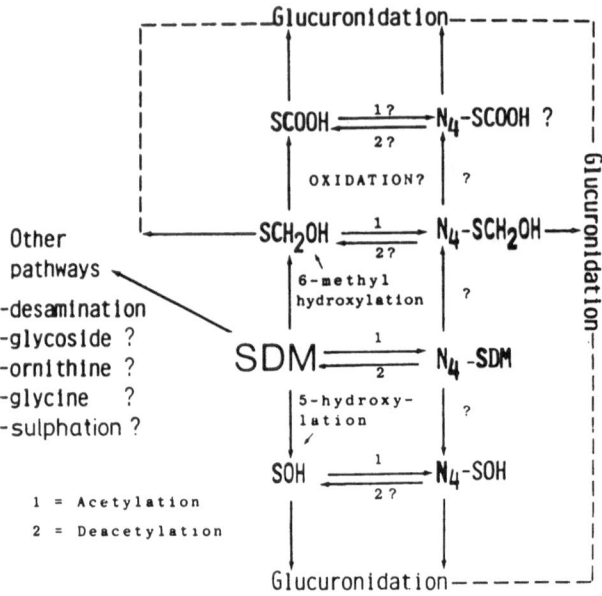

Figure 28.1   Metabolic pathways of sulphadimidine.

dominant over hydroxylation of the 6-methyl group. The elimination half-life of sulphadimidine varies between 5 and 14 h, independent of the dosage. The main metabolite in urine is the SOH and its glucuronide, accounting for 50% of the drugs present (Table 28.3).

Cows and calves
SDM is extensively converted to hydroxy derivatives and to a lesser extent it is acetylated. Hydroxylation of the 6-methyl group to form 6-hydroxymethylsulphadimidine dominates (1.5 times) hydroxylation of the 5 position. At high dose levels (100 mg/kg), a biphasic elimination SDM plasma concentration-time curve was observed with a steady state plasma concentration of SCH_2OH (6-15 µg/ml) during a period when the SDM plasma concentration exceeded 20 µg/ml. At high dosage a capacity-limited hydroxylation of SDM into SCH_2OH was obtained (Figure 28.3). The main metabolite in the urine was SCH_2OH accounting for 23-55% of the administered dose. An unknown metabolite (X) and

Table 28.1   Mean percentages[a] of   sulphadimidine   and   its
metabolites in plasma of different species

	Man[b]		Calf		Cow	
	(S)	(F)				
Dose mg/kg	12	12	10	100	10	100
SDM[c]	57.6	23.5	62.6	79.7	70.5	85.4
N$_4$ -SDM[c]	32.7	67.3	5.7	11.0	2.1	2.3
SCH$_2$OH[c]	–	–	30.9	8.6	22.4	9.7
SOH[c]	–	–	1.4	0.7	3.9	1.0
X(+gluc)[c]	–	–	–	–	3.4	2.2

	Goat	Horse	Pig	Poultry	Fish (Carp)
Dose mg/kg	100	20–200	20	100	560
SDM[c]	77.6	95.0	90.0	87.8	96.8
N$_4$ -SDM[c]	1.5	0.7	10.0	7.5	2.8
SCH$_2$OH[c]	7.2	0.5	–	4.5	0.4
SOH[c]	5.4	3.8	–	1.2	0.05
X(+gluc)[c]	8.5	–	–	–	–

a Percentage of AUC versus total AUC (= AUC parent + metabolites).
b S = Slow acetylator, F = Fast acetylator phenotype.
c Percent.

its   glucuronide   were   detected   in   plasma (Figure 28.3)
and/or in urine of cows, goats and horses (Tables 28.1 and
28.3).   The unknown metabolite (X) may be the further oxidation product of the 6-hydroxymethyl   metabolite   (Figure
28.2)   being tentatively identified as the compound 6-car-
boxysulphadimidine and its glucuronide.   The   renal   clearance   of   SDM was urine-flow correlated, and was half the
creatinine clearance (Table 28.4).

Table 28.2 Protein binding of sulphadimidine and its metabolites in different species

	Calf	Cow		Pig	Goat
SDM[a] μg/ml	<50	<50	>50	<100	<50
SDM	81.1	79.0	50.8	64.9	75.4
N₄-SDM	86.0	86.2	59.3	63.9	77.9
SCH₂OH	49.9	48.4	22.2	-	50.2
SOH	53.0	64.0	39.3	-	53.7
SOHgluc	-	-	67.4	-	-
X	x	x	89	-	94
Xgluc	x	x	22	-	91

	Horse		Fish	Man	Poultry
SDM[a] μg/ml	<50	>50	>100	<50	>50
SDM	65.0	51.0	41.2	88.6	49.9
N₄-SDM	55.4	46.0	14.7	92.5	45.1
SCH₂OH	-	15.1	33.8	60.8	51.2
SOH	59.2	38.3	-	-	29.0
SOHgluc	-	-	-	-	-
X	x	-	-	-	-
Xgluc	x	73	-	-	-

a Plasma concentration; - Not present; x Not determined.

Goats

Goats eliminate sulphadimidine very rapidly and predominantly by hydroxylation. The elimination half-life of the parent drug and metabolites in the dwarf goat is approximately 3 h. Recently it has been shown that hydroxylator phenotypes exist between goat breeds. Acetylation-deacetylation is a minor pathway. The unknown metabolite (X) and its glucuronide were detected in plasma and urine in considerable amounts (Table 28.1 and 28.3). Hydroxylation at the 5 position followed by glucuronidation is a minor pathway (Figure 28.4). In castrated male goats the

Table 28.3 Plasma elimination half-life, and urinary recovery of sulphadimidine and its metabolites expressed as
percentages of the dose administered (mean values) in different species

	Calf		Cow		Pig	Goat
Dose mg/kg	10	100	10	100	20	100
$T_{1/2}$ el h	3.5	15+5[b]	3.5	12+6.5[b]	9-11	2.7-3.8
Time period h	0-72	0-120	0-72	0-72	0-72	0-20
Total recovery[a]	84	88	86	72	52	98
SDM[a]	7	22	9.7	26	10.1	15.1
N_4-SDM[a]	13	34	7.2	9	41.7	4.5
SCH_2OH[a]	50	26	50.5	26	-	28.2
SOH[a]	14	6	18.0	8	-	30.9
X[a]	-	-	-	0.2	-	1.4
Xgluc[a]	-	-	4.8	2.3	-	18.2

	Horse	Fish (Carp)	Man[d] (S)	(F)	Poultry
Dose mg/kg	200	560	12	12	100
$T_{1/2}$ el h	9.5	17.5	7.7	1.6+5[b]	10+3.5[b]
Time period h	0-27	0-48	0-60	0-60	0-60
Total recovery[a]	25	64.4	88	87	42
SDM[a]	10.1(40.5)[c]	62.2	12.9	3.6	13.9
N_4-SDM[a]	1.4(5.6)[c]	1.8	62.5	74.1	12.1
SCH_2OH[a]	0.25(1.0)[c]	0.23	6.3	7.0	10.2
SOH[a]	12.7(51)[c]	0.18	3.5	0.75	5.8
X[a]	0.4(1.4)[c]	-	2.8	1.56	-
Xgluc[a]	-	-	-	-	-

- Not detected.
a Urinary recovery as percentage of the dose.
b Biphasic elimination-time curve (both elimination half-
  lives given).
c Relative percentage of the total recovered drug in 27 h.
d S = Slow acetylator, F = Fast acetylator phenotype.

Table 28.4 Renal clearance values of creatinine, unbound sulphadimidine and its unbound metabolites in different species

	Calf		Cow		Pig
Urine flow ml/min	5	5	15	15	0.45
pH urine	7.5	7.5	8	8	7.5
Dose mg/kg	10	100	10	100	20
Creatinine[a]	0.83	0.62	1.45	1.55	3.25
SDM[a]	0.37[b]	0.34[b]	0.89[b]	0.28[b]	0.40[b]
SCH_2OH[a]	2.45	1.59	3.57	3.38	–
SOH[a]	8.6	6.8	12.8	4.9	–
SOHgluc[a]	–	–	–	17.4	–
X[a]	–	–	–	–	–
Xgluc[a]	–	–	7.4	10.4	–
N_4–SDM[a]	17.3	6.1	25.4	7.4	10.0

	Goat	Horse	Fish	Man[c] (S)	(F)	Poultry
Urine flow ml/min	2.6	1.27	x	1.3	1.5	x
pH urine	8	8.5	x	6.4	6.6	x
Dose mg/kg	100	200	560	12	12	100
Creatinine[a]	2.5	0.68	x	1.9	1.9	x
SDM[a]	0.75	0.20	0.29	1.21	0.64	0.27
SCH_2OH[a]	7.7	1.9	0.22	x	x	4.8
SOH[a]	10.9	1.2	x	x	x	10.9
SOHgluc[a]	–	8.7	x	x	x	x
X[a]	0.34	2.6	x	x	x	x
Xgluc[a]	37.1	–	x	x	x	x
N_4–SDM[a]	15.2	2.9	0.39	11.6	8.5	3.5

a Renal clearance expressed as ml/kg per min.
b Urine flow related.
c S = Slow acetylator, F = Fast acetylator phenotype.
x Not determined.

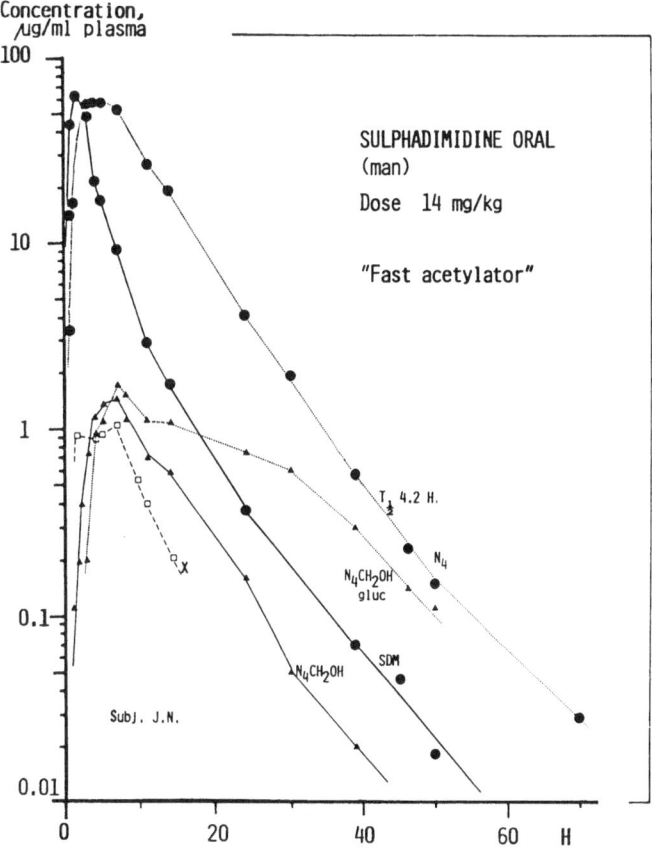

Figure 28.2 Plasma concentration-time curves of sulphadimidine (SDM), its N_4-acetyl (N_4), unknown (X) metabolite
and the N_4-acetyl derivative and its glucuronide of 6-
hydroxymethylsulphadimidine in a human volunteer after an
oral dose of 14 mg/kg ("fast acetylator" phenotype).

percentage of the hydroxy metabolites in plasma was significantly higher than in female goats. Disease states like
tickborne fever slow down the rate and yield of hydroxylation products and increases the half-life to 5 h[1].

Pigs
In pigs SDM is metabolized by acetylation into N_4-SDM; no
hydroxy metabolites could be detected in plasma, tissues
and urine (Table 28.3 and reference[8]). The elimination

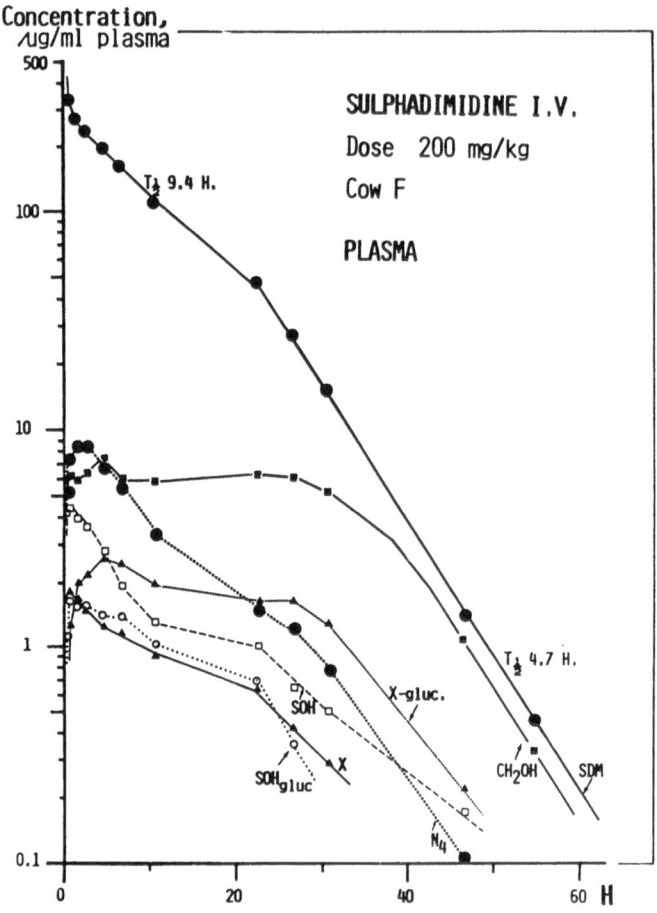

Figure 28.3   Plasma concentration-time curves of sulphadimidine (SDM), and its 6-methylhydroxy (CH₂OH), 5-hydroxy
(SOH) and its glucuronide (SOH₉₁ᵤᵴ), N₄-acetyl (N₄) and
unknown (X) metabolites in a cow after an intravenous dose
of 200 mg/kg.

half-life ranged from 9 to 11 h, because the acetylation-
deacetylation equilibrium favours the deacetylation, in
contrast to man.

Dogs
Because of the absence of the acetylation pathway, hydroxylation of sulphadimidine in dogs is the dominant pathway

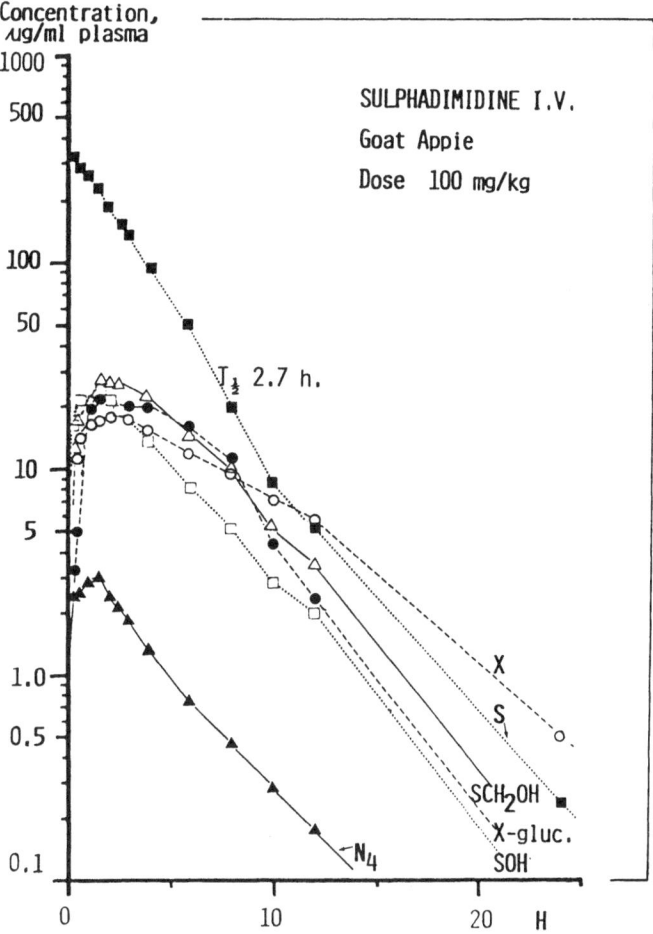

Figure 28.4   Plasma concentration-time curves of sulphadimidine (SDM), and its metabolites N₄-acetyl (N₄), 5-hydroxy (SOH), 6-hydroxymethyl (SCH₂OH), and unknown metabolite (X) with its glucuronide (Xgluc) following intravenous administration of 100 mg/kg to a castrated male dwarf goat.

(mainly CH_2OH), but 50% of the administered dose is still unaccounted for. Other metabolic pathways may be assumed to occur, for example, oxidation of the 6-hydroxymethyl metabolite and glucuronidation[11].

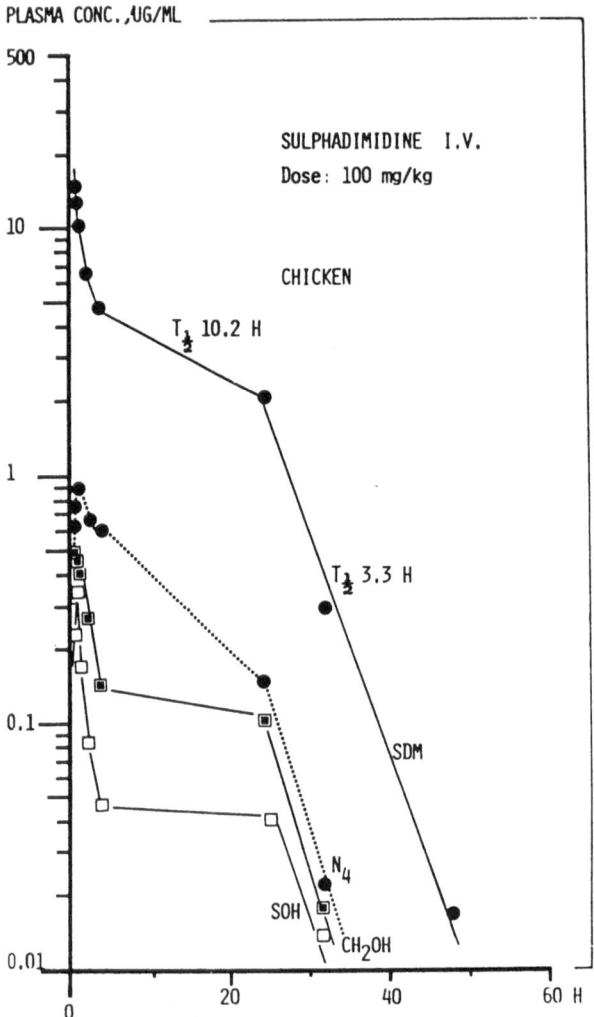

Figure 28.5 Plasma concentration-time curves of sulphadimidine (SDM), its metabolites N_4-acetylsulphadimidine
(N_4), 6-hydroxymethylsulphadimidine (CH_2OH) and 5-hy-
droxysulphadimidine(SOH) after an intravenous dose of 100
mg/kg sulphadimidine.

Poultry
Both hydroxylation and acetylation are relatively important pathways for metabolism of sulphadimidine, but approximately 57% of the administered dose is unaccounted for

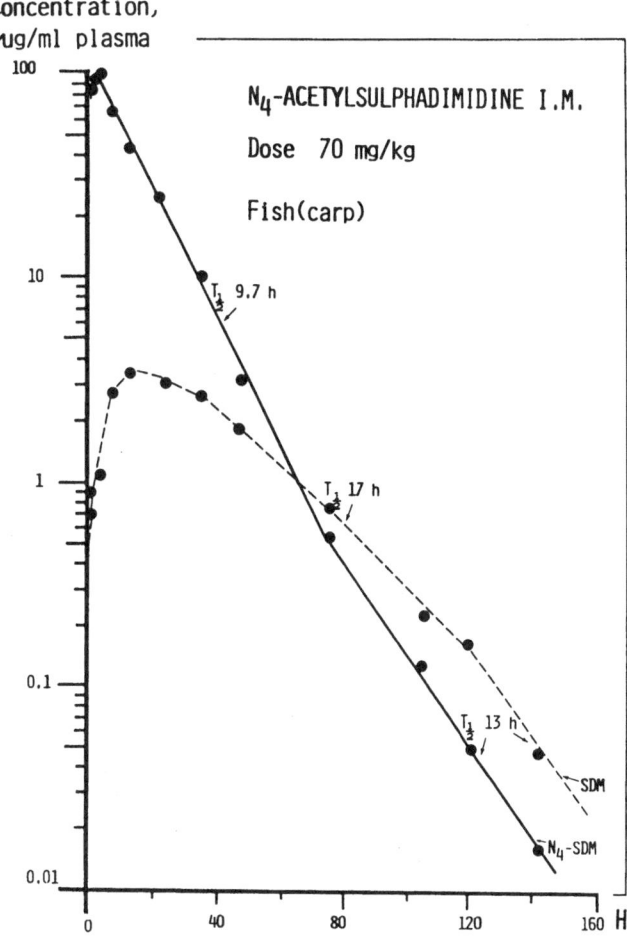

Figure 28.6 Plasma concentration-time curves of N_4-acetylsulphadimidine (N_4-SDM) and its metabolite sulphadimidine (SDM) following intramuscular administration of 70 mg/kg N_4-acetylsulphadimidine.

(Table 28.3). No glucuronides are formed and excreted in the faeces. A capacity-limited-like elimination pattern was noticed after intravenous dosage of 100 mg/kg (Figure 28.5). The renal clearance values for N_4-SDM and the hydroxy metabolites are ten to 50 times greater than that of SDM (Table 28.4).

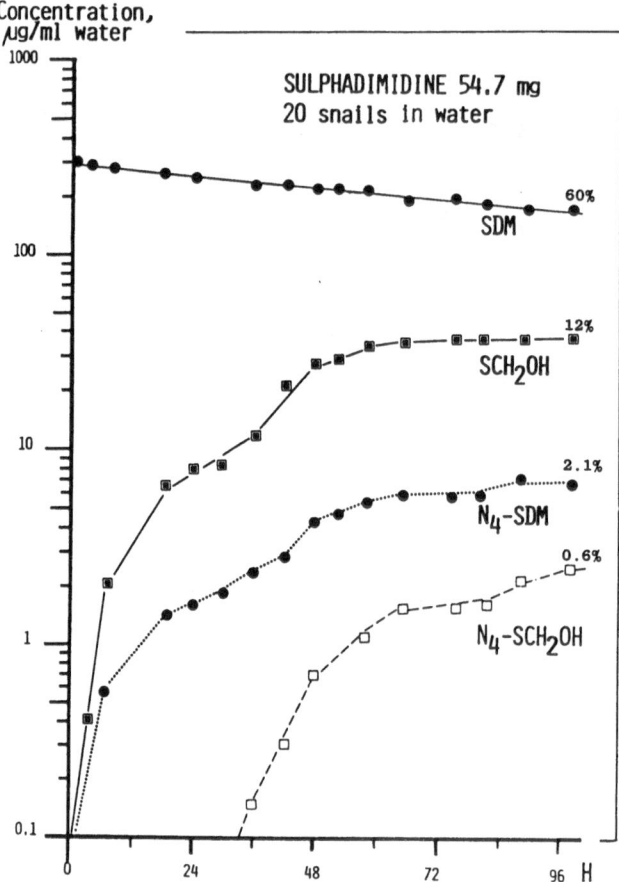

Figure 28.7 Concentration-time curves of sulphadimidine
(SDM) and cumulative concentration-time curves of its metabolites 6-hydroxymethyl (SCH$_2$OH), N$_4$-acetylsulphadimi-
dine and its N$_4$-acetyl metabolite of SCH$_2$OH (N$_4$-SCH$_2$OH) in
20 snails (C. hortensis) with an environmental dose of
54.7 mg sulphadimidine.

Fish (carp)
In the carp SDM is hydroxylated and acetylated to a small
extent. The clearance values of SDM, N$_4$-SDM and hydroxy
metabolites were equivalent and the elimination was predominantly by a passive diffusion process[4] (Table 28.4). An
acetylation-deacetylation equilibrium also exists in the
carp, as shown in Figure 28.6.

Turtles

The turtle (Cuora amboniensis) is able to acetylate and to hydroxylate sulphadimidine at the 6 position (SCH_2OH).

Molluscs

In snails 6-methyl group hydroxylation predominates over acetylation : within 4 days 12% of the administered SDM dose was converted into SCH_2OH and 2.1% into N_4-SDM. The hydroxylated metabolite was also acetylated (Figure 28.7).

DISCUSSION

Various metabolic pathways of sulphadimidine are found in different species, as illustrated in Figure 28.1. In mammals and poultry, all N_4-acetyl metabolites formed at low and high dosages, and hydroxy metabolites formed at low dosages, show plasma concentration-time curves running parallel with that of the parent compound, SDM. This observation indicates that the intrinsic elimination of metabolites is higher than that of the parent drug as shown in Table 28.4. The hydroxy metabolites are elimina- ted partly by glomerular filtration with some tubular reabsorption, and partly by tubular secretion, producing a net excretion of 50 times higher renal clearance than for the parent sulphadimidine. The N_4-acetyl and glucuronides are eliminated predominantly by tubular secretion (Table 28.4). In fish (carp) the plasma clearance of SDM and its metabolites occurs to a similar extent, presumably due to a passive diffusion process (glomerular filtration and presumably diffusion across the gills; Table 28.4). For turtles and molluscs no data are available. For mammals and birds the biotransformation of sulphadimidine yields metabolites which are excreted faster than the parent drug (Table 28.4). Thus hydroxylation and the subsequent glu- curonidation as well as acetylation, speeds up the elimi- nation of SDM (Figure 28.1).

In horses hydroxylation of the 5 position (SOH) predominates over that of the 6-methyl group (SCH_2OH). In goats, cows and calves, and poultry hydroxylation of the

6-methyl group (SCH$_2$OH) predominates over that of the 5 position (SOH). For the goat it was shown that the yield of hydroxylation products was higher in castrated dwarf males than in females. In dwarf goats the hydroxylation rate is greater than in cows; in the latter a capacity-limited hydroxylation of SDM into SCH$_2$OH was observed at a dosage of 100-200 mg/kg. A similar capacity-limited elimination of SDM was reported by Van Gogh[3] for goats (mixed breed) at a dosage of 200 mg/kg, for sulphadiazine in rabbits by Souich et al.[10] and for sulphamonomethoxine in pigs by Shimode et al.[9]. A capacity-limited elimination pattern was also noticed in laying-hens (Figure 28.5); this may be attributable to either capacity-limited metabolism or extensive reabsorption from the cloaca. In the latter, the urinary faecal flow may become the limiting factor in the elimination rate (especially at night) resulting in a "pseudo" capacity-limited elimination of SDM and its metabolites; this has been called chronopharmacokinetics. In poultry both hydroxylation and acetylation are relatively important, but even so 57% is undetected at high dosage. This was also noticed in pigeons[11], so, birds must possess additional metabolic pathways. Our data show clearly (Tables 28.3 and 28.4) that the rate and extent of hydroxylation as well as the overall renal clearance values of the hydroxy metabolites determine the elimination half-life whenever hydroxylation is predominant over acetylation (for example, in cows, calves, goats, horses).

When hydroxylation is absent or negligible, and SDM is acetylated, the position of the acetylation-deacetylation equilibrium[2] is important, as shown for man and pigs. The renal clearance values of N$_4$-SDM in the latter two species are the same (approximately 10 ml/kg per min; Table 28.4), but in man the equilibrium favours acetylation[11], while for pigs deacetylation predominates[8]. Hence, the amount of N$_4$-SDM formed and excreted per min (renal excretion rate) is higher in man than in pigs producing a shorter elimination half-life in the former (2-8.7 h, versus 9-11 h for pigs). The acetylation-deacetylation equilibrium is not affected by dosage; the same plasma concentration ratios of N_4-SDM to SDM in the equilibrium state were measured in cows at 10 and 200 mg/kg dose level (Table 28.1), even though the renal clearance of N_4-SDM was diminished at the high dosage of 100-200 mg/kg (Table 28.4). This is also observed for N_4-acetylsulphamonomethoxine in pigs[9], and N_4-acetylsulphamethoxazole in man[11]. It may be explained by precipitation of sulphonamides (crystalluria) or competitive inhibition between the tubular secretion of N_4-SDM and hydroxy metabolites[7,9-11]. At high SDM dosage, acetylation becomes relatively more important in the elimination process of SDM (Table 28.3).

Differences in elimination half-lives between species could not be related to differences in plasma protein binding (Tables 28.2 and 28.3).

In conclusion, differences in SDM elimination half-lives between species depend mainly on : (a) the extent and rate of hydroxylation, conjugation, and acetylation versus deacetylation (thus amount and composition of enzymes available), which differ between species, and is presumably related to the sulphonamide structure[10]; (b) the renal clearance values of the metabolites, which are usually constant between species; (c) the position of the acetylation-deacetylation equilibrium; (d) in ruminants, the dosage; (e) in birds, a faecal/urinary flow rate; (f) other factors affecting absorption and elimination of SDM including age, gender (affecting hydroxylation) of the animal, disease state of the animal, season, mode of application, and product formulation.

References
1. Anika, S.M., Nouws, J.F.M., Van Duin, C.T.M. and Van Miert, A.S.J.P.A.M. (1986). Tick-borne fever model : effects on pharmacokinetics of chemotherapeutic agents in the goat. In : Van Miert, A.S.J.P.A.M., Bogaert, M.G. and Debackere, M. (eds). Comparative Veterinary Pharmacology, Toxicology and Therapy, Proc. 3rd EAVPT Congress, Part I, Abstracts, p.216. Utrecht: EAVPT.
2. Bevill, R.F., Dittert, L.W. and Bourne, D.W.A. (1977). Disposition of sulfonamides in food-producing animals.

IV. Pharmacokinetics of sulfamezathine in cattle following administration of an intravenous dose and three
oral dosage forms. J. Pharmacol. Sci. 66:619-622.

3. Gogh. H. van (1980). Pharmacokinetics of nine sulfonamides in goats. J. Vet. Pharmacol. Ther. 3:69-81.

4. Haenen, O.L.M., Grondel, J.L. and Nouws, J.F.M.
(1986).   Pharmacokinetics of oxytetracycline, trimethoprim, sulphatroxazole and sulphadimidine in the
carp. In : Van Miert, A.S.J.P.A.M., Bogaert, M.G. and
Debackere, M. (eds). Comparative Veterinary, Pharmacology, Toxicology and Therapy, Proc. 3rd EAVPT
Congress. Part I. Abstracts, p.112. Utrecht : EAVPT.

5. Nielsen, P. (1973). The metabolism of four sulfonamides in cows. Biochem. J. 136:1039-1045.

6. Nouws. J.F.M., Vree, T.B. and Hekster, Y. (1985). In
vitro antimicrobial activity of hydroxy and N_4-acetyl
sulfonamide metabolites. Vet. Q. 7:70-72.

7. Nouws, J.F.M., Vree, T.B., Baakman, M., Driessens, F.,
Breukink. H.J. and Mevius, D. (1986). Age and dosage
dependency in the plasma disposition and the renal
clearance of sulfamethazine and its N_4-acetyl and
hydroxy metabolites in calves and cows. Am. J. Vet.
Res. 47:642-649.

8. Nouws, J.F.M., Vree, T.B., Baakman, M., Driessens, F.,
Vellenga, L. and Mevius, D. (1986). Pharmacokinetics,
renal clearance, tissue distribution and residue aspects of sulphadimidine and its N_4-acetyl metabolite
in pigs. Vet. Q. (in press).

9. Shimode, M., Shimizu, T., Kokue, E. and Hayama, T.
(1984).   Possibility of saturation in renal excretion
after high dose of intravenous sulfamonomethoxine in
pigs. Jap. J. Vet. Sci. 46:331-337.

10. Souich, P. du, McLean, A.J., Lalka, D., Vicuna, N.,
Chauhuri, E. and McNay, J.L. (1978). Sulfadiazine
handling in the rabbit. II. Mechanisms of nonlinear
kinetics of elimination. J. Pharmacol. Exp. Ther.
207:228-235.

11. Vree. T.B. and Hekster, Y.A. (1985). Pharmacokinetics
of sulfonamides revisited. Antibiot. Chemother. 34:
1-208.

12. Vree, T.B., Tijhuis, M., Baakman, M. and Hekster, Y.A.
(1983).   Analysis of N_4-trideuteroacetylsulphamera-
zine and its metabolites sulphamerazine and N_4-
acetylsulphamerazine in man by means of high-perfor-
mance liquid chromatography and mass spectrometry.
Biomed. Mass Spectrometry 10:114-119.

13. Vree, T.B., Tijhuis, M., Nouws, J.F.M. and Hekster,
Y.A. (1984). Identification, isolation, chromatography, and preliminary pharmacokinetics of 4-hydroxysul-
famerazine in dogs. Pharmacol. Weekbl., Sci. Ed. 6:
80-87.

29
Disposition and metabolism of ^{14}C-mebendazole in sheep and poultry

P. BÉNARD, V. BURGAT-SACAZE, F. MASSAT AND A. G. RICO

ABSTRACT

In sheep, guinea-fowl chicks and laying hen-pheasants, dosed orally with ^{14}C-mebendazole, radioactivity was distributed in several compartments. The terminal half-life was between 189.6 and 304.8 h in sheep and between 132.5 and 150.6 h in birds. Radioactivity was detected in all the tissues examined and rather high residual concentrations were present in the melanin-containing tissues and in the liver, 15 days (guinea-fowl chicks and hen-pheasants) and 30 days (sheep) after administration. In sheep liver a concentration of 1.23 ug unchanged mebendazole per g of wet tissue was measured 30 days after dosing.

INTRODUCTION

Mebendazole (MBDZ) is the generic name for methyl(5-benzoyl-1H-benzimidazol-2-yl)carbamate. It is an anthelmintic drug with a broad spectrum of activity. It affects numerous species of nematodes and cestodes, so it is widely used both in human medicine and veterinary practice.

In order to define the withdrawal time for different species, it was necessary to obtain metabolic data. The aim of this paper is to describe results obtained in three animal species : sheep, guinea-fowl chicks and hen-pheasants.

MATERIAL AND METHODS
Labelled compound

[14]C-mebendazole was prepared by Janssen Pharmaceutica Research Centre. It was labelled in the 2-position of the benzimidazole ring. The specific activity was 3 mCi.mmol^{-1}. The radiochemical purity was checked by thin-layer chromatography. It was found to be higher than 96%. ^{14}C-mebendazole was dispersed in an aqueous solution of Tween 80 with unlabelled mebendazole so that the final concentration was 5.15 mg.ml^{-1} and the volume activity 50 µCi.ml^{-1}. The radiochemical purity of the suspension was controlled before every administration.

Animals

The experiment was performed on sheep, guinea-fowl chicks and hen-pheasants. Ten sheep were housed in metabolic cages in order to collect separately faeces and urine every day. All the animals were dosed orally with 20 mg.kg^{-1} body weight labelled mebendazole. Blood samples were obtained from the jugular vein at regular times. The animals were killed 24 and 48 h and 4, 6, 10, 15 and 30 days after administration of the drug. Four lactating ewes were caged separately and milked twice a day; 16 guinea-fowl chicks and three hen-pheasants were also used in this study. They were fed orally and all animals were maintained under the same conditions. Blood samples were obtained from the jugular vein. The animals were killed 24 and 48 h and 3, 8, 10 and 15 days (guinea-fowl chicks) and 8, 10 and 15 days (hen-pheasants) after dosing.

Techniques

Whole-body autoradiography (WBA) was performed on sheep and birds according to Ullberg's technique[4]. In sheep, the technique was carried out to establish the distribution of radioactivity on two lambs killed 24 and 48 h after dosage and on the main organs of sheep slaughtered later. In sheep, WBA was performed on one animal each time.

Liquid scintillation counting was carried out on whole-blood, plasma, blood cells, urine, faeces, milk and most of the organs collected after slaughter. All the samples were prepared with an Oxidizer 306 Packard as described previously[1]. The results were expressed as µg of unchanged mebendazole per g of wet tissue. Separation of urinary radioactivity fractions was performed by thin-layer chromatography and radioactivity was detected either by autoradiography or by scanning (Berthold II).

RESULTS

Sheep

As illustrated in Figure 29.1, most of the detected radioactivity was present in the lumen of the digestive tract. Rather low activity was detected in all other organs except the melanin-containing tissues and the liver which concentrated high radioactivity.

The highest plasma concentration (approximately 2 µg.ml^{-1} of unchanged mebendazole) was observed between 24 and 30 h after administration. From a pharmacokinetic point of view, radioactivity was distributed in three compartments. The terminal half-life was 304.8 and 189.6 h on two animals (Figure 29.2). In the body, concentrations rapidly decreased except in the melanin-containing tissues and the liver. In bile, radioactivity was still detectable 10 days after dosing. In the liver, a concentration of 1.23 µg of unchanged mebendazole was still measurable (Figure 29.3) at 30 days.

Most of the radioactivity was excreted in faeces (73.1 ± 7.2%) and to a lesser extent in urine (10.8 ± 1.4%). In milk, very low concentrations (< 0.1 ppm) were present for 4 days. In urine, 13 metabolites were separated by thin-layer chromatography. Very low concentrations of parent compound were present. The main metabolite isolated was the methyl[5-(α-hydroxy-α-phenylmethyl)-1H benzimidazol-2-yl]carbamate which results from the

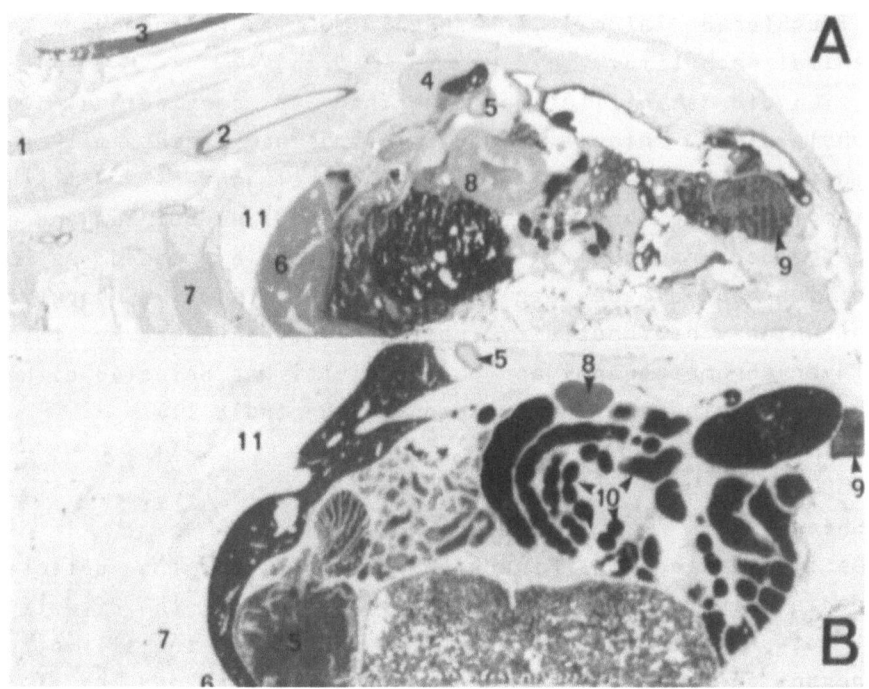

Figure 29.1 Whole body autoradiogram of lambs dosed with
^{14}C-mebendazole and killed 24 h (A) and 48 h (B) later.
1 = spinal cord; 2 = aorta; 3 = chord; 4 = spleen; 5 =
adrenal gland; 6 = liver; 7 = heart; 8 = kidney; 9 = urinary bladder; 10 = intestines; 11 = lungs.

reduction of the ketone grouping. Minor metabolites were
also present in urine; they resulted from carbamate
hydrolysis.

Guinea-fowl chicks
Whole-body autoradiography clearly indicated that
radioactivity was distributed throughout the body 24 h
after dosing (Figure 29.4). On the animal killed after 15
days, radioactivity was still detectable in the skin, the
uveal tract and the liver. Autoradiograms also
demonstrated the presence of radioactivity in bile in all
animals.
   From a kinetic point of view, the plasma concentration

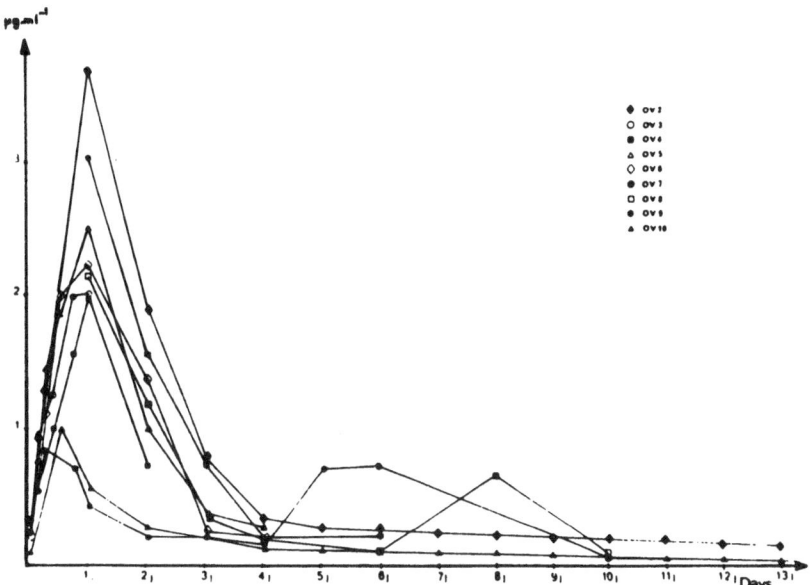

Figure 29.2 Plasma kinetics of radioactivity in sheep dosed with ^{14}C-mebendazole. Concentrations are expressed as µg mebendazole per ml of plasma.

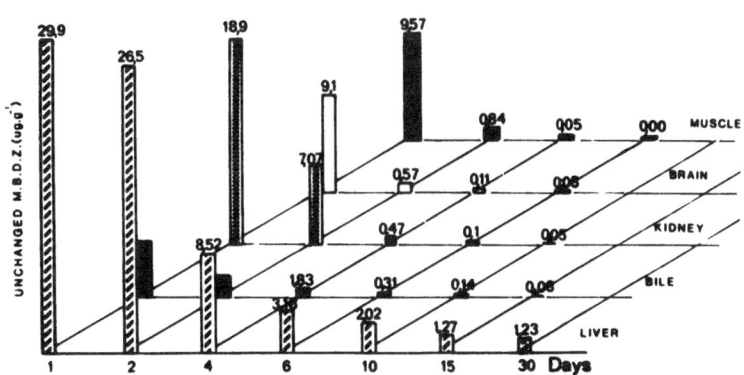

Figure 29.3 Residual concentrations of unchanged mebendazole in organs of sheep dosed with ^{14}C-mebendazole. Concentrations are expressed as µg parent drug per g of wet tissue.

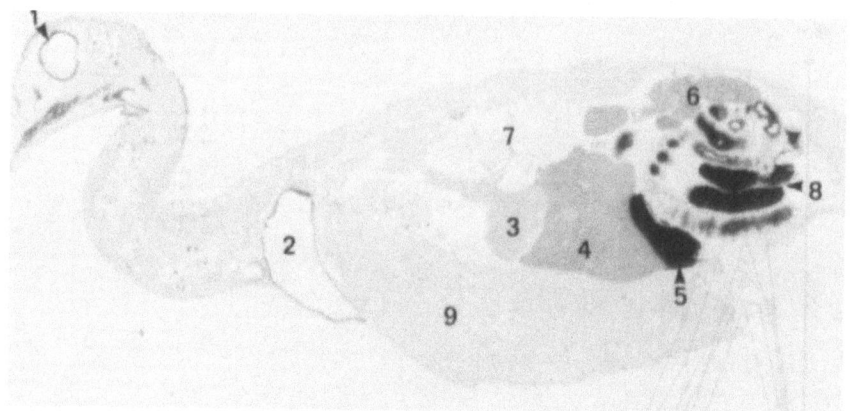

Figure 29.4   Whole body autoradiogram of a guinea-fowl
chick   sacrificed 24 h after feeding with ^{14}C-mebendazole.
1 = uveal tract; 2 = crop; 3 = blood; 4 = liver; 5 =   gall
bladder; 6 = kidney; 7 = lungs; 8 = caecum; 9 = muscles.

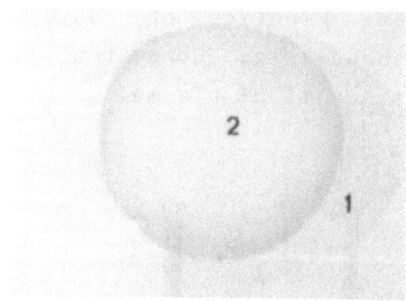

Figure 29.5 Autoradiogram of an egg collected 3 days
after administration of ^{14}C-mebendazole to a laying hen-
pheasant.

curve   demonstrated   that   the highest concentrations
occurred around the 24th h. The peak concentration was
between   3.5   and   5.5 $\mu g.ml^{-1}$.   Radioactivity was
distributed in at least two compartments; the half-life of
the slowest elimination phase was 150.6 h.
   By liquid scintillation counting, evaluation of the
residual levels in different organs confirmed that the
liver, the skin and the uveal tract concentrate the

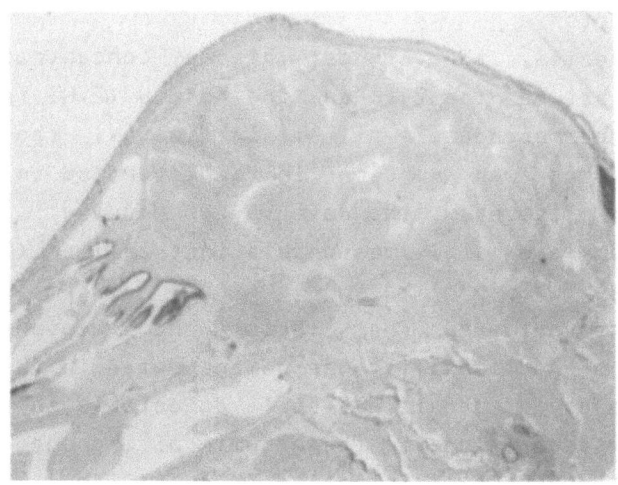

Figure 29.6 Whole body autoradiogram of the head of a
lamb killed 24 h after feeding with labelled mebendazole.

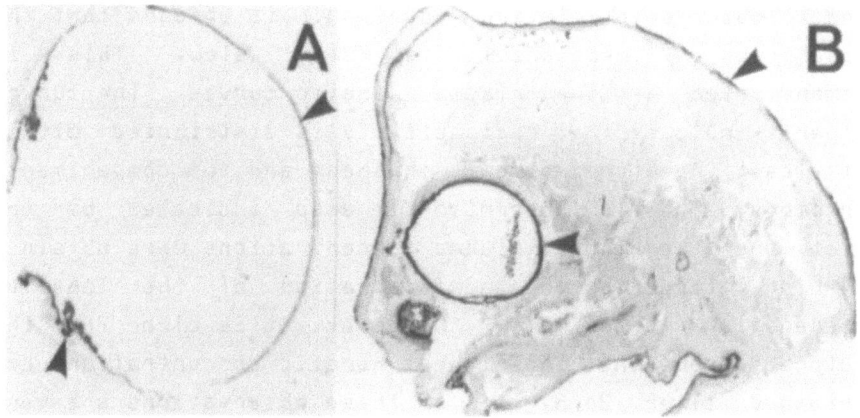

Figure 29.7 Enlargement of autoradiograms. Note the high
radioactive   content   in   melanin-containing   tissues
(arrows); (A) autoradiogram of the eye of a sheep killed
15 days after the administration of ^{14}C-mebendazole; (B)
autoradiogram of the head of a guinea-fowl chick killed 2
days after feeding with labelled mebendazole.

highest   activities.   In   the   liver,   the   residual
concentration   was   0.66 µg of unchanged mebendazole per g
of wet tissue (15 days).

Hen-pheasants

In this species, the highest plasma concentration was obtained between the 24th and the 48th h (2.01 to 2.23 µg of unchanged mebendazole.ml^{-1}). In tissues, the highest concentrations were present in the liver and in melanin-containing tissues. 15 days after dosing, residual activities were still measurable in the liver (0.45 ppm) and kidneys (0.21 ppm).

In eggs obtained from laying hen-pheasants, the presence of radioactivity was demonstrated in the albumin 24 h after dosing and it was still detectable in the yolk and to a lesser extent in the albumin of the egg collected 3 days after drug administration (Figure 29.5).

DISCUSSION

From the results obtained using whole-body autoradiography and liquid scintillation counting, it appears that the absorption of mebendazole is rather slow. This is demonstrated by the plasma kinetic curves. The curves clearly indicate that radioactivity is distributed within at least three compartments in sheep and two compartments in birds. The slow absorption is also indicated by the fact that the highest plasma concentrations were obtained 24 h or later after the administration of the labelled preparation to animals. Moreover, it is clear from the autoradiograms that the highest hepatic concentrations are obtained after 24 h. All of these observations are very consistent with a slow absorption pattern.

In the body, our results clearly show that in the first day after administration, radioactivity is present in all organs including the central nervous system (Figure 29.6). However, several tissues are able to concentrate mebendazole or its main metabolites; we have found in the three animal species studied that radioactivity persists for as long as 1 month in melanin-containing tissues (Figure 29.7) and in the liver of sheep. Persistence of residues in the liver is the consequence of prolonged biliary excretion which lasts 10 days in sheep and 15 days in guinea-fowl chicks. Such a long biliary excretion can be explained by an enterohepatic cycle. The long persistence of residues in the liver can also be explained by the presence of conjugated and covalently bound metabolites as demonstrated previously[2,3]. In the liver, the residual concentrations 15 days after administration are : 1.27 ppm in sheep. 0.70 ppm in guinea-fowl chicks and 0.50 ppm in hen-pheasants.

CONCLUSION

From a safety point of view. hepatic residues of mebendazole and its metabolites are most important since they are the most persistent. In order to define tolerance limits for this drug, one must consider toxicological data and the toxicological significance of these hepatic residues. Such an approach would seem to provide a rational basis for estimating the relative hazard of the residues compared to the parent drug.

References
1. Bénard. P., Rico. A.G., Braun, J.P., Burgat. V., Bonnaud. B. and Cousse. H. (1981). Picafibrate. Note II : Absorption, distribution et élimination chez le rat après marquage au carbone-14. Boll. Chim. Farm. 120:114-123.
2. Bénard. P., Burgat, V., Massat. F. and Rico, A.G. (1984). Metabolism of C-14-mebendazole in sheep. 9th European Congress on Drug Metabolism Workshop, Pont à Mousson, Abstract. P4.
3. Burgat-Sacaze. V. and Rico. A.G. (1984). Bioactivation and bound residues. Food Additives and Contaminants 2:121-129.
4. Ullberg. S. (1954). Studies on the distribution and fate of S-35-labelled benzylpenicillin in the body. Acta Radiol.. Suppl.118:1-110.

Diarrhoea

30
Modulation of intestinal ion absorption and secretion by enterotoxins, hormones and neurotransmitters

H. R. DE JONGE AND A. B. VAANDRAGER

ABSTRACT

The absorption of electrolytes and water by mammalian small intestine and proximal colon is primarily controlled by an electroneutral entry mechanism for Na^+ and Cl^- in the brush-border membrane of the enterocytes, consisting of parallel Na^+/H^+ and Cl^-/HCO_3^- exchangers coupled by circular proton movements. Enterotoxins produced by non-invasive micro-organisms (such as choleratoxin, heat-stable and heat-labile Escherichia coli toxin) and neurohumoral factors (such as acetylcholine, vasoactive intestinal peptide [VIP], prostaglandins, bradykinin) promote salt and water secretion by a dual action involving (1) blockade of the antiporters in the villus compartment and (2) Cl^- channel opening in the apical membrane of intestinal crypt cells, allowing Cl^- exit down an electrochemical gradient created by a basolateral $Na-K-Cl_2$ entry process. During Cl^- secretion, the accumulation of Na^+ and K^+ in the enterocyte is prevented by Na^+ exit through the Na^+/K^+-pump and K^+ exit through secretagogue-sensitive K^+ channels in the basolateral membrane.

Secretagogues act through at least three different mechanisms :

(1) a reversible activation of adenylate cyclase coupled to hormone receptors (VIP, PGE_2) in the basolateral membrane or a permanent activation of this enzyme through ADP-ribosylation of the coupling factor N_s (CT, LT), both leading to cyclic AMP accumulation;

(2) activation of guanylate cyclase in the brush-border membrane presumably by thiol-disulphide exchange (ST_A) and raising intramicrovillous cyclic GMP levels;

(3) receptor-mediated activation of a phosphatidylinositol specific phospholipase C in the basolateral membrane (such as acetylcholine) generating two products : inositoltri-phosphate (IP_3), initiating Ca^{2+} mobilization from internal stores; and diacylglycerol (DAG), an activator of Ca^{2+}/phospholipid-dependent protein kinase (C-kinase). The recent recognition of high-affinity receptors for cyclic nucleotides, DAG and Ca^{2+} in the intestinal brush-border as regulatory components of protein kinases suggest a causal relationship between protein phosphoryl-ation and modulation of ion transport systems in the apical membrane. Calcium may additionally inhibit Na^+/Cl^- entry in a more direct manner through binding to the Ca^{2+} receptor protein calmodulin.

New aspects of stimulus-secretion coupling discussed in this review include :

(1) the role of a 25,000 molecular weight proteolipid in the brush-border membrane as a key regulator of ion trans-port across the apical membrane, its phosphorylation by both cyclic GMP-dependent and cyclic AMP-dependent protein kinases and a possible link between its phosphorylation state and phosphatidylinositol metabolism ("PI-cycle") in intestinal microvilli;

(2) the identification of potential targets for pharmaco-logical intervention along the molecular pathways leading to secretion, potentially enabling the rational design of new antidiarrhoeal drugs.

INTRODUCTION

Diarrhoeal diseases constitute a major cause of morbidity and mortality on a global scale[19]. Plasmid-encoded heat-labile (LT) and heat-stable (ST) enterotoxigenic proteins secreted by Escherichia coli are the most frequent cause of non-inflammatory infectious diarrhoea in man and of neonatal diarrhoea in calves, lambs and piglets. Both toxins evoke excessive water and electrolyte secretion by triggering a physiological mechanism of stimulus-secretion coupling in the intestinal epithelium. In this chapter, the mode of action of each of these toxins is briefly discussed and its similarity to the action of neurohumoral regulators of intestinal secretion is emphasized. Moreover, recent insights into the mechanisms by which intracellular signals (cyclic nucleotides, Ca^{2+}) could modulate ion transport processes in the intestinal brush-border membrane are recapitulated.

HEAT-LABILE ESCHERICHIA COLI TOXINS

The heat-labile toxins, analogous to choleratoxin, are composed of five binding (B) subunits and one active (A) subunit. Following binding of B to surface receptors on the intestinal microvilli (ganglioside, and perhaps glyco-protein), the A subunit is injected into the cytoplasm and split by disulphide bond reduction into fragments A_1 and A_2. The A_1 peptide migrates towards the basolateral membrane and activates adenylate cyclase in an essentially irreversible manner by catalysing transfer of the ADP-ribosyl moiety of NAD^+ (nicotinamide adenine dinucleo-tide) to an arginine residue in the $alpha_s$ subunit of the coupling protein N_s (references [4,18] for recent reviews). Sustained activation of the cyclase leads to excessive production of cyclic AMP, an intracellular signal leading to electrolyte secretion. The spontaneous recovery from heat-labile and choleratoxin-provoked diarrhoea may there-fore only occur by turnover of cells or regulatory pro-teins. In contrast, some endogenous secretagogues, such as vasoactive intestinal peptide (VIP) and eicosanoids

(PGE$_2$) induce a less permanent activation of adenylate cyclase through binding to basolateral hormone receptors. Neurohumoral cascade mechanisms may potentiate toxin-evoked secretion. For example, heat-labile (and possibly heat-stable toxins also) could mobilize serotonin from enterochromaffin cells, initiating a neural reflex through a nicotinic ganglion to liberate a secretagogue (possibly VIP or acetylcholine) that acts on the enterocyte[1,13].

HEAT-STABLE ESCHERICHIA COLI TOXINS

Heat-stable enterotoxins are low-molecular weight peptides (18-72 amino acids) lacking a subunit structure. One cysteine-rich subclass (ST$_A$) binds to a protein receptor in the intestinal microvilli and triggers a rapid and reversible activation of a unique isoenzyme of guanylate cyclase (GC) embedded in the apical membrane[5,16]; Figure 30.1). Membrane-bound forms of guanylate cyclase in non-intestinal tissues seem to be insensitive to the toxin[25]. Both the structure and mechanism of action of ST$_A$ show a striking resemblance to a recently discovered family of peptide hormones, the atrial natriuretic factors (ANF)[21]. Recent evidence suggests that a reversible activation of particulate guanylate cyclase in non-intestinal tissues (smooth muscle, kidney, adrenal cells) forms the basis of their antihypertensive action[29]. Activation of guanylate cyclase by ST$_A$ or ANF is reproducible in isolated membranes in the absence of soluble proteins or co-factors, such as NAD$^+$, excluding a choleratoxin-like mechanism. Studies in our laboratory[7], and elsewhere[12], have also ruled out a cascade mechanism analogous to hormone-induced phospholipid turnover, but instead suggest a direct interaction between ST$_A$ and its receptor or guanylate cyclase itself presumably involving mixed disulphide formation. Our recent finding that bivalent metal ions (Cu^{2+}, Cd^{2+}, Zn^{2+}) and hemin were able to mimic ST$_A$-activation of the brush-border cyclase, whereas the action of all three compounds, but not basal guanylate cyclase activity, was inhibited by thiol-blocking and

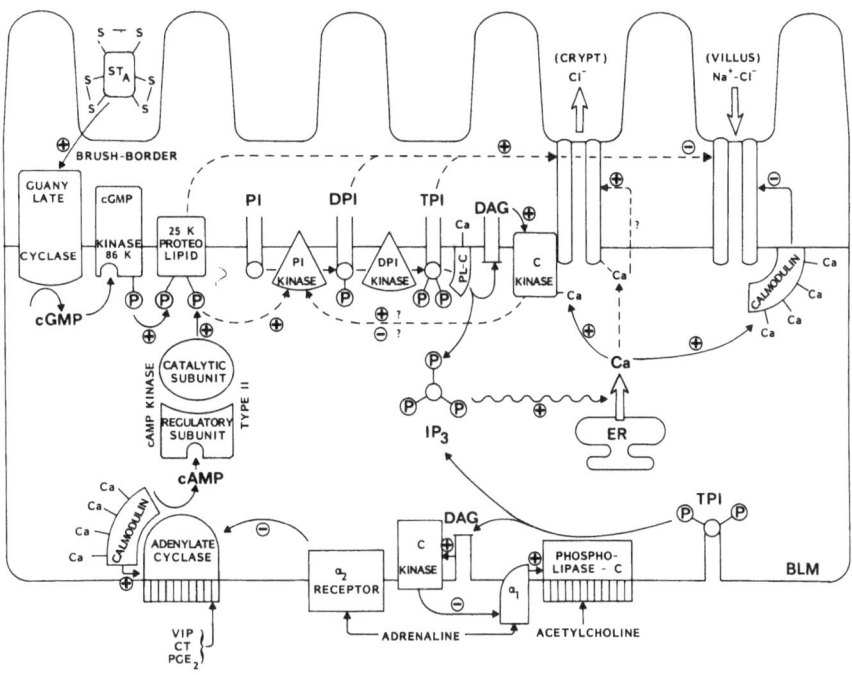

Figure 30.1 Model of stimulus-secretion coupling in intestinal epithelium. Details of the various secretory
mechanisms are explained in the text. ST$_A$, heat-stable
Escherichia coli toxin; CT, choleratoxin; PGE$_2$, prostaglandin E$_2$; VIP, vasoactive intestinal peptide; PI, phosphatidylinositol; DPI, phosphatidylinositol-4-phosphate;
TPI, phosphatidylinositol-4,5-biphosphate ; DAG, diacylglycerol; PL-C, phospholipase C; IP$_3$, inositol 1,4,5,-
triphosphate; BLM, basolateral membrane; ER, endoplasmic
reticulum : +, stimulation; -, inhibition.

disulphide-reducing agents, further indicates the role of
critical SH-groups in the activation mechanism. Inte-
restingly, ANF was unable to mimic the action of ST$_A$ on
guanylate cyclase and ion transport in rat intestine (H.R.
de Jonge, unpublished observation) but it reproduced
perfectly the blockade of NaCl entry by cyclic GMP in
teleost intestine (S.M. O'Grady and M. Field, personal
communication).

The other major subclass of heat-stable toxins, STs, initiates intestinal secretion exclusively in weaned piglets by a presently unknown mechanism distinct from adenylate or guanylate cyclase activation[30].

PHYSIOLOGICAL SECRETAGOGUES ACTING THROUGH CALCIUM

A number of endogenous secretagogues, such as acetylcholine, serotonin, neurotensin and bradykinin, do not directly change intestinal cyclic nucleotide levels but act primarily by a receptor-mediated activation of phospholipase C in the basolateral membrane of the enterocyte, leading to the rapid breakdown of polyphosphoinositides, a specific class of phospholipids[9]; see Figure 30.1. One of the products, inositoltriphosphate (IP$_3$), analogous to its role in other tissues, is likely to release Ca^{2+} from endoplasmic reticulum through an as yet unknown mechanism. By direct measurements of intracellular free Ca^{2+} levels in the colon carcinoma cell line HT-29 loaded with the fluorescent Ca^{2+} probe quin-2, we have recently obtained direct evidence for the triggering of internal Ca^{2+} mobilization by acetylcholine, neurotensin, adrenaline (acting through alpha$_1$-receptors) and bradykinin (see Figure 30.1). In contrast to recent observations in chicken enterocytes[2], no changes in intracellular Ca^{2+} levels were observed in response to PGE$_2$, VIP, cyclic AMP and cyclic GMP indicating that, at least in this secretory cell type, Ca^{2+} did not function as a third messenger.

The other product of phospholipid breakdown, diacylglycerol (DAG) stimulates a Ca^{2+}/phospholipid-dependent protein kinase (C-kinase) recently discovered in the cytosol and brush-border membranes of villous and crypt epithelium[9]. Direct activation of the enzyme in intact epithelium by phorbolesters and membrane-permeable diacylglycerols partially mimicked the secretory action of acetylcholine in rabbit ileum and colon[3,10], underscoring its importance in signal transduction.

Mucosal and submucosal prostaglandins, presumably generated from arachidonic acid released by Ca^{2+}-activation of phospholipase A_2, do not play a role in the acute phase of the secretory response to acetylcholine (0-2 min) but appeared to be responsible for the maintenance of the response during the next 5-10 min. This conclusion is based on our recent electrophysiological measurements in rat intestinal mucosa mounted in Ussing chambers and exposed to carbachol in the presence or absence of indomethacin (10^{-5}M), a specific blocker of prostaglandin synthesis. In this model system, prostaglandins were apparently not involved in the secretory response to VIP, cyclic nucleotides, substance P and bradykinin (H.R. de Jonge and J.A. Groot, manuscript in preparation).

A third mechanism contributing to acetylcholine-evoked secretion is the influx of extracellular Ca^{2+} through hormone-responsive and verapamil-sensitive Ca^{2+}-channels in the basolateral membrane. However, our recent measurements of Ca^{2+} transients in the HT-29 cell line have shown that, in comparison with other cell lines, such as fibroblasts, the hormone-induced Ca^{2+} signals in the colonocytes were remarkably resistant to extracellular Ca^{2+}-depletion. The secretory response to cyclic nucleotides in rabbit ileum was also found to be insensitive to Ca^{2+} depletion at the serosal side of the epithelium[11].

PHYSIOLOGICAL ANTISECRETAGOGUES

Noradrenaline, the principal sympathetic neurotransmitter producing absorption, is able to counteract the secretory response to acetylcholine, VIP, choleratoxin and heat-labile toxins (but not to cyclic nucleotides; H.R. de Jonge, unpublished observations) through binding to $alpha_2$-receptors on the enterocytes followed by blockade of adenylate cyclase through the inhibitory factor N_i[7,13,18]; (Figure 30.1). At least part of its antagonism of acetylcholine action may be explained by the involvement of prostaglandins in the secretory response to acetylcholine.

Other important antisecretory hormones and neurotransmitters include :

(1) angiotensin, presumably acting through noradrenaline
release[23];
(2) dopamine, acting through dopaminergic receptors different from peripheral DA_1 - or DA_2 -receptors[28];
(3) enkephalins, increasing basal absorption rates but not
blocking secretagogue actions, probably mediated through
delta-receptors in the submucous plexus[24].

Somatostatin and neuropeptides may also promote basal
absorption rates through as yet unknown mechanisms.

COUPLING MECHANISMS BETWEEN SECOND MESSENGERS AND ION
TRANSPORT SYSTEMS IN THE INTESTINAL BRUSH-BORDER
The major Ca^{2+}-, diacylglycerol (DAG)- and cyclic nucleo-
tide-sensitive electrolyte transport systems in the
enterocyte have been localized at the mucosal border and
include :

(1) an electroneutral Na-Cl co-transport process in the
villus cell, presumably composed of separate Na^+/H^+ and
Cl^-/CHO_3^- exchangers coupled by circular proton movements.
The blockade of one or both exchangers by Ca^{2+}, DAG or
cyclic nucleotide signals may lead to a reduced absorption
rate of NaCl and water in the villus compartment;
(2) an electrogenic Cl^- channel, presumably enriched in
intestinal crypt cells. The triggering of Cl^- channel
opening by cyclic AMP or Ca^{2+} constitutes the basis of
hormone-induced salt secretion in a number of other secretory epithelia[17]; however, a similar role for cyclic GMP
is unique for intestinal epithelium[9].

    The molecular mechanism involved in stimulus-secretion
coupling at the level of the brush-border membrane
constitutes a major area of research in our laboratory.
High-affinity receptors for intracellular signals identi-

fied in the apical membrane include :

(1) a unique isoenzyme of cyclic GMP-dependent protein kinase (G-kinase) structurally and immunologically different from soluble and particulate G-kinases in other
tissues[6,8,9];
(2) the type II isoenzyme of cyclic AMP-dependent protein
kinase (A-kinase[8,9]);
(3) Ca^{2+}/phospholipid-dependent protein kinase (C-kinase[9]);
(4) Ca^{2+}/calmodulin-dependent protein kinase[8];
(5) calmodulin, presumably forming a complex with the Na-
Cl cotransport system[14] (Figure 30.1);
(6) phospholipase C, triggered by micromolar amounts of
Ca^{2+} (Figure 30.1).

Most protein kinases were found capable of phosphorylating
a specific set of apical membrane proteins. The precise
role of each of these phosphoproteins in stimulus-
secretion coupling has still to be elucidated. However,
only the G-kinase showed an extremely limited substrate
specificity : apart from catalysing phosphate incorporation into its own structure (autophosphorylation; Figure
30.1), it was found capable of phosphorylating only one
other brush-border protein possessing a molecular weight
of 25,000[7-9]. The same protein also served as one of the
major substrates for A-kinase in the brush-border region, and might therefore play a crucial role in cyclic
nucleotide-provoked ion secretion.

STRUCTURE AND FUNCTION OF THE 25K PROTEIN COMPONENT OF THE
INTESTINAL BRUSH-BORDER
The 25K protein is a minor component of the brush-border
membrane, but also one of the major phosphoproteins
extractable by chloroform-methanol in the presence of HCl
(but not in its absence[8]), and should therefore by
classified as an acidic proteolipid. Mapping of its
phosphorylation sites by tryptic fingerprinting has

recently demonstrated that the same serine residues (possibly two) are recognized by both G- and A-kinase but not by endogenous Ca²⁺/calmodulin-kinase and C-kinase[7]. In this respect, the protein clearly differs from phospholamban, a 25K proteolipid regulating Ca²⁺-pump activity in heart membranes, which is phosphorylated on different sites by A-, C- and Ca²⁺/calmodulin kinases[22]. Analogous to phospholamban, the 25K protein might function as a regulatory subunit of an ion transport system or even be identical to the ion channel or carrier itself.

Preliminary results from phosphorylation studies with isolated brush-borders in our laboratory, however, suggest that cyclic GMP-dependent protein phosphorylation, presumably of the 25K proteolipid, triggers the phosphorylation of a phospholipid component of the apical membrane – in other words, it converts phosphatidylinositol (PI) into DPI (Figure 30.1). Similarly to DPI-modulation of a Ca²⁺-pump in skeletal muscle[27], the formation of DPI in the vicinity of the transporter might directly regulate its function. Alternatively, phosphoryl- ation of PI may start a cascade of other phospholipid transitions ("PI-cycle") very similar to hormone-induced PI turnover at the baso-lateral membrane (Figure 30.1). Enzymes involved in such lipid transition (such as PI-kinase and DPI-kinase; phospholipase C) were found to be integral components of the brush-border membrane (A.B. Vaandrager-manuscript in preparation). As shown in Figure 30.1, the main products of PI metabolism, that is, IP₃ and DAG, may promote Ca²⁺-mobilization and C-kinase activation at the brush-border region, analogous to the action of acetylcholine at the basolateral membrane. This concept, although still rather speculative, may elegantly explain several recent observations :

(1) the occurrence of a highly active polyphosphoinositide turnover in the apical membrane despite the apparent lack of hormone receptors at this subcellular region; the model in fact suggests that the action of first messengers at

the basolateral membrane is mimicked by second messengers
at the brush-border membrane;
(2) the reversal of cyclic nucleotide-provoked inhibition
of the Na-Cl entry pathway by calmodulin antagonists
(chlorpromazine, trifluoperazine[11,14]);
(3) the cyclic AMP-induced internal Ca^{2+}-mobilization measured in chicken villous cells by the quin-2 method[2].

Future research on PI metabolism in the brush-border and
analysis of the properties of the 25K proteolipid is
needed to further substantiate this model.

TARGETS FOR PHARMACOLOGICAL INTERVENTION IN SECRETORY
DIARRHOEA
A better knowledge of the molecular pathways leading to
excessive electrolyte and water secretion could potentially lead to the rational design of new antidiarrhoeal
drugs. Unfortunately, most regulatory components of the
absorptive and secretory pathways in the enterocyte are
not unique to the intestinal epithelium (compare $alpha_2$-,
delta- and dopamine receptors; adenylate and guanylate
cyclases; A-, G- and C-kinase; phospholipase A_2 and C;
cyclo-oxygenase). Moreover, transport systems involved in
secretion (Na-K-Cl_2 co-transport; Cl^--channels and
Ca^{2+}-sensitive channels) are also operating in other
epithelial tissues, such as kidney and trachea. Therefore,
the ideal antidiarrhoeal drug should be effective upon
oral administration and should be prevented of reaching
the circulation, for example, by rapid inactivation in the
liver or by entrapment in the intestinal lumen or epithelial cell layer. Compounds interacting from the luminal
site with secretory components of the brush-border membrane are potentially important candidates. With reference to the model shown in Figure 30.1, such compounds
may include : (1) Cl^- channel blockers; (2) anticalmodulin
drugs (such as trifluoperazine; calmidazolium); (3) inhibitors of PI metabolism in the brush-border membrane (such
as chlorpromazine); and (4) inhibitors of A-, G- and

C-kinase. Cyclic nucleotide receptor antagonists (such as Rp-cAMPS; compare reference[26]), and a novel class of potent and selective protein kinase inhibitors, the iso-quinoline sulphonamides[20] are presently being screened in our laboratory for antidiarrhoeal activity.

References
1. Cassuto, J., Siewert, A., Jodal, M. and Lundgren, O. (1982). The involvement of intramural nerves in choleratoxin-induced intestinal secretion. Acta Physiol. Scand. 117:195-202.
2. Chang, E.B. and Semrad, C.E. (1985). Calcium-mediated cyclic AMP inhibition of Na/H exchange in chicken small intestine. Gastroenterology 88:1345.
3. Chang, E.B., Wang, N.S. and Rao, M.C. (1985). Role of protein C-kinase in intestinal anion secretion. Gastroenterology 88:1345.
4. Coulson, C.J., Nassau, P.M. and Tait, R.M. (1984). The ADP-ribosyltransferase activity of choleratoxin and Escherichia coli heat-labile toxin. Biochem. Soc. Trans. 12:184-187.
5. De Jonge, H.R. (1975). The localization of guanylate cyclase in rat small intestinal epithelium. FEBS Lett. 53:237-242.
6. De Jonge, H.R. (1981). Cyclic GMP-dependent protein kinase in intestinal brush-borders. Adv. Cyclic Nucleotide Res. 14:315-333.
7. De Jonge, H.R. (1984). The mechanism of action of Escherichia coli heat-stable toxin. Biochem. Soc. Trans. 12:180-184.
8. De Jonge, H.R. (1984). Cyclic nucleotide-dependent protein phosphorylation in intestinal epithelium. Kroc Foundation Ser. 17:263-286.
9. De Jonge, H.R. and Lohmann, S.M. (1985). Mechanisms by which cyclic nucleotides and other intracellular mediators regulate secretion. Ciba Foundation Symp. 112:116-138.
10. Donowitz, M., Cheng, N. and Sharp, G.W.G. (1985). Role of protein kinase C in regulation of rat colonic active NaCl transport. Gastroenterology 88:1367.
11. Donowitz, M., Wicks, J., Madara, J.L. and Sharp, G.W. G. (1985). Studies on role of calmodulin in Ca^{2+} regulation of rabbit ileal Na and Cl transport. Am. J. Physiol. 248:G726-G740.
12. Dreyfus, L.A., Jaso-Friedmann, L. and Robertson, D.C. (1984). Characterization of the mechanism of action of Escherichia coli heat-stable enterotoxin. Infect. Immunol. 44:493-501.
13. Eklund, S., Jodal, M. and Lundgren, O. (1985). The enteric nervous system participates in the secretory response to the heat-stable enterotoxin of Escherichia coli in rats and cats. Neuroscience 14:673-681.
14. Fan, C.C. and Powell, D.W. (1983). Calcium/calmodulin inhibition of coupled NaCl transport in membrane

vesicles from rabbit ileal brush-border. Proc. Natl.
Acad. Sci. USA 80:5248-5252.

15. Field, M. and McColl, I. (1973). Ion transport in
rabbit ileal mucosa. III. Effects of catecholamines.
Am. J. Physiol. 225:852-857.

16. Field, M., Graf, L.H. Jr., Laird, W.S. and Smith, P.L.
(1978). Heat-stable enterotoxin of Escherichia coli :
in vitro effects on guanylate cyclase activity, cyclic
GMP concentration of ion transport in small intestine.
Proc. Natl. Acad. Sci. USA 75:2800-2805.

17. Frizzell, R.A., Field, M. and Schultz, S.G. (1979).
Sodium-coupled chloride transport by epithelial
tissues. Am. J. Physiol. 236:F1-F8.

18. Gill, D.M. and Woolkalis, M. (1985). Toxins which
activate adenylate cyclase. Ciba Foundation Symp.
112:57-73.

19. Guerrant, R.L. (1985). Microbial toxins and diarrhoeal diseases : introduction and overview. Ciba
Foundation Symp. 112:1-13.

20. Hidaka, H., Inagaki, M., Kawamoto, S. and Sasaki, Y.
(1984). Isoquinalinesulfonamides. Novel and potent
inhibitors of cyclic nucleotide dependent protein
kinase and protein kinase C. Biochemistry 23:
5036-5041.

21. Kangawa, K., Fukuda, A. and Matsuo, H. (1985). Structural identification of ß- and Ɣ-human atrial natriuretic polypeptides. Nature (London) 313:397-400.

22. Le Peuch, C.J., Haiech, J. and Demaille, J.G. (1979).
Concerted regulation of cardiac sarcoplasmic reticulum
calcium transport by cAMP-dependent and calcium-
calmodulin-dependent phosphorylation. Biochemistry
18:5150-5157.

23. Levels, N.R. (1985). Control of intestinal absorption
by the renin-angiotensin system. Am. J. Physiol.
249:G3-G15.

24. Miller, R.J., Brown, D.R., Chang, E.B. and Friel, D.D.
(1985). The pharmacological modification of secretory
responses. Ciba Foundation Symp. 112:155-174.

25. Rao, M.C., Guandalini, S., Smith, P.L. and Field, M.
(1980). Mode of action of heat-stable E. coli
enterotoxin : tissue and subcellular specificities and
role of cyclic GMP. Biochim. Biophys. Acta 632:35-46.

26. Van Haastert, P.J.M., Van Driel, R., Jastorff, B.,
Baraniak, J., Stec, W.J. and De Wit, R.J.W. (1984).
Competitive cAMP antagonists for cAMP-receptor
proteins. J. Biol. Chem. 259:10020-10024.

27. Varsanyi, M., Tölle, H.G., Heilmeyer, L.M.G. Jr., Dawson, R.M.C. and Irvine, R.F. (1983). Activation of
sarcoplasmic reticular Ca^{2+}-transport ATPase by phosphorylation of an associated phosphatidylinositol.
Embo J. 2:1543-1548.

28. Wahawisan, R., Gaginella, T.S. and Wallace, L.J.
(1985). Jejunal-ileal difference in dopaminergic but
not α-adrenergic anti-secretory effects. Am. J.
Physiol. 248:G332-G336.

29. Waldman, S.A., Rapoport, R.M. and Mucad, F. (1984).

Atrial natriuretic factor selectively activates particulate guanylate cyclase and elevates cyclic GMP in rat tissues. J. Biol. Chem. 259:14332-14334.

30. Weikel, C.S. and Guerrant, R.L. (1985). ST$_a$ enterotoxin of Escherichia coli : cyclic nucleotide-independent secretion. Ciba Foundation Symp. 112: 94-115.

31
Species and age-dependent factors governing the clinical severity of diarrhoea

R. A. ARGENZIO

ABSTRACT

Many of the species and age-dependent factors governing the severity of a diarrhoea can be explained by the development of colonic function. Compensatory responses by the colon for a small bowel diarrhoea are brought about by the aldosterone mechanism and by the microbial fermentation process. These two functions may be of importance in enterotoxigenic secretory diarrhoea and in small bowel malabsorptive disease. Similarly, in species where colonic function is quantitatively important, such as in non-ruminant herbivores, colonic malabsorption or secretion may result in serious fluid and energy losses, whereas in carnivores, colonic disease usually results in mild diarrhoea and weight loss is uncommon. The quantitative importance of the colon in fluid and energy absorption and in compensating for small bowel fluid losses is age-dependent and may explain to some degree the age-dependent resistance in some species to infectious diarrhoea.

INTRODUCTION

Loss of body fluids, electrolytes, and energy due to a given enteric infection differs substantially in the neonate and the adult animal. Although these age-dependent differences are in large part due to development of immunological factors and mucosal resistance, a second important factor which has been less well appreciated is development of colonic function. In diseases affecting primarily the small bowel, the compensatory response of the colon may be substantial and is mediated by (a) the aldosterone mechanism, and (b) microbial fermentation of carbohydrate. The efficacy of this compensatory response is dependent on colonic absorptive capacity and the development of microbial digestion, both age-dependent factors. On the other hand, the severity of a diarrhoea in diseases primarily affecting the colon will be greater in the older animal. This is because the adult colon, especially in non-ruminant herbivores and omnivores, normally handles much more fluid than the neonatal colon and loss of this fluid is significant.

This chapter describes the response of secretory and malabsorptive diarrhoeas affecting either the small or large bowel and some of the age-dependent factors involved in the severity of the response.

ENTEROSYSTEMIC CYCLE AND DEVELOPMENT OF COLONIC FUNCTION

Depending on the species and age of the animal, there are large differences in the amount of endogenous fluids handled daily by the intestine. In all species, these digestive secretions increase with age, but the relative amounts are much greater in herbivores. In adult non-ruminant herbivores (the pig will be included in this group), these daily secretions may equal the extracellular fluid volume. Most of these fluids are reabsorbed by the distal intestine and colon[6,11]. The proximal intestine becomes relatively inefficient in absorption after the animal is weaned. Prior to weaning, however, the small bowel may reabsorb up to 90% of these endogenous secretions[1]. This change in intestinal handling of fluid parallels the development of microbial fermentation digestion in the large intestine, which requires large amounts of buffered fluids for its operation. A similar pattern

is not seen in the ruminant and carnivore whose small
intestine remains relatively efficient.

These differences in intestinal function explain to a
degree why the relative dehydration and malnutrition caused by a small or large bowel diarrhoea differ substantially depending on the species and age of the animal affected. For example, small bowel involvement in the dog is
characterized by large volumes of stool and, if chronic,
weight loss is present, while large bowel involvement is
characterized by small stools and weight loss is uncommon[4]. In contrast, large bowel involvement in the pig or
horse may be characterized by a fatal loss of extracellular fluids, and if a more chronic condition is present,
weight loss can be expected[2].

MALABSORPTIVE DIARRHOEA : SMALL INTESTINE

Malabsorptive diarrhoea is commonly caused by enteric
viral infection. These agents cause villous atrophy in
various degrees of severity, resulting in both maldiges-
tion due to loss of surface enzymes and malabsorption due
to the loss of transport mechanisms. In the pig, both
rotavirus and coronavirus result in marked losses of lac-
tase and sucrase enzymes and failure of the intestinal mucosa to absorb glucose[5,7,12].

There is an age-dependent resistance to the severity of
enteric virus infection. Moon et al.[8] have shown that the
turnover rate of intestinal epithelium increases with age
in the pig, so that in older pigs, regeneration of the
villus could occur more rapidly. They have postulated
that this more rapid restoration of the villus in older
pigs may be responsible for the age-dependent resistance
to transmissible gastroenteritis virus (TGE).

However, an equally important feature in these malabsorptive diseases is the degree of compensation by the
colon. In the case of the pig coronavirus (TGE), the
colon is unaffected and could presumably compensate for
the small bowel malabsorption to some degree. It must be
kept in mind, however, that the milk lactose, or any

carbohydrate for that matter, cannot be digested and absorbed by the colonic epithelium. Rather, these carbo-
hydrates are fermented by microbial action to volatile
fatty acids (VFA), which can then be absorbed by the
colonic mucosa. Thus, the ability to compensate relies on
the development of microbial digestion. In pigs 1 week
old or less, both rotavirus and coronavirus infections
lead to severe diarrhoea with large amounts of lactose in
the stool[1,5]. However, in 3 weeks old infected pigs which
had been introduced to some solid feed, nearly all of the
unabsorbed lactose was converted to VFA and absorbed as
such. Thus, these older pigs had a very mild diarrhoea
and maintained their body weight, even though the small
bowel was severely affected[1]. These factors again point
out the importance of colonic compensation in older
animals.

MALABSORPTIVE DIARRHOEA : LARGE INTESTINE
An example of a colonic malabsorptive disease is swine
dysentery. This disease exclusively affects the large
bowel and results in malabsorption of ions and water;
hypersecretion is not evident[3]. In older pigs, the
dehydration can be severe, resulting in death in up to 60%
of the cases. Presumably, this reflects the fact that the
colon must reabsorb large amounts of endogenous secretions
to preserve the extracellular fluid volume in these
animals.

   Similar, acute diarrhoeas are seen in horses with colonic involvement[9]; however, in this species, endotoxin absorption and prostaglandin production may cause hypersecretion by the colon.

   In dogs, colonic inflammation usually results in chronic diarrhoea with small amounts of fluid lost. This can
be postulated to be due to two factors. First, cyclic AMP
does not seem to cause colonic secretion in the dog[10], so
that products of inflammation (such as prostaglandins) may
not be capable of activating colonic secretion in this
species. Secondly, a colonic malabsorption caused by

mucosal damage would not result in serious loss of fluids, due to the efficiency of small bowel absorption in this species.

Thus, there appears to be a great deal of species variation in the response to inflammation. Further study may provide a critical role for metabolites of arachidonic acid in these responses.

References
1. Argenzio, R.A., Moon, H.W., Kemeny, L.J. and Whipp, S. C. (1984). Colonic compensation in transmissible gastroenteritis of swine. Gastroenterology 86:1501-1509.
2. Argenzio, R.A. and Whitlock, R.H. (1980). Diseases of the colon, rectum, and anus in the horse, cow, and pig. In: Anderson, N.V. (ed.). Veterinary Gastroenterology,pp.523-552. Philadelphia: Lea and Febiger.
3. Argenzio, R.A., Whipp, S.C. and Glock, R.D. (1980). Pathophysiology of swine dysentery : colonic transport and permeability studies. J. Infect. Dis. 142: 676-684.
4. Burrows, C.F. (1980). Diseases of the colon, rectum, and anus in the dog and cat. In: Anderson, N.V. (ed.). Veterinary Gastroenterology, pp.553-592. Philadelphia: Lea and Febiger.
5. Graham, D.Y., Sackman, J.W. and Estes, M.K. (1984). Pathogenesis of rotavirus-induced diarrhoea. Dig. Dis. Sci. 29:1028-1035.
6. Hamilton, D.L. and Roe, W.E. (1977). Electrolyte levels and net fluid and electrolyte movements in the gastrointestinal tract of weanling swine. Can. J. Comp. Med. 41:241-250.
7. Kerzner, B., Kelly, M.H., Gall, D.G., Butler, D.G. and Hamilton, J.R. (1977). Transmissible gastroenteritis: sodium transport and the intestinal epithelium during the course of viral enteritis. Gastroenterology 72:457-461.
8. Moon, H.W., Kemeny, L.J., Lambert, G., Stark, S.L. and Booth, G.D. (1975). Age-dependent resistance to transmissible gastroenteritis of swine. Vet. Pathol. 12:434-445.
9. Palmer, J.E. (1984). Acute diarrhoeal diseases of the adult horse. Proc. American College of Veterinary Internal Medicine, Washington, DC, pp.247-250.
10. Robinson, J.W.L. (1976). Inhibition of transport processes in the dog colon. In: Robinson, J.W.L. (ed.). Intestinal Ion Transport, pp.187-198. Baltimore: University Park Press.
11. Schmall, L.M., Argenzio, R.A. and Whipp, S.C. (1982). Effects of intravenous Escherichia coli endotoxin on gastrointestinal function in the pony. In : Byars, T.G., Moore, J.W. and White, N.A. (eds). Proc. Equine Colic Research Symposium, Athens, Georgia, pp.157-164. University of Georgia : College of Veterinary Medi-

cine.
12. Shepperd, R.W., Gall, D.G., Butler, D.G. and Hamilton, J.R. (1979). Determinants of diarrhoea in viral en- teritis. Gastroenterology 76:20-24.

32
Antidiarrhoeal therapy

L. A. A. OOMS AND A.-D. DEGRYSE

ABSTRACT
A short review on the pharmacology of current antidiarrhoeal therapy is presented. Fluid replacement
therapy and symptomatic therapy are useful in the treatment of diarrhoea of varying origin. The pharmacology of
loperamide, alpha-2-agonists, anti-inflammatory drugs,
chlorpromazine, trifluoperazine, parasympatholytics and
serotonin-2-antagonists is discussed.

INTRODUCTION
Theoretically, diarrhoea can be classified into decreased
intestinal absorption, increased intestinal secretion,
decreased transit time and diarrhoea due to local blood
flow disturbances. The origin of diarrhoea can be located
in the small and/or large intestine. Usually, more than
one factor is involved; exceptionally it is restricted to
only small or large intestine.

FLUID REPLACEMENT THERAPY
Intravenous fluids are effective, but require maintenance
therapy. Oral rehydration in diarrhoea is viewed as a
practical and effective therapy, especially in secretory
diarrhoea. In the developing countries, oral rehydration
of man is established as pivotal by the World Health

Organization[40].

The coupled Na-organic solute (glucose or neutral amino acids) mechanism is still active in secretory diarrhoea. These two solutes increase the effective osmotic pressure in the intercellular spaces, thus creating a driving force for transepithelial water absorption. Rice water (the excess water in which whole rice has been cooked) is believed to supply amylose and amylopectin as carbohydrate sources (glucose is released by intraluminal digestion). In weanling pigs, diarrhoea induced with rotavirus followed by haemolytic enteropathogenic Escherichia coli, it was shown that the dietary regimen plays an important role in the treatment of diarrhoea. In piglets fed one-third of the nutrient intake either hourly or three times a day, the diarrhoea was shortened and the colonization of the E. coli and the shedding of rotavirus was less in comparison with the full dietary regimen[23].

SYMPTOMATIC TREATMENT OF DIARRHOEA
The symptomatic treatment of diarrhoeas of different origin can only be undertaken in animal species with substances reducing the occurrence in the absence of side-effects. Antidiarrhoeal specificity is defined as the ratio of the lowest dose producing undesirable effects, to the dose at which protection from diarrhoea occurs. The larger the ratio, the higher the anti-diarrhoeal specificity of a test compound. The data for different substances are summarized in Tables 32.1 and 32.2.

Loperamide
Loperamide (for extensive review, see [30] and [32]) has high antidiarrhoeal specificity, irrespective of the desired duration of such effects. Intravenous loperamide is capable of producing opiate-like CNS activity, although this activity occurred only at doses that are equal to or only slightly lower than the lethal dose[29]. Loperamide is by far the most specific of all known drugs producing

Table 32.1 Comparative pharmacological data on 20 compounds with antidiarrhoeal properties in rats : ED_{50} (mg/kg) for antidiarrhoeal activity and side-effects

	A	B	C	D	E	F
Anticholinergics						
1. Atropine	1.76	9.30	49.2	98.4	0.39[1]	–
2. Scopolamine	1.03	7.12	28.3	37.3	0.22[1]	–
3. Methylscopol- amine	3.52	14.1	37.3	74.6	2.67[1]	–
4. Propantheline	65.1	149.0	299.0	320.0	64.9[1]	–
5. Isopropamide	18.6	74.6	113.0	160.0	21.4[1]	–
Narcotic analgesics						
6. Phenazocine	6.65	15.3	23.0	40.0	8.18[2]	90.0
7. Dextromoramide	1.80	2.83	5.58	8.25	2.78[2]	71.8
8. Propoxyphene	25.0	50.1	90.0	101.0	48.2[2]	990.0
9. Anileridine	4.42	8.05	17.8	33.0	9.48[2]	175.0
10. Pethidine	16.3	30.2	52.5	87.0	54.5[2]	760.0
11. Fentanyl	0.19	0.49	0.96	1.60	0.86[2]	43.9
12. Methadone	2.19	6.38	12.6	16.9	14.2[2]	95.0
13. Codeine	2.85	10.8	28.8	70.0	56.5[2]	427.0
14. Morphine	1.52	5.21	30.9	60.7	33.6[2]	905.0
Antidiarrhoeals						
15. Diphenoxylate	0.15	0.54	1.41	4.77	12.8[2]	221.0
16. Difenoxine	0.04	0.16	0.31	0.91	4.06[2]	149.0
17. Nufenoxole	0.83	1.72	3.12	9.41	85.9[2]	105.0
18. Loperamide	0.15	0.29	0.61	1.81	160[2]	185.0
19. Clonidine	0.012	0.028	0.043	0.19	0.085[3]	–
20. Lidamidine	0.45	1.67	3.81	9.36	24.9[3]	184.0

Antidiarrhoeal activity by the castor oil test : A = lowest ED_{50}; B = ED_{50} 2 h; C = ED_{50} 4 h; D = ED_{50} 8 h.
Side effects : E = lowest ED_{50}; F = LD_{50}. The side effects limiting the antidiarrhoeal use of these drugs are : [1]mydriasis; [2]inhibition tail-withdrawal reaction; [3]autonomic side-effects.
– data not available.

Table 32.2 Comparative pharmacological data on 20 compounds with antidiarrhoeal properties in rats : antidiarrhoeal specificity, based on the data given in Table 32.1

	E/A	E/B	E/C	E/D	F/D
Anticholinergics					
1. Atropine	0.22	0.042	0.0079	0.0040	–
2. Scopolamine	0.21	0.031	0.0078	0.0059	–
3. Methylscopol-amine	0.76	0.19	0.072	0.036	–
4. Propantheline	1.00	0.44	0.22	0.20	–
5. Isopropamide	1.15	0.29	0.19	0.13	–
Narcotic analgesics					
6. Phenazocine	1.23	0.53	0.36	0.20	2.25
7. Dextromoramide	1.54	0.98	0.50	0.34	8.70
8. Propoxyphene	1.93	0.96	0.54	0.48	9.80
9. Anileridine	2.14	1.18	0.53	0.29	5.30
10. Pethidine	3.34	1.80	1.04	0.63	8.74
11. Fentanyl	4.53	1.76	0.90	0.54	27.4
12. Methadone	6.48	2.23	1.13	0.84	5.62
13. Codeine	19.9	5.24	1.97	0.81	6.10
14. Morphine	22.1	6.45	1.09	0.55	14.9
Antidiarrhoeals					
15. Diphenoxylate	85.3	23.7	9.08	2.68	46.3
16. Difenoxine	102.0	25.4	13.1	4.46	164.0
17. Nufenoxole	103.0	49.9	27.5	9.13	11.2
18. Loperamide	1067.0	552.0	262.0	88.4	102.0
19. Clonidine	7.08	3.04	1.97	0.45	–
20. Lidamidine	55.3	14.9	6.54	2.66	19.7

Antidiarrhoeal specificity – E/A : at peak effect; E/B : for a duration of action of 2 h; E/C : for a duration of action of 4 h; E/D : for a duration of action of 8 h; F/D: safety margin of antidiarrhoeal activity of 8 h.

antidiarrhoeal effects, irrespective of the desired duration of such effects (Table 32.1). In addition, loperamide also has a wide safety margin. High doses of loperamide are well tolerated over long periods of time, and do not lead to significant side-effects[2]. About 70% of orally administered ^{14}C-loperamide (1 mg/kg) in rats was absorbed by the intestine, 30% of which was secreted back into the intestinal cavity after demethylation while the remaining 40% was transferred to the liver, metabolized and largely excreted into the bile. In rats, unaltered loperamide was eliminated from the plasma with a half-life of 15 h. Only 1.4% of the dose was excreted in the urine up to 72 h. Although initial and maximum plasma levels were higher following intravenous administration than after oral administration, the elimination pattern was very similar.

Loperamide significantly inhibited the activity of the calmodulin-activated enzyme (calmodulin-activated phosphodiesterase activity) at concentrations as low as 5 µmol/l and reduced activity to levels observed in the absence of calmodulin between 50 and 100 µmol/l, suggesting that calmodulin had been completely inactivated. Morphine, diamorphine and dihydrocodeine and the opioid peptide metenkephalin had no effect. This was further supported by the inability of naloxone to reverse the inhibition of calmodulin by loperamide[26]. The order of potency of binding to calmodulin in the presence of calcium is : loperamide = diphenoxylate, chlorpromazine, promethazine, amitryptiline in order or decreasing potency. A positive correlation between calmodulin binding and antidiarrhoeal activity was demonstrated[43].

Loperamide reverses cholera (CT)-induced secretion (ligated colon loops in rats) without affecting adenylate cyclase and without affecting tissue cAMP levels (in man)[8]. Loperamide interferes with the secretory process at a point beyond the cAMP increase caused by activation of adenylate cyclase. The effect of loperamide on CT-induced secretion is blocked by naloxone without any effect on cAMP[34]. Loperamide prevents theophylline from inducing net chloride secretion, but does not signifi-

cantly affect the theophylline-dependent increase of Cl^-
exchange across the mucosal border[16]. Loperamide may
activate a separate Cl^- transport system across the
serosal border of the intestine ("morphine effect"). This
has also been demonstrated in the isolated rabbit colon
and rabbit ileum[28]. This increased Cl^- permeability could
reduce intestinal secretion by facilitating the net loss
of electrolytes from the mucosal epithelial cells into the
serosal bathing solution. Naloxone (10^{-6} M) prevents the
loperamide-induced increase in Cl^- movement across the
serosal border[16]. Also in the colon, loperamide reverses
the stimulated chloride secretion and produces an increase
in the chloride permeability of the serosal border. There
is also evidence of greater Na absorption and this further
enhances the antisecretory effect.

Using a triple lumen perfusion technique, it was shown
that loperamide (4 mg bolus followed by 3 mg/1 perfusate)
inhibited PGE_2 (5×10^{-4}M) induced secretion of Na, Cl and
water. Loperamide converted secretion to absorption in
three of six subjects and reduced mean water secretion by
$91.1 \pm 15.2\%$. In addition, loperamide given after the
PGE_2 reduced secretion[14]. Loperamide effectively antagonized prostaglandin (PGE_2, 5 mg orally) induced diarrhoea
in adult healthy male volunteers; also loperamide administered 30 min before PGE_2 prevented (4 mg orally) the PGE_2
induced diarrhoea. In patients undergoing pregnancy termination with prostaglandins ($PGF_{2\alpha}$) three oral doses of
4 mg loperamide at 6 h intervals prevented diarrhoea[18].
Also diarrhoea induced with other prostaglandin derivates
could be prevented by pretreatment with loperamide[22].
Loperamide did not reduce the prostaglandin-induced increase in net Cl secretion, although it prevented the inhibition of mucosal-to-serosal Na movement. Hence, loperamide does not alter cyclic adenosine 3',5'-monophosphate
levels induced by prostaglandins by a direct action at the
enterocyte, since in isolated enterocytes, neither basal
nor prostaglandin-stimulated cyclic AMP levels were affected by the drug[13]. Oral administration of 0.1-2 mg/kg

PGE$_2$ to rats produced a dose-dependent increase in the volume of intestinal contents. The fluid volume was reduced for 6-8 h and by 60-80% when the animals were pretreated with 1 mg/kg orally[18]. Loperamide also enhances normal absorption from glucose-electrolyte mixture in steady state perfusion technique. The mechanism of action is unknown.

The opposing action on fluid transport (guinea-pig colonic mucosa) of the laxative 1,8-dihydroxyanthraquinone by loperamide seems to be due to decreased paracellular permeability[39]. Bisacodyl and other diphenolic laxatives inhibit the Na$^+$-K$^+$-activated ATP-ase and increase cAMP content[35]. Bile acid (4 mM deoxycholic acid)-induced secretion in the rat caecum is associated with mucosal blunting, degranulation of goblet cells, crypt dilatation, increased inflammatory cells, submucosal oedema and vascular congestion. At 0.6 mg/kg, loperamide significantly decreased the secretion and also protected against these histological changes[10].

Loperamide inhibits the release of acetylcholine and prostaglandin produced by distention of the intestine (in vitro)[42]. Hence, loperamide inhibits the peristaltic movement principally by reducing the release of acetylcholine and prostaglandin, at least during circumferential distention of the intestinal wall in vitro. Also the release of acetylcholine from the intestine without distention was decreased after loperamide. Loperamide also blocked the smooth muscle stimulating action of prostaglandins, acetylcholine and histamine on gastrointestinal smooth muscle preparations[18]. Loperamide (administered enterally : 5 µg/kg/min or intravenously 1.5 µg/kg/min) significantly reduced the slow wave frequency and significantly increased the percentage of slow waves initiating fast wave activity. Naloxone (40 µg/kg/h) abolished interdigestive motor activity or reduced mean cycle duration and the mean motility index.

The mode of action of loperamide may involve a reduction in the quantity of intracellular free ionized

calcium   available   to   the   stimulus-release-coupling
mechanism (guinea-pig isolated ileum).   4-Aminopyridine,
which enhances calcium influx into the cell, antagonizes
the effect of naloxone[20]. Loperamide (intragastrically :
4 mg bolus in 2 ml) reversed these effects. In the small
intestine, morphine and loperamide seem to lock the small
intestinal circular muscles of all species studied into a
continuous segmentation pattern of motility (mixing) which
is non-propulsive and constipating. In rats (in vitro) it
was shown that the opiate-induced contractile response is
mediated by stereospecific, naloxone-sensitive, opiate
receptors and that the muscular response involves the
activation of a 5-HT (5-Hydroxytryptamine) neurone in the
nerve terminals of the colon[15].

Alpha-2-agonists
Alpha-2-receptor activation mediates the inhibition of a
number of gastrointestinal functions including gastric and
intestinal secretions. Alpha-2-adrenergic agonists also
enhance absorption. Alpha-2-receptors are present on the
enterocytes. These receptors mediate enterocyte fluid and
electrolyte transport[4]. Alpha-2-receptors are coupled to
inhibition of basal and hormone-stimulated adenylate
cyclase activity. Alpha-2-induced decrease in cellular
cAMP levels are mediated at least in part by decreased
cAMP synthesis[24]. In vitro in the rabbit intestine, both
clonidine and lidamidine increased sodium and chloride
absorption[7]. Perfusion of the pig jejunum with Escherichia
coli heat-stable enterotoxin reversed net absorption of
water and electrolytes to net secretion. Clonidine,
L-phenylephrine and morphine, added to the perfusate,
reduced the secretory response to enterotoxin and
stimulated absorption[1]. In dog jejunum, lidamidine
reduced intestinal secretion due to damage by deoxy-
cholate[11]. The antisecretory activity was related to the
ability of lidamidine to reduce intestinal villous damage
and enhance permeability changes[12]. Clonidine inhibited
the distention-induced peristaltic reflex in the isolated

guinea-pig ileum. For the inhibitory effects of alpha-2-
agonists, the pacemaker neurones of the enteric nervous
system as well as postganglionic neurones innervating
intestinal smooth muscles are involved[6]. Lidamidine
inhibited gastric emptying, but not intestinal transit[27].

Anti-inflammatory drugs

Prostaglandins are involved in secretion[38]. Acetylsali-
cylic acid given orally (100 mg/kg) 4 h before inoculation
of Escherichia coli heat-stable enterotoxin (ST) into
ligated loops in the distal part of the jejunum of calves
did not substantially alter the intestinal fluid response
to the toxin. Intravenous sodium salicylate administered
simultaneously with or 1 h after inoculation of ST significantly decreased fluid accumulation in loops with ST
dilutions of 1:25 or greater[41]. Quinacrine hydrochloride
and zomepirac sodium decreased secretion caused by Escherichia coli heat stable toxin in mice[38]. Indomethacin
decreased secretion in rabbits[36]. Flunixin meglumine
reduces the quantity of diarrhoeal fluid loss in calves
with colibacillosis[17]. Despite promising results in
selected situations, most anti-inflammatory drugs are
potentially dangerous, especially in dehydrated animals.

Chlorpromazine and trifluoperazine

Both substances act by inhibition of intracellular
calmodulin activity[5]. In piglets, secretion was induced
with Escherichia coli producing both heat-stable and
heat-labile toxins, and chlorpromazine (1-5 mg/kg) decreased the intestinal fluid losses. A similar effect was
obtained in spontaneous outbreaks of colibacillosis[25].

Parasympatholytics

Secretion induced with ampiphatic drugs (bile salts, fatty
acids) in dogs was reversed by the intravenous injection
of atropine[21]. Atropine also decreases Cl-secretion in
porcine enterocytes induced by Escherichia coli heat-
stabile enterotoxin.

Benzetimide, when combined with antibiotics in newborn calves and adult cattle cured diarrhoea more quickly than when antibiotics were given alone[37]. In another study benzetimide again shortened the duration of diarrhoea[9].

Serotonin-2-antagonists

Both in vitro and in vivo, it was shown that 5-HT increased the electrical activity of the rat jejunum. The increased potential difference and short circuit current resulted from a stimulation of electrogenic chloride secretion and by reducing NaCl absorption. Intestinal secretagogues, including cholinergic agonists and serotonin from the serosal side do not cause mucosal cAMP to increase and require extracellular calcium to produce a full electric response; these substances may act as calcium ionophores on the epithelial cells. Intravenous infusion in rabbits of 5-HT (20 μg/kg/min) resulted in highly significant net secretion of water and sodium in both jejunum and ileum. The addition of glucose to the perfusate completely abolished the serotonin effect. The effect was achieved without any detectable histological alterations in small bowel mucosa by light or electron microscopy[19]. In the dog small intestine, Burks[3] provided evidence that 5-HT excited intraneural cholinergic nerve elements since the intestinal contracting effect of 5-HT was blocked by tetrodotoxin, nicotinic depolarization and atropine, but not by TEA. After oral ingestion of 5-HTP (30 mg/kg), increased spiking (from 25% [control] to 50%) activity was observed on dog intestine during the first hour. A percentage of 90 to 95 is reached for the next 5 hours[33]. Piglets, 10 days old, infected by gastric tube with an Escherichia coli strain producing heat-stable and heat-labile enterotoxin and treated with a serotonin-2-antagonist survived while all controls died. Blind loops were created in the jejunum of pigs and injected with cholera toxin, and a significant reduction in secretion (ml/cm of intestine) was observed after treatment with a serotonin-2-antagonist[31].

References
1. Ahrens, F.A. and Zhu, B.L. (1982). Effects of epine-
   phrine, clonidine, L-phenylephrine, and morphine on
   intestinal secretion mediated by Escherichia coli
   heat-stable enterotoxin in pig jejunum. Can. J.
   Physiol. Pharmacol. 60:1680-1685.
2. Blaton, H., Niemegeers, C.J.E. and Marsboom, R.
   (1976). Preclinical animal studies of modern anti-
   diarrheals. Safety evaluation. In : Van Bever, W.
   and Lal, H. (eds). Modern Pharmacology-Toxicology.
   Vol. 7 : Synthetic Antidiarrheal drugs, pp.155-203.
   New York : Marcel Dekker Inc.
3. Burks, T.F. (1973). Mediation by 5-hydroxytryptamine
   of morphine stimulant actions in dog intestine. J.
   Pharmacol. Exp. Ther. 185:530-539.
4. Chang, E.B., Field, M. and Miller, R.J. (1983).
   Enterocyte alpha 2-adrenergic receptors : yohimbine
   and p-aminoclonidine binding relative to ion transport. Am. J. Physiol. 244:G76-G82.
5. Dobbins, J.W. and Binder, H.J. (1981). Pathophysiology of diarrhoea : alterations in fluid and electrolyte
   transport. Clin. Gastroent. 10:605-625.
6. Doherty, N.S. and Hancock, A.A. (1983). Role of al-
   pha-2 adrenergic receptors in the control of diarrhea
   and intestinal motility. J. Pharmacol. Exp. Ther.225:
   269-274.
7. Durbin, T., Rosenthal, L., McArthur, K., Anderson, D.
   and Dharmsathaphorn, K. (1982). Clonidine and lidamidine (WHR-1142) stimulate sodium and chloride
   absorption in the rabbit intestine. Gastroenterology
   82:1352-1358.
8. Farack, U.M., Kautz, U. and Loeschke, K. (1981).
   Loperamide reduces the intestinal secretion but not
   the mucosal cAMP accumulation induced by cholera
   toxin. Naunyn-Schmiedeberg's Arch. Pharmacol. 317:
   178-179.
9. Glawischnig, E., Pichler, P., Fehr, P. and Dourakas,
   E. (1974). Uber die Wirkung von Spasmentral bei
   Durchfallerkrankungen des Rindes. Dtsch. Tierarztl.
   Wochenschr. 81:549-604.
10. Gordon, S.J., Kinsey, M.D., Magan, S.J., Joseph, R.E.
    and Kowlessar, O.D. (1978). Effect of bile acid
    induced secretion in the rat caecum. Gastroentero-
    logy 74 (5) part 2:1040.
11. Gullikson, G.W., Dajani, E.Z. and Bianchi, R.G.
    (1981). Inhibition of intestinal secretion in the
    dog : a new approach for the management of diarrheal
    states. J. Pharmacol. Exp. Ther. 219:591-597.
12. Gullikson, G.W., Jasty, V. and Dajani, E.Z. (1981).
    Effect of lidamidine on deoxycholate-induced histo-
    logical and permeability changes in canine jejunum.
    The Pharmacologist 23:122.
13. Hardcastle, J., Hardcastle, P.T., Read, N.W. and
    Redfern, J.S. (1981). The action of loperamide in
    inhibiting prostaglandin-induced intestinal secretion
    in the rat. Br. J. Pharmacol. 74:563-569.

14. Hughes, S., Higgs, N.B. and Turnberg, L.A. (1983).
    Loperamide has antisecretory activity in vivo in human
    jejunum. Gut 24:A495.
15. Huidobro-Toro, J.P. and Leong Way, E. (1981). Contrac-
    tile effect of morphine and related opioid alkaloids,
    beta-endorphin and methionine enkephaline on the iso-
    lated colon from long evans rats. Br. J. Pharmacol.
    74:681-694.
16. Ilundain, A. and Naftalin, R.J. (1981). Opiates in-
    crease chloride permeability of the serosal border of
    the rabbit ileum. J. Physiol. 316:56-57.
17. Jones, E.W., Corley, L., Hamm, D. and Bush, L. (1977).
    Calf diarrhea : a brief resumé with observations on
    treatment and prevention. Bovine Pract. 12:48-54.
18. Karim, S.M.M. and Adaikan, P.G. (1977). The effect of
    loperamide on prostaglandin induced diarrhoea in rat
    and man. Prostaglandins 13:321-331.
19. Kisloff, B. and Moore, E.W. (1976). Effect of sero-
    tonin and water and electrolyte transport in the in
    vivo rabbit small intestine. Gastroenterology 71:
    1033-1038.
20. Kromer, W., Scheiblhuber, E. and Illes, P. (1980).
    Functional antagonism by calcium of an intrinsic
    opioid mechanism in the guinea-pig isolated ileum.
    Neuropharmacology 19:839-843.
21. Kvietys, P.R., Wilborn, W.H., Granger, D.N. and
    Cuccias, H. (1981). Effect of atropine on bile-oleic
    acid-induced alterations in dog jejunal hemodynamics,
    oxygenation and net transmucosal water movement.
    Gastroenterology 80:31-38.
22. Lange, A., Secher, N.J. and Amery, W. (1977). PGE$_2$
    induced secretion of fluid and electrolytes was
    reversed to absorption. Acta Med. Scand. 202:449-454.
23. Lecce, J.G., Clare, D.P., Balsbaugh, R.K. and Collier,
    D.N. (1983). Effect of dietary regimen on rotavirus-
    Escherichia coli weanling diarrhea of piglets. J.
    Clin. Microbiol. 17:689-695.
24. Limbird, L.E. (1983). Alpha-2-adrenergic systems :
    models for exploring hormonal inhibition of adenylate
    cyclase. TIPS 4:135-137.
25. Lonroth, I., Andren, B., Lange, S. et al. (1979).
    Chlorpromazine reverses diarrhea in piglets caused by
    enterotoxic Escherichia coli. Infect. Immun. 24:
    900-905.
26. Merritt, J.E., Brown, B.L. and Tomlinson, S. (1982).
    Loperamide and calmodulin. Lancet i:283-284.
27. Mir, G.N., Alioto, R.L., Sperow, J.W. et al. (1978).
    In vivo antimotility and antidiarrheal activity of
    lidamidine hydrochloride (WHR-1142A), a novel anti-
    diarrheal agent. Arzneim. Forsch. 28:1448-1454.
28. Naftalin, R.J. (1982). Control of small intestinal
    absorption and secretion by modulation of the mucosal
    and serosal border chloride permeability. In : Case,
    R.M., Garner, A., Turnberg, L.A. and Young, J.A.
    (eds). Electrolytes and Water Transport Across the
    Gastrointestinal Epithelia, pp.277-285. New York : Ra-

ven Press.

29. Niemegeers, C.J.E., McGuire, J.L., Heykants, J.J.P. and Janssen, P.A.J. (1979). Experimental dissociation between opiate-like and antidiarrheal drugs. J. Pharmacol. Exp. Ther. 210:327-333.

30. Ooms, L. (1983). Alterations in intestinal fluid movement. Scand. J. Gastroenterol. 18 (Suppl. 84): 65-77.

31. Ooms, L. and Degryse, A. (1982). Antiserotonergic compounds in secretory diarrhea. Funds for Sci. Med. Res. 496-502.

32. Ooms, L.A.A., Degryse, A.-D. and Janssen, P.A.J. (1984). Mechanisms of action of loperamide. Scand. J. Gastroenterol. 19 (Suppl. 96):145-155.

33. Ruckebusch, Y., Buéno, L. and Fioramonti, J. (1981). Workshop : stress and serotonin in animals and man. Janssen Pharmaceutica. Beerse, Belgium.

34. Sandhu, B. (1981). Loperamide and cholera secretion. Clinical Res. Rev. 1 (Suppl. 1):155-159.

35. Schreiner, J., Nell, G. and Loeschke, K. (1980). Effect of diphenolic laxatives on Na^+-K^+-activated ATPase and cyclic nucleotide content of rat colon mucosa in vivo. Naunyn-Schmiedeberg's Arch. Pharmacol. 313:249-255.

36. Smith, P.L., Blumberg, J.B., Stoff, J.S. and Field, M. (1981). Antisecretory effects of indomethacin on rabbit ileal mucosa in vitro. Gastroenterol. 80:356-365.

37. Symoens, J., Geerts, H. and Van Gestel, J. (1974). Benzetimide in the treatment of diarrhoea in newborn calves and adult cattle. Vet. Rec. 94:180-183.

38. Thomas, D.D. and Knoop, F.C. (1982). The effect of calcium and prostaglandin inhibitors on the intestinal fluid response to heat-stable enterotoxin of Escherichia coli. J. Infect. Dis. 145:141-147.

39. Verhaeren, E.H.C., Dreessen, M.J. and Lemli, J.A. (1981). Influence of 1,8-dihydroxyanthraquinone and loperamide on the paracellular permeability across colonic mucosa. J. Pharm. Pharmacol. 33:526-528.

40. WHO Diarrheal Disease Control Programme (1979). WHO Wkly Epidem. Rec. 54:121-123.

41. Wise, C.M., Knight, A.P., Lucas, M.J., Morris, C.J., Ellis, R.P. and Phillips, R.W. (1983). Effects of salicylates on intestinal secretion in calves given (intestinal loops) Escherichia coli heat-stable enterotoxin. Am. J. Vet. Res. 44:2221-2225.

42. Yagasaki, O., Suzuki, H. and Sohji, Y. (1978). Effects of loperamide on acetylcholine and prostaglandin release from isolated guinea pig ileum. Jap. J. Pharmacol. 28:873-882.

43. Zavecz, J.H., Jackson, T.E., Limp, G.L. and Yellin, T.O. (1982). Relationship between anti-diarrheal activity and binding to calmodulin. Eur. J. Pharmacol. 78:376-377.

33
The effects of veterinary drugs based on humic acids in the treatment of enteritis in young animals

S. GOLBS, M. KUEHNERT AND V. FUCHS

ABSTRACT

The breeding of young pigs and cattle presents a number of difficulties due to an increased occurrence of diseases, especially those of the gastrointestinal tract - for example, in calves and piglets - in conventional as well as industrial circumstances.

In the German Democratic Republic humic acids have been used for more than 15 years as agents for the therapy, prophylaxis and metaphylaxis of infectious and non-infectious gastrointestinal diseases (particularly in pigs and ruminants). In these clinical cases the chemical, biochemical and physicochemical properties, as well as their broad spectrum of pharmacological effects, are utilized.

Experiments on laboratory animals and clinical tests in practice showed that humic acids are a valuable supplement to the present conventional therapeutic methods against enteritis of calves, pigs and several species of zoo animals.

INTRODUCTION

Due to the increased gastrointestinal diseases, especially in calves and pigs, the breeding of young livestock has problems in conventional as well as industrial cattle breeding farms and zoo animals[1].

For more than 15 years humic acids as basic active substances have been used in the German Democratic Republic for the treatment of infectious and non-infectious gastro-intestinal diseases.

Experiments on laboratory animals and clinical tests in practice have shown that humic acids contained as solitary active substances in the veterinary medicaments Kalumat and Sulumin ara a valuable supplement to the present therapeutic methods against enteric diseases.

In these cases the chemical, biochemical and physico-chemical properties of humic acids as well as their broad spectrum of pharmacological effects have been used.

MATERIALS AND METHODS

About 70% of the earth's organic bound carbon is found in fossil fuel (coal, oil, peat and natural gases). Up to 8-10% of it belongs to the group of humic substances, but only 1% is present as cellulose and less than 0.001% is available as biologically active substances used for medical purposes - for example, antibiotics and hormones. Humic acids are polyvalent macromolecules composed of a large number of basic components. These substances are three-dimensional molecules with molecular mass between 10,000 and 200,000.

The peripheral zones consist of partially modified metabolites of organic structures resulting from protein, fatty acid and carbohydrate metabolism[3]. Core and periphery are bound mainly by phenolic groups (the substitution pattern is usually lignin-like, flavonoid-like or chinoid-like). Functional groups are found in the peripheral zones (hydroxyl-free, carbonyl-free, carboxyl-free phenolic as well as amino, and sulphydryl groups).

Humic acids are weak polyvalent organic acids with a tendency to form complexes (absorption, ion exchange, mainly concerning cationoid groups, such as metals). For pharmaceutical use highly concentrated humic acids are available.

The clinical and pharmacological effects of humic acids, which can be derived from their chemical properties and from the wellknown pharmacological and toxicological effects, may be summarized as follows[3] :

(1) antiphlogistic, astringent and analgesic effects;
(2) adsorption effect as well as resorption-reducing effect particularly concerning cationic compounds;
(3) antimicrobial effects on the basis of the presence of phenolic-chinoid groups;
(4) detoxifying effects with pesticides[4].

RESULTS AND DISCUSSION

The most favourable use of these pharmacodynamic properties may be by combination of several products of humic acids, as found in the veterinary drugs Kalumat and Sulumin (humic acids in form of an acid depending primarily on the molecular mass have antimicrobial properties as well as antiphlogistical effects; on the other hand, the alkaline salts of the humic acids have both adsorptive and metabolism-regulating effects).

Kalumat in the treatment of enteritis in calves and zoo animals

The composition of Kalumat is as follows : humocarb 90%; highly concentrated humic acids 5%; and aluminium/magnesium silicate 5%. Its use is for the prevention and treatment of infectious and non-infectious enteritis in calves and zoo animals. Administration is oral.

Various clinical tests showed that Kalumat is more effective in comparison to the conventional chemotherapy[3].

After the oral administration of Kalumat the frequency of enteritis was reduced by more than 30%. Moreover, the costs of used drugs were decreased by about 60%, and body weight was increased by nearly 7%.

In summary, therefore Kalumat is highly effective and extremely well tolerated, when applied orally and can therefore be used successfully in therapy and prevention

of specific (such as Escherichia coli) infections, and
unspecific (for example, dyspepsia) enteritis in calves
and zoo animals (such as elephants, tigers, horses, and
monkeys).

It is possible to substitute the conventional treatment
with chemotherapy on the basis of humic acids as a
solitary active substance, the drug must be used at an
early stage.

Sulumin in the treatment of diarrhoea in suckling pigs and young pigs

Worldwide the breeding of pigs is connected with many
types of gastrointestinal diseases, such as virus
diarrhoea, E. coli diseases, colitoxicosis and dyspepsia.
In most cases mortality and morbidity is very high,
especially in virus diarrhoea and E. coli infections.
Some authors have even described rates of morbidity up to
100%[1,2].

In the German Democratic Republic Sulumin is the newest
of the veterinary medicaments based on humic acids as a
complex agent. Its composition is as follows : highly
concentrated humic acids 70%: Fe^{2+} 1.5%: Na-carboxymethyl-
cellulose 28.5%. Its use is for the prevention and treatment of infectious and non-infectious enteritis especially
E. coli diseases and virus diarrhoea in baby pigs, piglets
and young pigs. Administration is oral.

The scheme of dosage, which showed the optimum results
of treatment in various enteritic diseases of pigs, could
be ascertained on the basis of laboratory tests and
clinical investigations in practice (Tables 33.1 and
33.2).

In clinical tests on sick animals the efficacy of
Sulumin on morbidity, mortality, frequency of enteritis,
development of body weight, effect of iron contained in
the drug, and the possibility of side-effects, was mainly
examined.

Table 33.3 shows that the frequency of enteritis was
reduced in more than 50% of patients. The development of

Table 33.1   Dosage of Sulumin in suckling pigs

Escherichia coli disease	500-750 mg/kg body weight, twice a day, for 3 days
Virus diarrhoea	350-500 mg/kg body weight, twice a day, for 3 days (maximum 1000 mg/kg body weight)
Chronic TGE	500-750 mg/kg body weight, for 5-10 days
Dyspepsia	500-750 mg/kg body weight, for 5-10 days
Infectious necrotic enteritis	500-750 mg/kg body weight, for 5-10 days

----

Table 33.2   Dosage of Sulumin in piglets and young pigs

Colitoxicosis	interval dosage : 500-1000-500 mg/kg body weight, for 10 days, in difficult cases, maximum 2000 mg/kg body weight
Dyspepsia	500-750 mg/kg body weight, for 5-10 days

----

body weight in the Sulumin group showed better progress and, furthermore, the rate of mortality in the case of virus diarrhoea was decreased from 24% to 0.5%.

Results on the influence of Sulumin on the metabolism of trace elements showed that plasma levels of iron, copper and zinc moved in the physiological range. Analogous effects were found in the following haematological parameters : erythrocytes, haemoglobin and haematocrit.

Table 33.3 Frequency of enteritis and development of body
weight in piglets during preventive oral administration of
Sulumin (400 mg/kg body weight)

Group	n	Frequency (%) of enteritis	Development of body weight (kg) start	end
Control	53	93	4.80±0.15	11.62±3.36
Sulumin	43	44	5.28±0.11	14.27±8.77

CONCLUSIONS

In summary, Kalumat is highly effective and extremely well
tolerated, when applied orally, and can therefore be used
successfully in the treatment of specific (E. coli) and
non-specific (dyspepsia) enteritis in calves and several
zoo animals.

   Sulumin has similar effects to Kalumat in the treatment
of infectious bacterial diseases (E. coli, Clostridia per-
fringens), virus diarrhoea (coronavirus and rotaviruses)
and dyspepsia in piglets and young pigs.

References
1. Elze, K. (1982). Über den Einsatz von Huminsäuren zur
   Profylaxe und Therapie von Durchfällen bei Zootieren.
   Internat. Symp. Erkrankungen Zootiere, Veszprem,
   Ungarn.
2. Golbs, S. (1983). Experimentelle Untersuchungen zur
   pharmakologischen Wirksamkeit und zur Pharmakodynamik
   von Huminsäuren unter besonderer Berücksichtigung koer-
   gistischer Effekte und ihrer therapeutischen und pro-
   phylaktischen Nutzung beim Schwein. Prom. B. Leipzig :
   Karl-Marx-Universität.
3. Golbs, S. and Kuehnert, M. (1983). Huminsäurenanwendung
   in Therapie, Pro- und Metaphylaxe in der Veterinärmedi-
   zin. Z. Physiother. 35:151-158.
4. Golbs, S., Kuehnert, M. and Fuchs, V. (1984). Beein-
   flussung der akuten Toxizität von ausgewählten Pesti-
   ziden durch Huminsäuren. Z. Ges. Hyg. 30:720-723.
5. Schnitzer, M. and Khan, S.U. (1972). Humic Substances
   in the Environment. New York : Marcel Dekker, Inc.

Clinical Toxicology

34
Drug reactions leading to toxicity

A. DE RICK

ABSTRACT

Clinically relevant drug interactions leading to toxicity are discussed with emphasis on the mechanism of action and clinical implications. No attempts are made to cover the whole field of drug interactions. Instead, the problems are illustrated by examples of pharmacodynamic and pharmacokinetic interactions described in the literature of veterinary and human medicine.

INTRODUCTION

Multiple drug therapy is often used and this may lead to drug interactions. Drug interactions change the expected relation between the dose administered and the effect obtained. This can involve the concentration of the drug at the site of action (pharmacokinetic interactions) or the sensitivity of the target organs (pharmacodynamic interactions).

There is extensive information on "potential" drug interactions. However, well-documented clinically relevant interactions are less numerous. Several reasons for this discrepancy can be cited. Drug interactions are often studied in vitro. A typical illustration is drug interaction at the level of serum protein binding : concentrations used in vitro are often higher than those occurring in vivo in the clinical situation. Even if altered serum protein binding occurs in vivo, it may not have the expected consequences. When, for example, the free fraction of a drug with a large volume of distribution is increased, the displaced molecules will redistribute outside the plasma compartment. As a result, even a marked increase in free drug fraction will only lead to a small change of free concentration, and no alteration of the effect will be seen. An increased elimination of free drug too tends to counteract the increase of free concentration. In vivo interactions are often studied in experimental conditions. Such experiments are predictive only if they mimic the clinical situation and if they relate to dosage regimens that are used in the clinic. Another problem is the difficulty of differentiating effects of drugs in normal animals from those with disease in the clinical situation.

Interactions can decrease or increase the efficacy of a drug so that exaggerated responses and toxicity can occur. Clinically relevant interactions leading to toxicity will mainly be seen for drugs with a steep dose-response curve.

In this chapter some of the clinically relevant drug interactions, leading to toxicity, will be discussed. Pharmacodynamic as well as pharmacokinetic interactions at the level of drug distribution and drug metabolism will be illustrated. No attempt will be made to cover the whole field as detailed information is available in recent reviews[4,5,7,9,12].

PHARMACODYNAMIC INTERACTIONS
Diuretics are commonly administered together with digoxin in the treatment of congestive heart failure. A drug interaction which causes an emergency seen in human medical practice is digitalis toxicity precipitated by the use of potassium-losing diuretics (for example, furosemide)[4]. Digitalis glycosides inhibit Na^+-K^+-membrane ATPase and this results in a decrease in intracellular potassium. Diuretic-induced hypokalaemia

may precipitate digitalis toxicity. It is generally accepted that hypokalaemia and potassium loss induced by diuretics are able to sensitize the myocardium to the arrhythmogenic effects of digitalis in man[11]. Thus, dosage of concurrently administered cardiac glycosides may require adjustment in patients treated with potassium-losing diuretics.

In dogs also it is known that furosemide may induce digitalis toxicity[10]. However, in the dog the mechanisms of interplay between digitalis, hypokalaemia and potassium loss are not clear. Binnion[2] showed that neither acutely nor chronically induced hypokalaemia sensitized the dog heart to digitalis-induced arrhythmias. These data were obtained in anaesthetized dogs. More recently this view was substantiated in awake dogs and in a more clinical setting of experiments[8]. In this latter study, clinical signs of digitalis toxicosis occurred when furosemide was added to chronically digitalized dogs but in the absence of changes in serum potassium concentration. Another important finding in this study was the increase in the steady-state serum digoxin concentrations caused by the furosemide treatment. Thus, in the dog the digoxin-furosemide interaction seems not to be purely pharmaco-dynamic. Whatever the underlying mechanisms of this interaction, the following recommendations can be made for the veterinary clinician. Chronic mitral valve insuffi-ciency is the most common cause of heart failure in the dog. These dogs are often presented as class III patients and respond well in most cases to diuretic treatment alone. Therefore it is advisable to commence therapy with diuretics, without the use of digitalis glycosides. When digoxin and furosemide are used concomitantly, the recommended dose of furosemide should not be exceeded (especially in anorexic dogs) and the effectiveness of alternate-day administration should be investigated. When furosemide is given parenterally, the administered dose should be lower by 30-50% than the oral dose as the bioavailability after oral administration is lower.

The most commonly administered drugs in veterinary medicine are undoubtedly the antibacterials. Many interactions affecting their activity against pathogens are known (for example, synergistic and antagonistic combinations of antibiotics). Interactions between antibiotics or between an antibiotic and other agents can also decrease their safety[5,7,12]. The aminoglycosides (streptomycin, neomycin, kanamycin, gentamycin) have a potential for ototoxicity, nephrotoxicity and neuromuscular blockade. These toxic effects can be additive with combinations of the aminoglycosides. The combination of aminoglycosides with other neuromuscular blockers, including anaesthetics, can result in respiratory failure and reduced cardiac output. Parenterally administered tetracycline may interact with the inhalation anaesthetic methoxyflurane to produce lethal nephrotoxicity.

PHARMACOKINETIC INTERACTIONS
Pharmacokinetic interactions leading to toxicity can take place at different levels, for example, absorption, distribution and elimination.

Absorption
Interactions due to effects on drug absorption which can lead to toxicity are rare in both human and veterinary medicine. Enhancement of digitalis toxicity has been recorded in animals treated with stool softeners[9].

Distribution
Drugs can alter each other's distribution. In the literature on human research much has been written about interactions of drugs at the level of the serum albumin binding, especially for the coumarin-based anticoagulants. These agents are highly bound to plasma proteins. Non-steroidal anti-inflammatory agents (NSAIDS), among other drugs, can decrease the protein binding of the coumarin anticoagulant and potentiate its effect. In

veterinary medicine coumarin anticoagulants are less commonly used therapeutic agents. In horses, however, they are used in the treatment of navicular disease. Moreover, poisoning of domestic animals by warfarin does occur quite frequently. In both cases the effects of warfarin could be expected to be more severe when plasma protein binding is decreased by concomitant therapy with non-steroidal anti-inflammatory agents such as phenylbutazone.

Recently, much work has been done on the binding of drugs to another plasma constituent, alpha$_1$-acid glycoprotein, an acute phase reactant[1]. Inflammatory diseases and administration of enzyme-inducing agents can increase the alpha$_1$-acid glycoprotein concentration in plasma and lead to an enhanced binding of mainly basic drugs. However, toxic effects due to decreased binding of drugs on this protein have not been reported.

A clinically relevant interaction where distribution phenomena are, at least in part, involved is that of digoxin and quinidine. Although quinidine and digoxin have been used concomitantly for many years in both human and veterinary medicine, an interaction between these two drugs was only detected a few years ago[1,3]. In human patients quinidine causes an increase in serum digoxin concentration in about 90% of cases. The increase may be accompanied by digitalis intoxication. In dogs the findings were similar. Serum digoxin concentrations increase as a consequence of two main factors : (a) a displacement of digoxin from tissue stores leading to a reduced volume of distribution (about 30%), and (b) a reduction in renal and non-renal elimination resulting in a reduced total clearance of digoxin. The first effect is responsible for the initial rise in serum digoxin seen in most studies when quinidine treatment is commenced; and the second, a fall in clearance, maintains the elevated level for as long as the two drugs are administered (see below). Skeletal muscles are quantitatively the most important binding sites for digoxin. The reduction of the volume of distribution is mainly due to a displacement of digoxin from its skeletal muscle binding sites by quinidine.

Elimination

A number of different drugs can affect each other's elimination. Interactions leading to toxicity are to be expected when the elimination of one drug is diminished by the other. This will be illustrated by the interaction between chloramphenicol and other agents, and between digoxin and quinidine.

Chloramphenicol is still widely used in veterinary medicine and it is well known for its ability to inhibit mitochondrial protein synthesis. This inhibition results in a reduced metabolism of several other drugs. Pentobarbitone sleeping time in chloramphenicol-treated dogs and cats is markedly prolonged due to reduced oxidative metabolism of the barbiturate. This effect may last for 2-3 weeks after the last dose of chloramphenicol. Another well-known interaction involves chloramphenicol and the antiepileptic drug phenytoin. Phenytoin intoxication has been seen in both human and canine patients receiving chloramphenicol. Intoxication can occur even after a few days of topical treatment with chloramphenicol in eye drops. Chloramphenicol inhibits the metabolism of phenytoin and this results in higher steady-state concentrations of phenytoin. A reduction of phenytoin dosage should be considered if phenytoin and chloramphenicol are given concurrently. The most prudent recommendation, however, is that concurrent use of these drugs be avoided. Moreover, phenytoin cannot be recommended as a suitable anticonvulsant drug in the dog, for several reasons. The bioavailability after oral administration is highly variable in the dog (15-75%). It has a short half-life in the dog (about 4 h), making multiple dosing necessary. Phenytoin stimulates its own degradation in the dog[6], a process that occurs in humans only at high dosages. It is also a drug that is difficult to use without plasma concentration determinations because of its zero-order kinetics. These experimental data support the impression of many clinicians that phenytoin is not the first choice drug for anticonvulsant therapy in the dog[3].

Quinidine, as already mentioned, not only decreases the volume of distribution of digoxin, but also inhibits the elimination of digoxin. The latter is responsible for the sustained elevation of the steady-state plasma concentrations of digoxin when quinidine is added to the treatment. Indeed, the steady-state concentrations of a drug are dependent on the dose, the dosing interval, the bioavailable fraction and the total body clearance. Quinidine has no important influence on the bioavailability of digoxin. Thus, the increased steady-state concentrations are due to a reduction in total body clearance. The increase in the steady-state concentrations of digoxin by quinidine can lead to digitalis toxicity as has been seen in humans and dogs. For rational therapy with digoxin-quinidine, it is necessary to understand the mechanisms underlying the adverse reactions. The pharmacokinetic data available, however, are of limited help. A frequent observation is that the rise in serum digoxin concentration as a result of quinidine co-administration is unpredictable and that the rise is largest in those subjects with the highest concentrations of digoxin and, therefore, in those most at risk. Regular monitoring of the clinical symptoms, ECG and serum digoxin concentrations is regarded as mandatory. Another possibility is not to use digoxin but digitoxin, as no interaction is seen between quinidine and digitoxin in the dog. The use of new antiarrhythmic drugs instead of quinidine can also be considered. However, it should be borne in mind that these drugs too (for example, verapamil) can interact with digoxin.

CONCLUSIONS

There is a wide variety of mechanisms responsible for drug

interactions. A number of adverse drug interactions are of practical importance to veterinary clinicians. Knowing the principles which underlie the mechanisms of drug interactions may help to minimize the incidence of adverse effects. Neverless, these data are not always sufficient for the clinician to adjust the dosage regimen in individual cases.

References
1. Belpaire, F.M., Braeckman, R.A. and Bogaert, M.G. (1984). Binding of oxprenolol and propranolol to serum, albumin and alpha₁-acid glycoprotein in man and other species. Biochem. Pharmacol. 33:2065-2069.
2. Binnion, P.F. (1975). Hypokalaemia and digoxin-induced arrhythmias. Lancet i:343.
3. Bunch, S.E. (1983). Anticonvulsant drug therapy in companion animals. In : Kirk, R.W. (ed.). Current veterinary therapy VIII, pp.746-754. Philadelphia : W.B. Saunders Company.
4. D'Arcy, F.P. (1983). Clinically relevant interactions with important classes of drugs. In : Noack, E., Ledwoch, W. and Schrey, A. (eds). Adverse Drug Interactions, pp.271-285. München : Universitäts-druckerei und Verlag, Dr. C. Wolf und Sohn.
5. Davis, L.E. (1979). Important interactions of anti-biotic drugs. J. Am. Vet. Med. Assoc. 175:729.
6. Frey, H.H. and Lösher, W. (1980). Clinical pharmaco-kinetics of phenytoin in the dog : a reevaluation. Am. J. Vet. Res. 41:1635-1638.
7. Paul, J.W. (1982). Drug interactions. Mod. Vet. Pract. 63:780-785.
8. Pedersoli, W.M. and Nachreiner, R.F. (1980). Serum digoxin concentrations in dogs before and during concomitant administration of furosemide. J. Vet. Pharmacol. Ther. 3:1-7.
9. Reilly, P.E.B. and Isaacs, J.P. (1983). Adverse drug interactions of importance in veterinary practice. Vet. Rec. 112:29-33.
10. Ross, J.N.Jr. (1983). Heart failure. In : Ettinger, S.J. (ed.). Textbook of Veterinary Internal Medicine. Diseases of the Dog and Cat, 2nd ed., pp.901-932. Philadelphia : W.B. Saunders Company.
11. Steiness, E. and Olesen, K.H. (1976). Cardiac arrhythmias induced by hypokalaemia and potassium loss during maintenance digoxin therapy. Br. Heart J. 38:167-172.
12. Stowe, C.M. (1984). Antimicrobial drug interactions. J. Am. Vet. Med. Assoc. 185:1137-1141.
13. Woodcock, B.G. and Rietbrock, N. (1982). Digitalis-quinidine interactions. TIPS 3:118-122.

35
Clinical toxicology of an antibiotic ionophore (monensin) in ponies and horses; diagnostic markers and therapeutic considerations

J. F. AMEND, R. L. NICHELSON, L. R. FREELAND, R. S. KING,
F. M. MALLON AND W. W. STROUP

ABSTRACT

Toxicity of the ionophorous antibiotic monensin has been documented in a number of species, with the horse showing greatest sensitivity. This study examined haemodynamic, renal, erythrocytic, and biochemical variables to determine mechanisms of equine monensin toxicosis, and potential therapy. Horse and pony mares were fitted with catheters for blood and urine collection, then given monensin orally. Other studies were carried out in anaesthetized ponies, which received an intravenous dose of monensin. Cardiovascular effects included pressor and positive inotropic responses, myocardial lesions post-mortem, and increased pericardial fluid CK and LDH. Renal disturbances noted were rises in BUN and in clearance of phosphorus and potassium, decline in urine pH, and elevated urine N-acetylglucosaminidase. Erythrocytic responses included a rise in unconjugated serum bilirubin, increased red cell osmotic fragility, and altered blood gas variables.

INTRODUCTION

Ionophorous antibiotics of the carboxylic class, of which monensin is one example, are used in substantial quantities in the production of poultry and beef cattle.

Their efficacy as poultry coccidiostats[6] and promoters of feed efficiency in beef cattle[3] is well documented. First approved for use in food animals, monensin has a longer history of application and evaluation than related ionophores. It has, therefore, been more fully described in terms of its actions, and in certain cases, of its toxic manifestations[4] than other members of the group. As described in reports documenting feed-mixing accidents involving excessive dosage[5], or exposure of inappropriate species[8], monensin, and potentially other carboxylic ionophores, possess a capacity for toxicity when used inappropriately. In particular, the horse shows little tolerance to monensin[1]. The separate studies reported here were performed to further define mechanisms of monensin toxicity in the equine, to determine clinicopa- thological variables of diagnostic significance, and to search for therapeutic approaches helpful to clinicians confronted with ionophorous antibiotic toxicosis in the horse.

MATERIALS AND METHODS

Ten adult horses and 30 adult ponies were experimental subjects. Each was procured, housed, and handled according to guidelines established by National Institutes of Health (USA) and the American Physiological Society. Horses (mares) were fitted with jugular venous catheters (Medicut Cannula, Sherwood Medical, St. Louis, Missouri) and Foley bladder catheters (Bardex, C.R. Bard, Murray Hill, New Jersey). Each then received 3 mg/kg crystalline monensin orally, in ethanol vehicle, and was monitored for 48 h. Euthanasia (T-61 Euthanasia solution, American Hoechst, Somerville, New Jersey) was then performed. Pony mares were similarly prepared and monitored for 36 h, then euthanatized. Blood and urine samples were taken every 4 h, with control samples drawn immediately prior to administration of monensin. A number of ponies and horses were studied in identical sham protocols using ethanol vehicle. Certain ponies and horses were prepared with arterial catheters for blood pressure measurement, and sampling for blood gases. In a few cases, left ventricular pressure (Mikro-tip catheter pressure transducer, Millar Instruments Inc., Houston, Texas) and dP/dt max (Beckman R611, Beckman Instruments Inc., Schiller Park, Illinois) were measured. Venous blood was examined for red cell osmotic fragility and blood gas analyses (Model 713 Blood Gas Analyzer, Instrumentation Laboratories, Lexington, Massachusetts) and serum was collected for a range of biochemical variables (Sequential Multiple Analysis Computer [SMAC 20]. Technicon Inc., Tarrytown, New York). Arterial blood gases and acid-base values were also measured. Urine samples were used to determine volume and pH, and urine electrolytes were measured to allow electrolyte clearance calculations. Urine N-acetylglucosaminidase (NAG), a renal tubular lysosomal enzyme, was measured as an index of renal injury[7].

A second group of ponies was used to study cardiopulmonary effects of monensin when given by intravenous infusion. These ponies were anesthetized with a combination of xylazine (0.5 mg/kg; Rompun, Bayvet Division, Miles Laboratories, Shawnee, Kansas), ketamine hydrochloride (2.5 mg/kg; Ketaset, Bristol Laboratories, Syracuse, New York), and glyceryl guaiacolate (50 mg/kg; Gecolate, Summit Hill Laboratories, Avalon, New Jersey), and were maintained in anaesthesia with halothane (USP, American Hospital Supply Corp., Scientific Products Division, Evanston, Illinois), 2-4% as required, vaporized in 100% O_2. Catheters were placed for venous sampling (red blood count fragilities and blood gases), and for intravenous administration of monensin. An arterial catheter was inserted for blood gas and blood pressure monitoring. In certain cases a catheter was passed into the left ventricle for determination of left ventricular pressure and dP/dt max. A ureter was catheterized for collection of urine and measurement of volume, pH, and NAG. A Wright's respirometer (Ohio Medical Products,

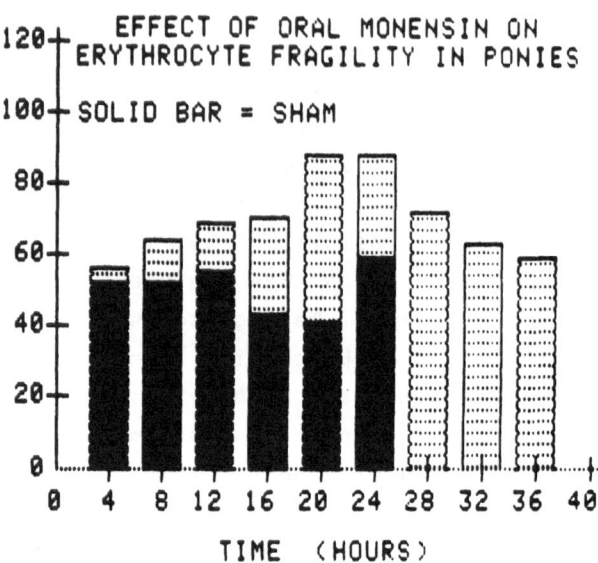

Figure 35.1 Erythrocyte osmotic fragility in sham-treated (solid bars) and monensin-treated (dotted open bars) ponies. The concentration of saline at which these measurements of haemolysis were made was 0.50%. Haemolytic responses of cells from sham-treated ponies ranged from 40 to 58% haemolysis, while cells from monensin-treated ponies showed progressive increase in haemolysis (peaking at 85% at 20-24 h).

Atlanta, Georgia) was used to measure minute ventilation prior to and following administration of monensin. Each pony received an intravenous dose of 200 μg/kg crystalline monensin. Sham procedures were performed in which ponies were given intravenous ethanol vehicle alone. Necropsy, histopathology, and pericardial fluid enzyme analyses were performed postmortem.

RESULTS AND DISCUSSION
Horses and ponies responded to oral monensin with haemodynamic stimulation, including increases in heart rate, systolic and diastolic arterial pressures, and dP/dt max. An haemolytic effect of monensin was observed, as

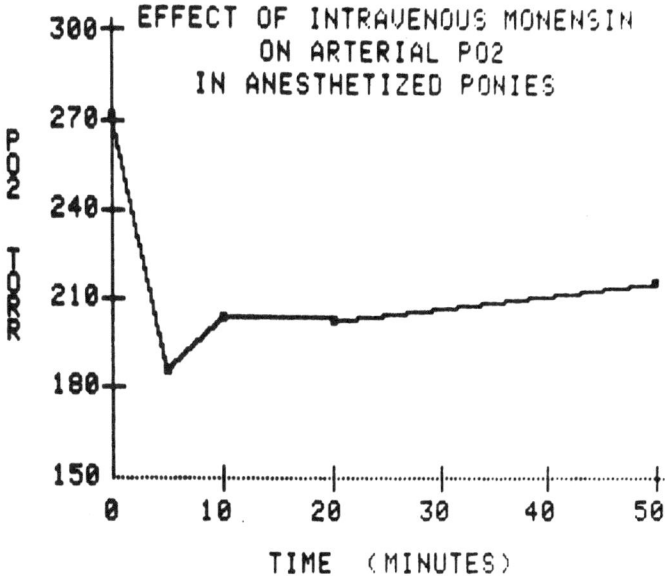

Figure 35.2   Intravenous monensin (200 µg/kg) caused a reduction in arterial pO_2 of nearly 100 torr within 5 min;
the control value of 270 torr reflects the fact that halothane anaesthetic was vaporized in 100% O_2. Although some
recovery of pO_2 occurred, the control level was never restored, in spite of profound hyperventilation.

indicated   by   rising   indirect   bilirubin,   and increased
plasma   haemoglobin.   Increases   in   erythrocyte   osmotic
fragility   also occurred following monensin (Figure 35.1).
In anaesthetized ponies, osmotic fragility of red cells
rose immediately after injection of monensin, and remained
elevated for the duration of the experiment.

     Blood gas changes in anaesthetized ponies comprised
depression   of pO_2, a rise in pCO_2 and fall in pH. Figure
35.2 illustrates the disturbance in pO_2 in these anaesthetized   animals.   Minute   ventilation   was, paradoxically,
dramatically elevated, but this change in ventilation was
not   effective   in   compensating   for   the disturbances in
blood gas variables.

     Urine volume was transiently increased after monensin,
and   this   appeared   to be related to a rise in arterial

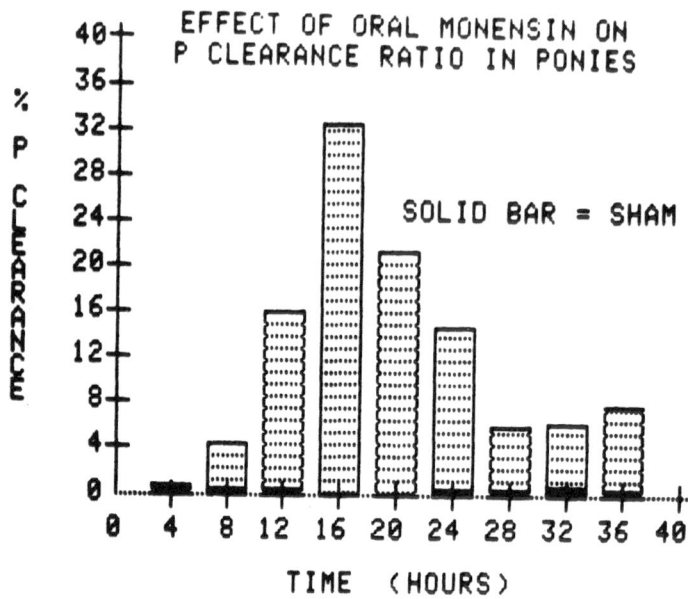

Figure 35.3 Phosphorus clearance ratio was profoundly elevated (dotted bars) by 16 h following oral monensin. This response was maintained throughout the remainder of the experimental period. A low phosphorus clearance ratio (sham treatment: solid bars) is normal for equine animals, thus the magnitude of phosphorus clearance ratio response was substantial.

blood pressure, which may have resulted in increased renal filtration. Serum potassium was similarly transiently depressed, and there was a delayed fall in serum phosphorus. Clearance ratios for potassium and phosphorus were significantly elevated. Of the two, phosphorus clearance ratio was most profoundly affected, as shown in Figure 35.3. Urine pH changed from alkaline to acid as the effects of monensin developed. Both conscious and anaesthetized ponies and horses responded to monensin with increases in urine N-acetylglucosaminidase (NAG). The NAG response is illustrated in Figure 35.4.

Postmortem gross and histopathology demonstrated myocardial lesions typical of those reported by others[2],

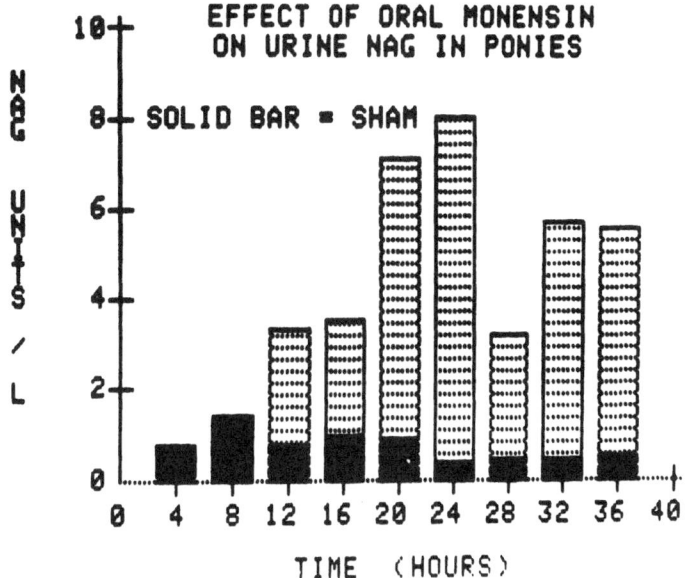

Figure 35.4 Confirmation of proximal renal tubular injury following monensin was demonstrated by the increase in urine N-acetylglucosaminidase (dotted bars). Solid bars show that urine NAG in sham-treated ponies rarely exceeded 1 unit/litre, while the maximum NAG response in monensin-treated ponies was 8 units/litre at 24 h.

and pericardial fluid CK enzyme levels were grossly increased (Figure 35.5). This increase resulted from the MB, or myocardial isoenzyme, fraction. Similarly, pericardial LDH was increased, with LDH₁ the predominant isoenzyme.

CONCLUSIONS

The severe myocardial lesions of equine monensin toxicosis seem to arise from a combination of increased cardiac work, electrolyte imbalance secondary to proximal renal tubular malfunction, and compromise in oxygen transport secondary to disturbed erythrocyte function. Diagnostic variables of importance may include elevated indirect bilirubin, depressed serum potassium and phosphorus (and

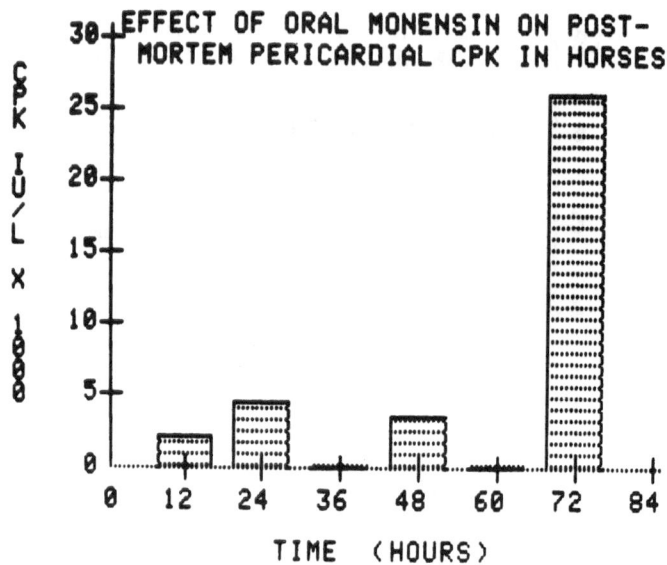

Figure 35.5 Pericardial CPK, obtained from samples taken immediately after euthanasia, was profoundly elevated in horses in which the duration of exposure to monensin was 72 h or more. Smaller increases were observed in peri- cardial fluid from horses which were euthanized with briefer exposure periods.

increased clearance of these electrolytes), decreased urine pH and elevated urine NAG, and at postmortem, myocardial lesions together with increased pericardial fluid CK-MB and LDH, concentrations. Therapeutic conside- rations should include pharmacological means of reducing cardiac work, fluid and electrolyte replacement with po- tassium and phosphorus supplementation, and probably supportive oxygen administration.

Acknowledgements
Supported in part by a grant from Eli Lilly and Co., Indianapolis, Indiana, the Agricultural Research Division, University of Nebraska-Lincoln, Lincoln, Nebraska, US and the Atlantic Veterinary College, University of Prince Edward Island, Charlottetown, Canada.

References
1. Matsuoka, T. (1976). Evaluation of monensin toxicity in the horse. J. Am. Vet. Med. Ass. 169:1098-1100.
2. Mollenhauer, N.N., Rowe, L.D. and Witzel, D.A. (1981). Ultrastructural observations in ponies after treatment with monensin. Am. J. Vet. Res. 42:35-40.
3. Raun, A.P., Cooley, C.O., Potter, E.L. et al. (1976). Effect of monensin on feed efficiency of feedlot cattle. J. Anim. Sci. 43:670-677.
4. Schlafer, M., Romson, J.L. and Kane, P. (1980). Potential adverse actions of the ionophore monensin. Fed. Proc. 39:694.
5. Schweitzer, D., Kimberling, C., Spraker, T. et al. (1984). Accidental monensin sodium intoxication of feedlot cattle. J. Am. Vet. Med. Ass. 184:1273-1276.
6. Shumard, R.F. and Callender, M.E. (1968). Monensin, a new biologically active compound. VI. Anticoccidial Activity. Antimicrob. Agent Chemother.:369.
7. Tucker, S.M., Pierce, R.J. and Price, R.C. (1980). Characterization of human N-acetyl-B-D-glucosaminidase as an indicator of tissue damage in disease. Helv. Chim. Acta 102:29-40.
8. Whitlock, R.N., White, N.A., Rowland, G.N. and Plue, R. (1979). Monensin toxicosis in horses : Clinical manifestations. Proc. 24th Ann. Mtg. A.A.E.P., pp. 473-486.

36
Mycotoxins and mycotoxicoses in Europe

J. LEIBETSEDER

ABSTRACT

Because of the moderate climate, fusariotoxins (zearalenone, vomitoxin) and ochratoxin are the most frequently
occurring mycotoxins in Europe. Aflatoxins are detected
almost solely in feed imported from tropical or subtropical areas. Mycotoxins often cause clinical symptoms in
livestock and tremendous economic losses in animal production. The main symptoms of mycotoxicoses are described.
The possibility of diagnosing and preventing intoxication
is considered.

INTRODUCTION

After the identification of toxins occurring in certain
plants and animals and the subsequent provisions for
avoiding intoxication by these substances, the environmental toxins caused by advancing technology are of
greatest importance at present. In addition, it must not
be ignored that even today naturally occurring toxins
create not only major economic losses in the animal
production by disease or decreased performance but also
risks for human health. Since classification of the
etiology of "turkey X disease" 25 years ago the mycotoxins
became very important amongst naturally occurring toxic
substances. Intensive research during the last two

decades has shown that about 30-40% of all fungal species occurring world wide are able to produce toxic secondary metabolites called mycotoxins under certain conditions. At present more than 100 toxins are chemically defined but there exists a much greater number of toxins not yet identified[6]. Mycotoxicosis is poisoning by the ingestion of toxins of fungal origin. The wide variety of the chemical structure of the toxins complicates their quantitative determination. Identical toxins can be synthesized by different fungal species, and different toxins can cause similar symptoms in man and animals. The toxins affect the synthesis of cell membranes, DNA-synthesis, transcription of the genetic code, and protein synthesis. Some of them are also carcinogenic or muta-genic. The mainly affected organs are : gastrointestinal tract, urinary tract, nervous system, haematopoietic system, genital tract, skin, and liver. In chronic intoxication the symptoms are often not very clear, but a deterioration of performance and reduced feed conversion can be observed.

NATURAL OCCURRENCE IN EUROPE

Besides the rarely occurring mycotoxicoses like ergotism, facial eczema in ruminants, slobber syndrome etc. only the frequently seen mycotoxicoses are discussed : fusario-toxicosis, ochratoxicosis and aflatoxicosis. Due to the preconditions of toxin synthesis (type and moisture of the substrate, temperature, microbiological ecosystem, insects) fusariotoxins and ochratoxins figure large in all European countries. whereas aflatoxins are synthesized only under hot and humid conditions. Aflatoxicosis is therefore a problem in the mediterranean area and in countries using contaminated feed imported from tropical or subtropical areas (Table 36.1).

FUSARIOTOXICOSIS

On the basis of the chemical structure as well as the toxic effects, two groups of fusariotoxins exist which

Table 36.1 2752 feed samples of a survey analysed since
1979   at   the   Institute   of   Nutrition,   University   of
Veterinary Medicine, Vienna (A = number of samples, B, C,
D = percentage of samples containing < 0.1, 0.1-1.0 and >
1 ppm respectively)

Feeds	Zearalenone				Vomitoxin			
	A	B	C	D	A	B	C	D
Maize	755	22.1	7.3	1.9	661	8.5	40.8	16.9
Barley	134	12.7	3.0	0	86	3.5	18.6	2.3
Oat	268	12.3	4.1	0	196	6.6	23.0	7.6
Rye	16	50.0	0	0	12	8.3	25.0	0
Wheat	204	19.1	10.3	1.5	112	10.7	50.9	13.4
Corn silage	183	49.1	13.7	0	157	7.0	44.6	19.1
Mixed feed	214	15.9	5.6	0.9	252	10.7	35.7	12.3
Others	70	17.1	2.9	1.4	64	9.4	9.4	0

Feeds	Ochratoxin A				Aflatoxins			
	A	B	C	D	A	B	C	D
Maize	26	7.7	3.8	0	15	0	0	0
Barley	32	15.6	0	0	4	0	0	0
Oat	37	32.4	5.4	0	9	0	0	0
Rye	10	10.0	0	0	9	0	0	0
Wheat	35	5.7	0	0	15	0	0	0
Corn silage	7	28.6	0	0	4	0	0	0
Peanut meal	–	–	–	–	48	10.4	18.7	47.9
Mixed feed	23	13.0	0	0	75	16.0	8.0	5.3
Others	6	0	0	0	58	6.9	5.2	1.7

occur   separately   or   together : zearalenone   and   its
derivatives; and trichothecenes.

Zearalenone
Zearalenone causes an oestrogenic syndrome   primarily
involving the genital system. This toxin can be produced

by various Fusarium species commonly infecting maize but also other cereals. In all European countries investigated for mycotoxins, zearalenone could be detected in concentrations ranging from 0.04 to 175 ppm². The frequency of contaminations varies from 2 to about 50% of the analysed samples due to the weather conditions in different years. The sensitivity of various animal species differs : oestrogenic effects could be observed in swine (1 ppm), cows (5 ppm) and other farm and experimental animals at different concentrations.

The gross changes include tumefaction of the vulva, enlargement of the mammary glands, hypertrophy of the nipples and increased size and weight of the uterus. Microscopic changes include oedema and hyperplasia of the uterus due to increased thickening of the myometrium, ductular proliferation of the mammary gland, and squamous metaplasia of the cervix and vagina. Prepubertal animals show ovarian hypoplasia and lack Graafian follicular development, while in adult females cystic degenerations of ovarian follicles are observed. In male swine reports indicate atrophic changes in the gross appearance of the testicles together with oedematous swelling of the prepuce as well as stimulation of mammary gland development. The semen quality seems to be affected as well. The consequence of these changes is a reduced or absent fertility.

Trichothecenes
Trichothecenes are sesquiterpenoids. Usually they are divided into four groups (A-D). The main toxins of these groups are :

group A : T-2 toxin, HT-2 toxin, neosolaniol, diacetoxy-
    scirpenol, monoacetoxyscirpenol, T-2 tetraol, scirpen-
    triol
group B : nivalenol, fusarenon-X, trichothecin, deoxy-
    nivalenol (vomitoxin)
group C : verrucarin A, roridin A

group D : crotocin

At present more than 40 different trichothecenes are
chemically defined. Under natural conditions only T-2,
diacetoxyscirpenol (DAS), nivalenol, T-2 tetraol, neosolaniol and deoxynivalenol (vomitoxin) could be
detected in feedstuffs. Trichothecenes are associated
with human and animal intoxications throughout the world
("staggering grains toxicosis", alimentary toxic aleukia,
stachybotryotoxicosis, "red mould disease", "mouldy corn
toxicosis"). The toxicological characteristics of trichothecenes are : lesions in the oral cavity and the
digestive tract characterized by intense inflammation,
haemorrhage and necrosis of the mucous membranes as well
as of the skin, vomiting and feed refusal, diarrhoea,
neural disturbances and abnormal positioning, degeneration
and haemorrhage in many tissues and organs, destruction of
the haematopoietic system with a marked reduction in
erythrocyte counts and a severe depression of leukocyte
and thrombocyte counts leading to a progressive
leukopenia, and immunosuppressive effects. Some of them
(nivalenol and fusarenon-x) are mutagenic. Trichothecenes
can be synthesized by the same species of Fusarium
producing zearalenone. Additionally, some others are able
to form trichothecenes. The most frequently contaminated
grain is maize, again in countries where maize is grown,
but all other cereals can be contaminated too. At first
T-2 and DAS were found more frequently but since methods
for determining vomitoxin have become available this toxin
seems to be the most frequently occurring of the
trichothecenes. Acute intoxications by trichothecenes
take place only rarely today but chronic intoxications of
farm animals are numerous and cause tremendous economic
losses in pig and broiler production. Toxicological
studies and field experiences indicate that animals can
take feed containing 0.1 ppm vomitoxin without distinct
risks for health and performance[5].

OCHRATOXICOSIS

Ochratoxicosis produced by Penicillium and Aspergillus spp. became an important mycotoxin because of the nephrotoxic effects in man and animals. The renal disorder is structurally characterized by tubular degeneration accompanied by interstitial fibrosis, whereas the predominant functional change is impairment of tubular activity. In kidneys showing pronounced changes the weight can be increased by 25%. The proximal tubules are frequently atrophic and the tubular basement membrane is thickened. Many glomeruli are totally hyalinized and cysts are noted in the cortex. Clinical symptoms are polydipsia and polyuria but also gastroenteritis and growth retardation. Under natural conditions ochratoxicosis is a chronic disease with a very low mortality. However, an acute syndrome including renal damage identical to mycotoxic nephropathy has been observed, mainly in newly weaned pigs, called "perirenal oedema". In addition to the symptoms already mentioned, subcutaneous oedema, ataxia, stiff arched back, and distention of the paralumbar abdominal wall were observed. The mortality is 40-90% within 1-2 days. Ochratoxin poisoning is not only recognized in pigs but also in poultry. As well as the renal lesions and the changes in the gastrointestinal tract the liver is severely affected in poultry. Pathological changes are fatty liver, focal haemorrhages, necrosis and marked vacuolation of hepatocytes. The concentration of ochratoxin residues is much higher in the liver of chicks than in the muscular tissue and corresponds well with the concentration of the kidney and the blood concentration. Especially in the Scandinavian countries, Poland, Yugoslavia and Austria ochratoxin was detected in foodstuffs and feedstuffs at concentrations which are able to affect human and animal health[4]. Residues in kidneys of pigs might cause a risk for consumers, so that the determination of ochratoxin in kidneys is indicated when kidneys show pathological changes. The tolerance level in the feed is 0.1 ppm.

AFLATOXICOSIS

At present knowledge concerning aflatoxin is the greatest amongst mycotoxins. The great importance of aflatoxin is justified by its carcinogenicity. The symptoms of aflatoxicosis range from none to acute or chronic disease with diagnostic characteristics which vary with the species, the amount of toxin consumed, and the length of time over which it was ingested. In acute poisoning a sudden loss of appetite, nervous symptoms, and a high and rapid mortality occur. Pathological changes are gastro-enteritis, haemorrhages in many tissues and organs and severe lesions in a number of parenchymal organs especially in the liver and kidneys and proliferation of the bile duct.

Liver tumours are probably induced by chronic aflatoxin intake. In general, aflatoxin contamination of home-grown products occurs only in the southern part of Europe, whereas in middle and northern Europe aflatoxin problems originate from imported feedstuffs especially from peanut products. Some European countries have already regulated the maximum allowance of aflatoxin by law which is in general 0.05 ppm in single feedstuffs and 0.02 ppm in concentrates for dairy cows. Dairy cows are the most critical species because toxin metabolites are excreted with the milk and cause a risk for human health.

DIAGNOSIS, TREATMENT AND PREVENTION

Diagnosis of chronic mycotoxicoses is difficult because of non-specific symptoms. The microbiological status of the feed is not closely correlated with the mycotoxin content[3]. Mycotoxicoses can be definitely diagnosed by mycotoxin determination in the feed. Only symptomatic treatments (increase of protein and vitamins in rations) are available. Methods for detoxification of feed applicable in practice are very few and only effective against aflatoxin. The most effective measures against mycotoxicosis are the reduction of fungal growth in the field (growing crop varieties suitable for climate conditions, crop rotation), careful harvesting, quick and adequate preservation after harvesting (drying, ensiling), correct storing, periodic cleaning and disinfection of feed containers and feeding equipment[1].

References
1. Leibetseder, J. (1982). Kenntnisse und Empfehlungen zur Mykotoxin-Problematik. In : Akt. Them. Tierernähr. Veredelungswirtschaft. Zusammenfassung der Vorträge der wissenschaftlichen Tagung der Lohmann Tierernährung GmbH. In Cuxhaven vom 21. und 22. Oktober 1981, pp.73-81.
2. Müller, H.-M. (1978). Zearalenon - ein östrogen wirksames Mykotoxin. Übers. Tierernähr. 6:265-300.
3. Neuhold, F. (1982). Untersuchungen über den Zusammenhang zwischen mikrobiologischem Status und Mykotoxingehalt von Futtermitteln. Diss. Vet. med. Univ. Vienna.
4. Schuh, M. and Schweighardt, H. (1981). Ochratoxin A - ein nephrotoxisch wirkendes Mykotoxin. Übers. Tierernähr. 9:33-70.
5. Schweighardt, H. and Schuh, M. (1981). Desoxynivalenol - ein bedeutendes Trichothecen. Übers. Tierernähr. 9:11-32.
6. Wyllie, T.D. and Morehouse, L.G. (eds). (1977, vol. I), (1978, vol. II, III) : Mycotoxic fungi, Mycotoxins, Mycotoxicoses. New York : Marcel Dekker, Inc.

Pathophysiological Models in Pharmacology Miscellaneous

37
Role of animal disease models in evaluating the efficacy of antimicrobial agents

T. E. POWERS, K. J. VARMA AND J. D. POWERS

ABSTRACT

The advantages of the use of animal infectious disease models in determining the efficacy of antimicrobial agents are discussed. They are of particular interest in veterinary medicine as the antibiotic can be studied in the same species, where it will be used clinically. A good infectious disease model should fulfill several criteria. In our laboratory, we developed Streptococcus zooepidemicus disease models in beagle dogs and horses. The results are shortly discussed.

INTRODUCTION

Animal disease models of target animal species are useful in determining the in vivo pharmacological efficacy and dosage regimens of antimicrobial agents. These animal models offer several advantages : (a) preinfection data can be collected; (b) all animals can be maintained under similar conditions; (c) one can conduct disposition studies of drugs in actual disease conditions, thereby eliminating the need for extrapolation; (d) use of controls is expedited; (e) they are of particular use in veterinary medicine since we can use the same species in which the drug will be used clinically; (f) they serve as a well-controlled method for dosage titration studies,

enabling us to better bridge the gap between in vitro and
clinical studies.

OBJECTIVES OF RESEARCH

Our research in the area of animal disease models over the
last 12 years has had as its objectives : (a) the development and characterization of several specific infectious animal disease models in dogs and horses; (b) to
study the efficacy of several antibiotics in the treatment
of the experimentally induced diseases; (c) to study the
pharmacokinetics of antibiotics in the healthy and disea-
sed states; (d) to correlate if possible the pharmacokinetic parameters with the efficacy of the drugs.

Animal disease models may be classified as :

(1) Those that mimic natural disease :
    a) in local infections;
    b) in systemic infections.
(2) Those that show a similar disease state in different
    species of animal.
(3) Those that are a challenge to death.

In this chapter type (1) models of systemic and local
infection are discussed.

The desirable properties of a good disease model to
prove efficacy of antimicrobial agents are that : (1) it
is caused preferably by a single pathogen; (2) it should
produce clinically observable signs of disease in an acute
and chronic phase; (3) it should run a course of several
days (10-20); (4) it should be readily susceptible to
therapy by the commonly available antibiotics; (5) it
should be consistently reproducible.

LABORATORY MODELS

In our laboratory we have developed Gram-positive
(Streptococcus zooepidemicus) disease models in beagle
dogs and horses[3,4,7,8].

Dogs

In a systemic Strep. zooepidemicus model, 6-8 month old beagle dogs were challenged with the microorganisms by the intravenous route. Various clinical parameters were monitored during the course of disease in order to characterize it well. These clinical parameters included daily blood culture tests, haematological examinations, body temperature and general condition.

The disease signs were scored subjectively by three clinicians daily[3]. This subjective scoring of degree of illness (health index on a scale of 0-40) was broken down as follows :

Lameness	0-15
Size of lymph nodes	0-08
Colour of mucous membranes	0-05
Degree of alertness	0-04
Condition of haircoat	0-04
Degree of dehydration	0-04

To determine the influence of blood level upon the efficacy, three graded steady-state levels of the antibiotics were usually employed which corresponded to two to four times the minimum inhibitory concentration (MIC), equal to the MIC, and half to a quarter of the MIC. For intermittent level studies we attempted to have the peak blood levels well exceeding the MIC, equal to the MIC, and below the MIC.

In another experiment, intermittent intravenous dosing with potassium penicillin G was studied. Doses that were studied were 10,000 IU/0.45 kg, 1000 IU/0.45 kg, or 100 IU/0.45 kg. All doses were effective. The very low dose of 100 IU/0.45 kg was also effective even though blood levels with the latter doses remained above the MIC for only 20 min.

Our conclusions from these studies were that :

(1) Streptococcus zooepidemicus is a well-characterized and consistently reproducible viable model for drug efficacy studies.

(2) Repeat kinetic studies were not different from single injection kinetic studies.

(3) The disease process did not change the kinetics of the drugs studied.

(4) Most antibiotics required blood levels that were equal to or four times the in vitro MIC.

(5) Gentamicin was not effective in vivo even at four times the in vitro MIC.

(6) Intermittent therapy with trough levels below the MIC were effective with penicillin G.

(7) Initiation of therapy as early as 12 h before experimental infection gave no additional benefits.

In a local infection model, sterilized tissue cages, with perforated holes, were implanted subcutaneously in beagle dogs[1]. Fibrous tissue grows around the cage and through the perforated holes to the inside of the cage so that the entire wall of the cavity becomes lined with connective tissue. The fluid inside the cavity does not come in contact with the cage itself but instead is in a true tissue space lined on all sides by tissues that are supplied with a vascular system. After 3 weeks the tissue fluid which can be withdrawn from these tissue cages is similar in composition to interstitial fluid. These tissue cages were then infected with Strep. zooepidemicus and the number of viable pathogens, degree of inflammation, fever and number of viable leukocytes in tissue cage fluid were recorded during the course of the disease[3].

A constant intravenous infusion of potassium penicillin G was injected so as to maintain blood levels of once the MIC and a half the MIC of Strep. zooepidemicus. This resulted in decreases in the number of pathogens in the tissue cage fluid after 72 h as compared to the control animals. In the untreated control only 3.3% of leukocytes were viable at the end of 44 h, whereas in case of once the MIC and a half the MIC groups, 96.5 and 47.5% of leukocytes were viable after 44 h.

Horses

A reproducible experimental disease model in horses using Strep. zooepidemicus was also developed[6,7]. The disease was characterized by depression, pyrexia, anorexia, abnormal lung sounds, inflammation of joints, moderate to severe lameness, gradual loss of condition and emaciation. The disease state had no effect on serum glucose, sodium, potassium, chloride, urea nitrogen, creatinine, uric acid, calcium, phosphorus and the enzymes serum glutamic-pyruvic transaminase (SGPT) and serum glutamic-oxaloacetic transaminase (SGOT). However, alkaline phosphatase showed a gradual decline. The serum iron levels dropped markedly and remained low to the last day of observation (postinfection day 13). The elevation of rectal temperatures and white blood cell counts related well with clinical observations. The serum iron levels proved very valuable in predicting the severity of clinical signs and often dropped before the onset of clinical signs and pyrexia.

In another disease model in horses, virulent Strep. equi were inoculated nasopharyngeally[2]. Animals with evidence of previous exposure to Strep. equi (positive dermal response), with one exception, developed minimal or no sign of disease after inoculation. In contrast Strep. equi skin test negative horses developed predictable and severe clinical signs of infection after their inoculation, including shedding of organisms from nasal discharges and ruptured mandibular lymph nodes. Results of this study indicated that resistance to virulent Strep. equi infection is correlated with existing immune responses to streptococcal antigens. In susceptible horses, recovery from infection was accompanied by the acquisition of a positive skin test response to Strep. equi antigen.

CONCLUSIONS

Our conclusion is that when well-characterized and

standardized infectious disease models are available, they should be used as one of the required well-controlled studies for determining both the pharmacokinetics and the efficacy of new developing antimicrobial agents.

Acknowledgements

This research was supported in part by FDA contracts number 223-74-7194 and 223-79-7054.

References
1. Garg, R., Powers, T. and Powers, J. (1978). Role of tissue cage models for studying the disposition of drugs in tissue. Abstract, Proc. Conf. of Res. Workers in Anim. Disease, November 1978.
2. Nara, P.L., Krakowka, S., Powers, T.E. and Garg, R.C. (1983). Experimental Streptococcus equi infection in the horse : correlation with in vivo and in vitro immune responses. Am. J. Vet. Res. 44:529-534.
3. Powers, T.E., Powers, J.D., Garg, R.C., Scialli, V.T. and Hajjans, G.H. (1980). Trimethoprim and sulfadiazine : experimental infection in beagles. Am. J. Vet. Res. 41:1117-1122.
4. Powers, T.E., Garg, R.C., Gabel, A.A. and Kohn, C.W. (1981). Experimental Streptococcus zooepidemicus infection model in horses. Proc. Am. Coll. Vet. Intern. Med., 21.
5. Powers, T.E., Varma, K.J. and Powers, J.D. (1984). Selecting therapeutic concentrations : minimum inhibitory concentrations vs. sub- or supra-minimum inhibitory concentrations. J. Am. Vet. Med. Assoc. 185: 1062-1067.
6. Powers, J.D., Powers, T.E., Varma, K.J., Gabel, A.A. and Spurlock, S.L. (1984). A health index to clinically evaluate a Strep. disease model in the horse. J. Vet. Pharm. Ther. 7:213-217.
7. Varma, K.J., Spurlock, S.L. and Powers, T.E. (1984). Standardization of an experimental disease model of Streptococcus zooepidemicus in equines. J. Vet. Pharm. Ther. 7:183-188.
8. Varma, K.J., Powers, T.E., Garg, R.C. and Spurlock, S.L. (1982). Experimental infectious models in horses. Pharm. Toxicol. Vet. INRA, Publ. Paris, Les Colloques de l' INRA 8:485-486.

38
Effects of disease states on drug binding to serum proteins

A. L. ARONSON, S. A. BAI, J. E. RIVIERE AND D. P. AUCOIN

ABSTRACT

The effect of disease on the serum protein binding of phenytoin and propranolol, model drugs for weak acids and bases, respectively, was studied in dogs. Our preliminary investigations showed that, as in humans, the binding of organic bases is increased in diseases associated with stress and inflammation. The implication of this finding is that larger doses of basic drugs, such as propranolol, quinidine, lidocaine, chlorpromazine and procainamide, may be required if the patient has a concurrent disease associated with inflammation.

INTRODUCTION

Drug dosage is usually selected on the basis of the weight or surface area of a patient. Many factors can influence the pharmacological/therapeutic response expected from an intended dosage; some of these factors are illustrated in Figure 38.1. Patient compliance problems, whether intentional or non-intentional, and errors in dose affect the dose that is actually administered to the patient. Once a dose is given one can encounter bioavailability problems related to the drug formulation or to gastrointestinal factors, including content and motility, if the drug is dosed orally. Individual patient

```
Intended dosage
        │       compliance
        │       errors in dose
        ▼
Administered dosage
        │       bioavailability
        │       distribution
        │       rate of biotransformation
        │           and excretion
        ▼
Plasma concentration
        │       protein binding
        │       displacement by another drug
        │           or endogenous substances
        ▼
Plasma water concentration
        │
        ▼
Concentration at receptor sites
        │
        ▼
Pharmacological/Therapeutic effect
```

Figure 40.1   Some   factors   influencing   dose-effect
relationships.

variations   in   cardiac   output,   rate   of   drug
biotransformation, hepatic and renal function, whether due
to age, genetic variation, concurrent administration of
other drugs, or to the presence of disease, can have a
marked effect on the plasma or serum concentration and
pharmacological/therapeutic response produced by a given
dose.

   Experience has shown that the pharmacological/therapeu-
tic response correlates much more closely with serum or
plasma concentrations of drug than with the dose of the
drug. Thus monitoring plasma concentrations has been
advocated especially for drugs with a narrow therapeutic
range and narrow margin of safety[7].   These include
antibiotics (such as aminoglycosides), anticonvulsants
(such   as   phenobarbitone,   phenytoin,   primidone),
bronchodilators (such as theophylline) and cardiac drugs
(such as digoxin, digitoxin, lidocaine, procainamide,

propranolol and quinidine).

However, serum concentrations are not perfect indices of the pharmacological/therapeutic response. It is well-documented in humans that disease states can significantly influence the binding of drugs to serum proteins[3,4,6,8,9]. In contrast, there is little information concerning the effects of disease states on the binding of drugs to serum proteins in animals. It is critical to know the degree to which a drug is bound to serum proteins and to what extent this may be altered by disease. Information of this kind is essential for therapeutic drug monitoring (TDM) and pharmacokinetic consultation. The total (bound + free) concentration of a drug may provide misleading information, because the intensity of a drug's action is related to its concentration in plasma water (also referred to as free or unbound drug). Thus, any change in the extent of binding of a drug, especially if it is highly bound to serum proteins, may have marked effects on the intensity of a drug's action. In addition, the extent to which a drug is bound to serum proteins will influence its pharmacokinetics by altering its clearance and/or apparent volume of distribution.

In serum, albumin and alpha-1-acid glycoprotein are the two major proteins involved in binding the majority of drugs. In general, albumin is involved in binding drugs that are weak acids while alpha-1-acid glycoprotein is involved in binding many drugs that are weak bases. The concentration of albumin in healthy subjects is high relative to the therapeutic concentration of most drugs, thus binding sites generally are not saturated. However, in hepatic or renal dysfunction, hypoalbuminaemia may occur and contribute appreciably to a decrease in the bound fraction of many acidic drugs[8]. Alpha-1-acid glycoprotein is known as an acute-phase reactant. The concentration of this protein (normally about 25 to 50 times less than albumin in serum) has been shown to increase 2- to 3-fold in humans with acute stresses such as surgery, trauma, cancer, myocardial infarct and inflammation[4]. It also has been shown that chronic administration of phenobarbitone leads to significant increases of base-binding proteins in the serum of dogs[1]. Thus it may be expected that the binding of basic drugs will increase in conditions associated with increases in this binding protein.

The purpose of this study was to evaluate the effects that defined disease states have on the binding of two model drugs : phenytoin as a model for weak acids, and propranolol as model for weak bases. These drugs have, respectively, been shown to bind predominantly to albumin and alpha-1-acid glycoprotein.

Materials and methods

Serum from dogs with defined disease states was divided into two 1 ml aliquots. Binding to serum proteins in vitro was determined by equilibrium dialysis[1,2]. Unlabelled propranolol (Ayerst Laboratories, New York) and ^{3}H-propranolol (Amersham Corporation, Arlington Heights, Illinois) were added to one aliquot to obtain a final concentration of 50 ng/ml. Unlabelled phenytoin (Sigma, St Louis, Missouri) and ^{14}C-phenytoin (Amersham Corporation, Arlington Heights) were added to the other aliquot to obtain a final concentration of 10 µg/ml. Each aliquot was dialysed against 1 ml phosphate buffer (pH, 7.4; ionic strenght, 0.111). Dialysis was carried out in Lucite dialysis chambers (Fisher Scientific Company, Springfield, New Jersey) that were gently rocked for 18 hours at 37 °C.

The percentage of serum-bound drug was calculated from the amount of radioactivity (DPM) in 50 µl aliquots of serum (s) and dialysate (d) :

$$\% \ bound = \frac{DPM_s - DPM_d}{DPM_s} \times 100$$

RESULTS AND DISCUSSION
In this chapter we present preliminary findings, and in future investigations we intend to study the effect of disease states on drug binding to serum proteins in several species. Our studies to date on canine patients suffering from renal dysfunction and inflammatory diseases are presented.

Renal dysfunction patients
One of the most thoroughly studied conditions causing altered drug binding in humans is that due to renal diseases[6]. The binding of virtually all acidic drugs (for example, phenytoin, salicylates, benzylpenicillin, dicloxacillin, phenobarbitone, thiopentone, phenyl-butazone) that are primarily bound to albumin is decreased in chronic renal disease, often by a factor of two or three. Factors responsible include loss of protein through the kidneys resulting in hypoalbuminaemia and the presence of endogenous inhibitors such as fatty acids in uraemic plasma. In contrast, out of six basic drugs studied, only triamterene had decreased protein binding from patients with poor renal function.

We investigated the binding of propranolol and phenytoin in vitro to proteins in serum obtained from dogs with chronic renal disease (CRD) and in dogs partially (75-80%) nephrectomized experimentally (Table 38.1). There was little effect on the unbound fraction of either drug. This may have been expected for propranolol, but not for phenytoin. The finding may be due to the fact that all of the dogs had serum albumin concentrations within the normal range except for one of the chronic renal disease patients with a value of 1.2 g/dl. Serum creatinine concentrations were normal in the partially nephrectomized patients, but ranged up to 10 mg/dl in the chronic renal disease patients.

Inflammatory disease patients
The binding of basic drugs appears to increase in several

Table 38.1 Effect of chronic renal disease (CRD) and experimental partial nephrectomy (PN) in dogs on the binding of propranolol and phenytoin to serum proteins

---

| | Percentage of unbound* | |
	Propranolol	Phenytoin
Control (n = 12)	21.1 (3.4)	35.4 (3.3)
CRD (n = 4)	17.6 (3.2)	33.3 (4.0)
PN (n = 6)	17.1 (1.6)	38.6 (4.6)

---

* mean (SD)

disease states associated with inflammation and stress, for example, myocardial infarction, postsurgical, ulcerative colitis and Crohn's disease, burns and trauma[3,6]. In such disease states it has been found that the concentration of alpha-1-acid glycoprotein is increased. The binding of basic drugs to this protein is expected to increase in these conditions. Indeed, this has been observed for propranolol and quinidine in human patients with Crohn's disease and rheumatoid arthritis. The binding correlated with the plasma concentration of alpha-1-acid-glycoprotein.

We have investigated propranolol and phenytoin binding in vitro in several canine patients suffering from inflammatory diseases including meningitis, pleuritis, pancreatitis and fever of indeterminate origin (Table 38.2). The binding of phenytoin increased slightly in these patients, but the effect was not significant. However, the binding of propranolol was significantly increased in these patients (6.7% unbound) as compared to control dogs (21.1% unbound). Serum alpha-1-acid glycoprotein concentrations were not measured, but the data suggest that, as in humans, the concentration of this protein was probably increased in patients with inflammatory disease.

We believe these data strongly suggest that it will be

Table 38.2 Effect of inflammatory disease in dogs on the binding of propranolol and phenytoin to serum proteins

| | Percentage of unbound* | |
	Propranolol	Phenytoin
Control (n = 12)	21.1 (3.4)	35.4 (3.3)
Inflammatory disease (n = 6)	6.7 (2.1)**	27.8 (8.9)

* mean (SD)

** p < 0.01

necessary to increase the dose of basic drugs that bind to alpha-1-acid glycoprotein (for example, propranolol, quinidine, lidocaine, chlorpromazine) in order to achieve the desired therapeutic effect if the patient also is suffering concurrently from stress or an inflammatory condition.

A case of rapidly progressing acute renal failure illustrates a problem in studying the effects of disease

Table 38.3 Effect of time-course of acute renal failure in a dog on the binding of propranolol and phenytoin to serum proteins

Date	12 February 1985	28 February 1985	1 March 1985
Albumin, g/dl	2.5	2.0	1.9
Total protein, g/dl	6.1	4.9	4.5
BUN, mg/dl	60	128	101
Creatinine, mg/dl	4.4	8.9	7.3
Percentage of free propranolol	5	32	33
Percentage of free phenytoin	31	43	56

on the binding of drugs to serum proteins (Table 38.3). Serum albumin and total protein concentrations fell while BUN and creatinine concentrations rose rapidly over a period of 2 weeks. The marked increase in the free fraction of both propranolol and phenytoin may be due to reduced synthesis or to the loss of their binding proteins via the kidneys. Obviously, any drug kinetic study performed at any given time with such rapidly changing functional parameters would apply only to that time. Daily therapeutic drug monitoring with determination of unbound drug may be required to optimize therapy.

References
1. Bai, S.A. and Abramson, F.P. (1982). Interactions of phenobarbital with propranolol in the dog. 1. Plasma protein binding. J. Pharmacol. Exp. Ther. 222:589-594.
2. Ehrnebro, M., Augrell, S. and Boreus, L.O. (1971). Age differences in drug binding by plasma proteins. Studies on human foetuses, neonates and adults. Eur. J. Clin. Pharmacol. 3:189-193.
3. Jusko, W.J. (1976). Pharmacokinetics in disease states changing protein binding. In: Benet, L.E. (ed.). The Effect of Disease States on Drug Pharmacokinetics, pp.99-124. Washington, DC : American Pharmaceutical Association.
4. Piafsky, K.M. (1978). Increased plasma protein binding of propranolol and chlorpromazine mediated by disease-induced elevations of plasma acid glycoprotein. New Engl. J. Med. 299:1435-1439.
5. Piafsky, K.M. (1980). Disease-induced changes in the plasma binding of basic drugs. Clin. Pharmacokinet. 5:246-262.
6. Piafsky, K.M. (1983). Disease-induced changes in the plasma binding of basic drugs. In: Gibaldi, M. and Prescott, L. (eds). Handbook of Clinical Pharmacokinetics, Section III. pp.70-88. New York : ADIS Health Science Press.
7. Pribor, H.C., Morrell, G. and Scherr, G.H. (1980). Drug Monitoring and Pharmacokinetic Data, p.18. Park Forest South, Illinois : Pathotox Publishing Inc.
8. Reidenberg, M.M. and Drayer, D.E. (1984). Alteration of drug-protein binding in renal disease. Clin. Pharmacokinet. 9 (Suppl. 1):18-26.
9. Tillement, J.P., Lhoste, F. and Giudicelli, J.F. (1983). Diseases and drug protein binding. In: Gibaldi, M. and Prescott, L. (eds). Handbook of Clinical Pharmacokinetics, Section III, pp.57-69. New York : ADIS Health Science Press.

39
Tickborne fever: efficacy and effects on pharmacokinetics of some chemotherapeutic agents in the goat

S. M. ANIKA, J. F. M. NOUWS, T. B. VREE, C. T. M. VAN DUIN.
J. NIEUWENUIJS AND A.S.J.P.A.M. VAN MIERT

ABSTRACT

The tickborne fever model developed in dwarf goats and used in this study has an acute character : fever, dullness, anorexia, tachycardia, a moderate inhibition of rumen contractions, leucopenia and a decreased serum alkaline phosphatase activity. The model can be of great value in testing the therapeutic efficacy and pharmaco-kinetics of chemotherapeutic agents in rickettsial infec-tions. The dwarf goats receiving oxytetracycline, chlor-amphenicol or trimethoprim (plus sulphonamides) showed improvement, whereas ampicillin and spiramycin were ineffective. Furthermore, marked changes in drug metabo-lism were observed in tickborne fever-infected goats treated with chloramphenicol or sulphadimidine; the elimination half-life values of these drugs and of oxytetracycline were significantly prolonged. The pharmacokinetics of ampicillin, spiramycin and sulpha-methylphenazole did not show marked differences between healthy and tickborne fever-infected animals.

INTRODUCTION

Tetracyclines are dramatically effective in rickettsial infections[1,3], including tickborne fever (TBF) in rumi-nants[16]. These drugs are usually merely rickettsiostatic, whereas less information is available about the effectiveness of other chemotherapeutic agents. Tickborne fever is caused by Ehrlichia phagocytophila, which invades neutrophils and – to a lesser degree – monocytes[20]. Characteristic tickborne fever inclusion bodies can be found in the peripheral neutrophils during febrile episodes. In dwarf goats, tickborne fever is characterized by high fever, dullness, anorexia, tachycardia, a moderate inhibition of rumen motility, leucopenia, decreased serum alkaline phosphatase activity (ALP) and a marked decline in plasma zinc and iron concentrations[16]. The clinical effects may cause therapeutic problems if fever alters the absorption, distribution, biotransformation and/or excretion of drugs being administered to treat this disease[7,12,13]. In the present study, experimentally infected dwarf goats were treated with chloramphenicol, ampicillin, spiramycin, trimethoprim plus sulphadimidine and sulphamethylphenazole (TSS) and oxytetracycline in groups of four or five animals each, to study the pharmacokinetics of these drugs and to evaluate the effectiveness of the doses administered using ALP, white blood cell count (WBC), parasitaemia and body temperature as parameters.

MATERIAL AND METHODS
Animals
Twenty-five healthy dwarf goats, female and castrated males, were used (mean body weight ± SE : 37 ± 1.7 kg). All goats were kept indoors and fed a diet of hay and pelleted concentrate; water was provided ad libitum.

Drugs
The drugs used were : sodium ampicillin (Penbritin[R], 20 mg.kg^{-1}), chloramphenicol (Amicol[R] Forte, 50 mg.kg^{-1}), spiramycin (Suanovil[R], 20 mg.kg^{-1}), oxytetracycline (Engemycine[R], 10 mg.kg^{-1}) and sulphamethylphenazole (Vesulong[R], 50 mg.kg^{-1}) plus sulphadimidine (50 mg.kg^{-1}) and trimethoprim (20 mg.kg^{-1}). All drugs were given by injection

into the jugular vein. Moreover, spiramycin was also studied after intramuscular injection into the thigh.

Experimental procedures

The animals were trained to stand quietly during actual recording sessions by repeatedly placing them in the experimental cage for several hours at a time. Thereafter, they were allocated into several groups : I = ampicillin (n = 5), II = spiramycin (n = 5), III = chloramphenicol (n = 5), IV = oxytetracyline (n = 5), and V = TTS (n = 5). Firstly, experiments were performed with single doses of the drugs given intravenously to goats free from any infection; experiments with infected animals were carried out 6 weeks later. The goats were infected by intravenous inoculation of 2 ml of a stabilate, which was prepared by a method described earlier[16]. On postinfection day 4 (PID$_4$) the same dose levels of drugs were administered. Of the five goats in group II, III and V, four were treated. The remaining three infected animals served as untreated controls (group VI). Blood samples were obtained before infection, immediately before treatment and at 2, 4, 6, 8, 12, 18, 24 and 48 hours posttreatment (by caudal puncture of the vena jugularis). White blood cell counts, parasitaemia and ALP activity were determined using methods described previously[16,21].

Fever

The procedure for recording rectal temperature was the same as earlier described[14]. A fever index (FI$_8$), proportional to the area between the response curve and the baseline temperature — with the response plotted so that five units on the ordinate represent a change of 1 °C and so that two units on the abscissa represent 1 hour — was calculated for a period of 8 h following drug administration on PID$_4$; ten units of FI are therefore equivalent to a 1 °C change lasting 1 h.

Drug analysis
Heparinized jugular blood samples were collected at :
0.16, 0.33, 0.5, 0.75, 1.0, 1.5, 2, 3, 4, 6, 8, 12, 18,
24, 36 and 48 h after drug administration. Concentrations
in these samples were determined by methods previously
described [6,8,10,11].

Pharmacokinetic and statistical analysis.
Results were expressed as mean $\pm$ SEM. In values compared
from the same goats between control and later values of
any group, the paired t-test was used. In comparisons
made between two groups, an independent t-test was used.
The "null" hypothesis was rejected at the 5% level.
Pharmacokinetic analysis[2] was performed by standard procedures employing preprogrammed calculators.

RESULTS AND DISCUSSION
The mean rectal temperature in the goats before they were
infected was 38.5 $\pm$ 0.2 °C, whereas the mean preinfection
values of ALP activity and WBC counts were 377 IU.l^{-1} and
9.2 $\pm$ 0.6.10^9.l^{-1}, respectively. These values agree with
those reported earlier[12,13]. After infection, the level
of ALP activity showed a progressive fall in all goats
(PID$_4$: 50.7 $\pm$ 2.7% from baseline values), whereas WBC
counts demonstrated a decline in the number of circulating
white blood cells (PID$_4$: 53.7 $\pm$ 6.3 % from baseline).
Similar changes were observed in a previous study[16].
After a sudden rectal temperature rise on the 3rd day of
infection, a plateau of 40.5-41.5 °C was maintained over a
period of 3-6 days (on PID$_4$, 0 h : 40.8 $\pm$ 0.1 °C, n = 25),
followed by a rapid fall to normal body temperature.
Concurrently, tachycardia and a moderate inhibition of
rumen contractions were observed[16].

Efficacy studies
Rectal temperature seemed to be the most effective
parameter to check the effectiveness of chemotherapeutic
agents (Table 39.1 and 39.2). TSS, oxytetracycline and

Table 39.1 Tickborne fever : effects of some chemotherapeutic agents on fever index, serum ALP activity and WBC
counts in dwarf goats

	Ampicillin	Spiramycin	Chloram-phenicol
	(I)	(II)	(III)
Fever index			
(PID$_4$ - 8 h)	163.6±13.5	170.3±14.6	107.9±4.2*
ALP			
Mean baseline	128.3	372	302.3
(IU.1^{-1})			
PID$_4$ (% change)	43.2±2.8	46.9±6.9	48.8±3.4
PID$_5$ (% change)	37.6±2.3	37.4±9.3	38.9±1.9
PID$_6$ (% change)	37.3±4.6	35.9±4.2	31.7±1.4
WBC			
Baseline	8.7±1.9	8.4±1.0	11.1±0.3
(10^9.1^{-1})			
PID$_4$ - 0 h (% change)	42.4±7.5	31.9±5.4	30.3±7.4
PID$_4$ - 8 h (% change)	33.5±8.4	30.6±5.6	33.3±9.6
PID$_4$ - 12 h (% change)	37.9±7.1	32.8±6.3	43.5±8.3
PID$_5$ - 18 h (% change)	30.0±3.8+	32.7±4.5	46.1±8.6*+
PID$_4$ - 24 h (% change)	33.6±6.9	31.9±3.3	43.2±7.6*

* p < 0.05, independent t-test
+ p < 0.05, paired t-test
PID : Postinfection day

chloramphenicol showed significant effects, whereas
neither ampicillin nor spiramycin (intramuscular) were

Table 39.2 Tickborne fever : effects of some chemotherapeutic agents on fever index, serum ALP activity and WBC
counts in dwarf goats

	Oxytetracy-cline (IV)	TSS (V)	Control (VI)
Fever index			
(PID$_4$ – 8 h)	92.3±10.7*	42.9±20.1*	213.3±22.5
ALP			
Mean baseline			
(IU.l^{-1})	392	272	172.7
PID$_4$ (% change)	58.7±8.6	45.5±2.6	64.3±11.7
PID$_5$ (% change)	54.8±4.0	38.9±2.5	47.7±8.6
PID$_6$ (% change)	50.3±3.8	40.3±2.6	43.8±12.7
WBC			
Baseline			
(10^9.l^{-1})	9.1±1.1	10.8±1.3	11.5±2.6
PID$_4$ – 0 h			
(% change)	78.3±1.7	36.8±3.9	36.0±5.2
PID$_4$ – 8 h			
(% change)	64.4±7.6$^+$	35.8±4.5	30.2±1.0
PID$_4$ – 12 h			
(% change)	81.4±5.5	35.2±1.2	30.9±4.8
PID$_4$ – 18 h			
(% change)	88.2±2.2$^+$	32.4±3.1	30.7±3.4*
PID$_4$ – 24 h			
(% change)	75.7±1.5	30.6±2.2	27.0±1.2*$^+$

* $p < 0.05$, independent t-test
$^+$ $p < 0.05$, paired t-test
PID : Postinfection day

effective. Moreover, in groups I, II and VI goats,
febrile reactions persisted for several days (PID$_5$ –PID$_7$).

Temperature relapses were not observed after oxytetracycline administration in contrast to the goats from group III (PID_3-PID_4). The fast temperature effect of TSS in addition to a shortlived relapse (on PID_3) suggest that trimethoprim is probably the active compound, because sulphonamides are not rickettsiostatic[5]. The characteristic inclusions of tickborne fever were most prominent in the neutrophils on the 3rd and 4th day of infection.

Approximately 8 h after oxytetracycline administration (PID_4), pycnotic spots were observed within these infected cells, whereas the other drugs did not induce this phenomenon. In most groups, the number of infected cells varied from 12 to 36% on PID_3, with somewhat lower values in the oxytetracycline-treated group. Therefore, it was not surprising that most drugs had no marked effects on the decline of WBC counts (Table 39.1 and 39.2). The fall in ALP activity appears to be correlated with the drop in WBC counts. Likewise, similar changes have been demonstrated in goats after bacterial toxin administration[15, 17, 18], in veal calves with salmonellosis[4] and in febrile horses due to Streptococcus zooepidemicus infection[19]. Therefore, the relationship between ALP activity and white blood cells requires more detailed investigations.

Pharmacokinetic studies

Table 39.3 shows the mean elimination half-life, plasma protein binding and total body clearance values for the chemotherapeutic agents tested in healthy dwarf goats. In the infected groups, treated with chloramphenicol, sulphadimidine or oxytetracycline half-life values were significantly ($p < 0.05$) prolonged. With ampicillin, both volume of distribution (V_d area in $l.kg^{-1}$) and the peripheral compartment (V_2 in $l.kg^{-1}$) were significantly greater during the febrile episode : 0.73 ± 0.05 $l.kg^{-1}$ and 0.04 ± 0.003 $l.kg^{-1}$ versus 1.04 ± 0.11 $l.kg^{-1}$ and 0.08 ± 0.012 $l.kg^{-1}$, respectively. Febrile goats treated with chloramphenicol, showed a greater peripheral compartment

Table 39.3 Tickborne fever in goats : some pharmacokinetic data ($t_{1/2}$ ß, h; protein binding, %; Cl, $l.kg^{-1}.h^{-1}$) of chemotherapeutic agents after intravenous administration into the jugular vein; A : Spiramycin; B : Oxytetracycline; C : Chloramphenicol; D : Ampicillin; E : Sulphamethylphenazole; F : Sulphadimidine; G : Trimethoprim

	A	B	C
$t_{1/2}$ ß			
−	13.1±2.6	6.1±0.58	1.49±0.16
+	ND	7.3±0.33*	1.94±0.25*
Protein binding			
−	ND	66.7±1.3	46.5±1.3
+	ND	69.6±1.4	45.7±3.0
Cl			
−	0.3±0.02	0.13±0.01	0.40±0.04
+	ND	0.10±0.01*	0.36±0.05

	D	E	F	G
$t_{1/2}$ ß				
−	0.92±0.08	33.4±3.7	2.9±0.31	1.9±0.27
+	1.1±0.05	37.4±1.6	5.1±0.7*	1.8±0.44
Protein binding				
−	44.1±2.8	98.0±0.3	75.4±3.4	ND
+	48.2±1.6	90.5±2.1*	59.3±4.0*	ND
Cl				
−	0.56±0.03	−	0.06±0.01	0.95±0.1
	0.67±0.07	−	0.02±0.004*	1.46±0.09*

− before infection , + after infection

* $p < 0.05$

for this agent as well (0.33 ± 0.05 l.kg^{-1} versus 0.19 ± 0.03 l.kg^{-1}). With oxytetracycline the AUC value (h.µg.ml^{-1}) increased from 82.4 ± 7.4 to 103.1 ± 6.4 in infected animals.

The pharmacokinetics of spiramycin (intramuscular) did not show significant differences between healthy and tickborne fever-infected goats. Blood concentrations and the clearance of trimethoprim significantly changed in tickborne fever-infected goats (Table 39.3); the mean AUC value was 39.1% less than in the control experiments. In the infected animals marked changes in drug metabolism were observed in the groups treated with chloramphenicol or sulphadimidine. In the control experiments chloramphenicol was rapidly conjugated with glucuronic acid, whereas during fever this major metabolite could not be detected. Biotransformation of sulphadimidine involved acetylation, hydroxylation and glucuronidation. In general, biotransformation processes of drugs speed up elimination. In particular the acetylated and glucuronidated metabolites of sulphadimidine contribute to this acceleration process, because they are excreted by tubular secretion. The SCH$_2$OH and SOH metabolites are excreted approximately six times faster than sulphadimidine itself[7]. This explains the relatively short elimination half-life of sulphadimidine in healthy dwarf goats in contrast to other species such as the horse, the pig and the cow[9]. In the tickborne fever-infected dwarf goats, hydroxylation into SCH$_2$OH and SOH metabolites was dramatically reduced (-57.6% and -63.6% respectively[7]). Acetylation decreased to a lesser extent (-22.1%), whereas the glucuronidated SOH metabolite was hardly detectable. The diminished metabolic capacity resulted in a decreased total body clearance and in a prolongation of its half-life (Table 39.3). Sulphamethylphenazole was acetylated, but no significant differences were found between healthy and febrile episodes (3.1 ± 0.4% versus 2.9 ± 0.2%).

Thus, during fever a complex pattern emerges of retardation of certain biochemical pathways. At the present time, sufficient data are not available to permit clear understanding of how fever affects drug metabolism and/or excretion in tickborne fever-infected goats. It was suggested[20] that the parasite only penetrates polymorphonuclear leucocytes and monocytes; up till now there is no evidence for tickborne fever-induced lesions within the liver and/or kidneys. Studies concerning the effects of tickborne fever-infection on renal clearance values and the alteration in overall metabolism of drugs related to liver function tests are in progress.

CONCLUSION

The tickborne fever model used in this study has an acute character. In dwarf goats the disease is characterized by fever, dullness, anorexia, tachycardia, a moderate inhibition of rumen contractions, leucopaenia and a decreased serum alkaline phosphatase activity. This model can be of great value in testing the therapeutic efficacy and pharmacokinetics of chemotherapeutic agents in rickettsial infections. The goats receiving oxytetracycline, chloramphenicol or trimethoprim (plus sulphonamides) showed improvement, whereas ampicillin and spiramycin were ineffective. Furthermore, marked changes in drug metabolism were observed in tickborne fever-infected goats treated with chloramphenicol or sulphadimidine; the half-life values of these drugs and of oxytetracycline were significantly prolonged. The pharmacokinetics of spiramycin, ampicillin and sulphamethylphenazole did not show marked differences between healthy and tickborne fever-infected animals.

References
1. Anigstein, L. (1964). Chemotherapy of rickettsial infection. In : Schnitzer, R.J. and Hawking, F. (eds). Experimental Chemotherapy vol. III, pp.481-525. New York : Academic Press.
2. Baggot, J.D. (1977). Principles of Drug Disposition in Domestic Animals. 1st ed. Philadelphia : W.B. Saunders Company.
3. Buhles, W.C., Huxsoll, D.L. and Ristic, M. (1974). Tropical canine pancytopaenia : clinical, haemato-

logic and serologic response of dogs to Ehrlichia canis infections, tetracycline therapy and challenge inoculations. J. Infect. Dis. 130:357-367.

4. Groothuis, D.G. (1983). Pharmacokinetics of some antimicrobial drugs in veal calves and their activity in relation to Salmonella dublin infections. Utrecht : PhD thesis.

5. Hudson, J.R. (1950). The recognition of tick-borne fever as a disease of cattle. Br. Vet. J. 106:3-17.

6. Nouws, J.F.M. (1984). Irritation, bioavailability, and residue aspects of 10 oxytetracycline formulations administered i.m. to pigs. Vet. Q. 6:80-84.

7. Nouws, J.F.M., Anika, S.M., Van Miert, A.S.J.P.A.M., Vree, T.B., Baakman, M. and Van Duin, C.T.M. (1986). Effect of tick-borne fever on the disposition of sulphadimidine and its metabolites in plasma of goats. Res. Vet. Sci.(in press).

8. Nouws, J.F.M., Van Ginneken, C.A.M., Hekman, P. and Ziv, G. (1982). Comparative plasma ampicillin levels and bioavailability of 5 parenteral ampicillin formulations in ruminant calves. Vet. Q. 4:62-71.

9. Nouws, J.F.M., Vree, T.B., Breukink, H.J., Van Miert, A.S.J.P.A.M. and Grondel, J. (1986). Pharmacokinetics, hydroxylation and acetylation of sulphadimidine in different species of mammals, birds, fish, reptiles, and molluscs. In : Van Miert, A.S.J.P.A.M., Bogaert, M.G. and Debackere, M. (eds). Comparative Veterinary Pharmacology, Toxicology and Therapy. Proc. 3rd EAVPT Congress, Part II, Invited lectures. Lancaster : MTP Press.

10. Nouws, J.F.M. and Ziv, G. (1979). Distribution and residues of macrolide antibiotics in normal dairy cows. Arch. Lebensmittelhyg. 30:202-208.

11. Van Gogh, H. (1980). Pharmacokinetics of nine sulphonamides in goats. J. Vet. Pharmacol. Ther. 3:69-81.

12. Van Miert, A.S.J.P.A.M. (1984). La febbre e le modificazioni ematologiche, ematochimiche e funzionali organiche ad essa associate nella capra ed in altre specie animali. Rassegna Sci. Vet. 3:296-314.

13. Van Miert, A.S.J.P.A.M. (1985). Fever and associated clinical haematologic and blood biochemical changes in the goat and other animal species. Vet. Q. 7:200-216.

14. Van Miert, A.S.J.P.A.M., Van der Wal-Komproe. L.E. and Van Duin, C.T.M. (1977). Effects of antipyretic agents on fever and ruminal stasis induced by endotoxins in conscious goats. Arch. Int. Pharmacodyn. Ther. 225:39-50.

15. Van Miert, A.S.J.P.A.M., Van Duin, C.T.M. and Schotman, A.J.H. (1984). Comparative observations of fever and associated clinical haematological and blood biochemical changes after i.v. administration of staphylococcal enterotoxins B and F (toxic shock syndrome Toxin-1) in goats. Infect. Immun. 46: 354-360.

16. Van Miert, A.S.J.P.A.M., Van Duin, C.T.M., Schotman, A.J.H. and Franssen, F.F. (1984). Clinical, haema-

tological and blood biochemical changes in goats after experimental infection with tick-borne fever. Vet. Parasitol. 16:225-233.

17. Van Miert, A.S.J.P.A.M., Van Duin, C.T.M., Verheijden, J.H.M. and Schotman, A.J.H. (1982). Endotoxin-induced fever and associated haematological and blood biochemical changes in the goat. The effect of repeated administration and the influence of flurbiprofen. Res. Vet. Sci. 33:248-255.

18. Van Miert, A.S.J.P.A.M., Van Duin, C.T.M., Verheijden, J.H.M. and Schotman, A.J.H. (1983). Staphylococcal enterotoxin B and E. coli endotoxin : comparative observations in goats on fever and associated clinical haematologic and blood biochemical changes after i.v. and intramammary administration. Am. J. Vet. Res. 44:955-963.

19. Varma, K.J., Powers, T.E., Carg, R.C., Spurlock, S.L. and Powers, J.D. (1983). Efficacy of penicillin against Streptococcus zooepidemicus infection model in the horse. In : Ruckebusch, Y., Toutain, P.L. and Koritz, G.D. (eds). Veterinary Pharmacology and Toxicology. Proc. 2nd EAVPT Congress, pp.429-436. Lancaster : MTP Press.

20. Woldehiwet, Z. (1983). Tick-borne fever : a review. Vet. Res. Commun. 6:163-175.

21. Woldehiwet, Z. and Scott, G.R. (1982). Immunological studies on tick-borne fever in sheep. J. Comp. Pathol. 92:457-467.

40
Statistical methods for evaluation of drug efficacy in animal models

J. D. POWERS AND T. E. POWERS

ABSTRACT

Animal disease models are used to simulate a naturally occurring disease state and/or to evaluate drug efficacy. A numerical rating system allows the clinician to express subtle differences he is observing: a rating system with a wide range of possible scores can furthermore statistically be handled as a continuous variable in longitudinal studies across time. A health index possessing the following properties — reproducible rating between clinicians, measuring existing differences and easy to use — provides such a rating system. Two health indices, developed for the Streptococcus zooepidemicus model in the beagle dog and the horse, respectively, are discussed.

INTRODUCTION

Animal disease models are primarily used to evaluate drug efficacy and/or to simulate a naturally occurring disease state. In either case it is necessary to quantitatively evaluate the results of the investigation. This evaluation occurs at two levels : (a) measuring the response of the individual subject at any point in time, and (b) measuring efficacy over time in groups of subjects receiving different treatments.

To restrict this quantification to only a few categories such as improved, no change, or deterioration imposes several limitations: for example, it increases the number of subjects needed to detect a difference and forces the evaluating clinician to report gross impressions only. Hence a numerical rating system which provides the clinician with a method of expressing the subtle differences his experienced eye preceives is preferable both to him and to the statistician who must evaluate the results. Furthermore, a rating system which has a broad range can be statistically handled as a continuous variable in longitudinal studies across time. This, in most cases, permits the use of parametric procedures such as analysis of variance and/or regression.

A health index to evaluate an animal disease model would provide such a rating system. However, to be of value, this index must possess the following properties :

(1) reproducible ratings between clinicians;
(2) measure differences when they exist;
(3) easy to use.

In our laboratory, two such indices have been developed. The first was constructed to be used with a Streptococcus zooepidemicus model in the beagle dog[1] and the second index evaluates a similar model in the horse[2].

CONSTRUCTION OF A HEALTH INDEX

The construction of a health index can only be achieved by the cooperative efforts of the clinician, the pharmacologist and the statistician. The clinician and pharmacologist must communicate verbally to the statistician those characteristics which their trained eyes observe which result in an ordering of a group of subjects, with respect to degree of illness. In turn, the statistician must convert these observations into a numbering system which has the following properties :

(1) Reproducible scores between clinicians : if the sco-

Table 40.1   Health index for beta-haemolytic streptococcal
disease model in the dog

Clinical sign   Description   Score given
----
(1) Lameness (0-15)
    (a) Is unable to get up and move and has
        painful limb joints   13-15
    (b) Can get up with difficulty, feels pain on
        walking, and has inflamed leg joints   10-12
    (c) Can get up easily, moves with staggering,
        leg and joints are painful on palpation   7-9
    (d) Shows some lameness and has abnormal gait   4-6
    (e) Almost no lameness, no inflammation, and no
        pain in joints even on palpation   0-3
(2) Size of lymph nodes (0-8)
    (a) Size more than double normal size   6-8
    (b) Almost double normal size   3-5
    (c) Normal to slight enlargement   0-2
(3) Colour of mucous membranes (0-5)
    (a) Pale and cyanotic   4-5
    (b) Pale   2-3
    (c) Pink or whitish pink   0-1
(4) Degree of alertness (0-4)
    (a) No response to surroundings, lying listless
        in a prostrate manner   4
    (b) Unconcerned to surroundings but has healthier
        posture   3
    (c) Not getting up on subjective approach but does
        move the tail   2
    (d) Active on approach shows playing behaviour,
        moves tail, and shakes head and ears   0-1
(5) Condition of hair coat (0-4)
    (a) Looks dull with falling of hair   3-4
    (b) Loss of shine, looking rough but no loss of
        hair   2
    (c) Shiny compact hair coat with no falling off   0-1

(6) Degree of dehydration (0-4)

(a) Skin just adherent with subcutaneous tissue   3-4

(b) Can get a skin fold, stays for some time on
   releasing the fold   2

(c) Can get a skin fold which disappears immediately with the release of fold   0-1

----

ring system is given to two or more "equally competent" clinicians, with a minimal amount of training,
these clinicians will independently rate the same
subject with similar scores. By "equally competent"
it is meant that the clinician has experience in
evaluating each of the components which comprise the
health index. A clear example of this would be the
small animal clinician attempting to evaluate the
degree of lameness in a horse or bloatedness in a cow.
This clinician's eye is not called upon to rate such
syndromes in his professional activities and hence is
not expected to do so with the same expertise of an
equinine or food animal clinician, respectively.

(2) Measure differences when they exist. This property is
most easily described by considering two "equally"
sick subjects and at least one subject which is "less"
ill and one which is clinically "quite" ill. The
desired property would dictate that the two "equally"
sick subjects would receive similar scores, whereas
the remaining two patients would be assigned scores
different from the first two and different from each
other.

(3) Easy to use indicates that with little or no instruc-
tion a qualified clinician is capable of translating
his professional expertise into a score appropriate
for the condition of the given patient.

STATISTICAL EVALUATION
Traditionally, efficacy studies compare treatment groups
across time. This permits the investigator to compare

Table 40.2 Health index for beta-haemolytic streptococcal disease model in the horse

---

Clinical sign	Score

General appearance

Normal	0
Depression slight but discernible (responsiveness, head position and involvement, "eye" and hair coat)	1
Head down, but responds to noise or menace	2
Head down with poor response	3
Very depressed, stares, little or no response	4
Down most of the time	5

Nasal and ocular exudate

Normal, ocular	0
Ocular serous	1
Ocular purulent	2
Normal, nasal	0
Nasal serous	1
Nasal purulent (small)	2
Nasal purulent (large)	3

Respiratory examination

Normal	0
Harsh tracheal sounds	1
Hyperpnoea	1
Slight respiratory distress at rest	1
Abnormal lung sounds	2
Cough elicited by pressure on trachea or larynx	2
Spontaneous cough	3
Moist, coarse rales in a third or more of lung field	4
Easily detected respiratory distress at rest and unable to exercise or walk more than 15 m slowly	5
Significant area of consolidation or evidence of pleural effusion	6

Lameness

Normal (no lameness)	0
Detectable at trot only	1
Detectable at walk	2
Bears only 50% weight on lame leg, or stiff and unwilling to walk except if urged	3
Drags or jumps to carry lame leg	4
Down all the time except when urged to stand	5
Down and unable to raise head	6

Swollen joints, etc.

One joint swollen (independent of lameness)	1
Each additional joint swollen or painful	0,1,2,3, 4,5,6,7
Bursa of withers affected	1
Other abscesses	0,1,2,3

----

responses across both time and treatment groups. Further, the interaction between groups and time is usually of major importance to the pharmacologist. The only efficient statistical equipment which results in these three evaluations is an analysis of variance (ANOVA). Clearly broad categories of clinical ratings such as improved, not improved or no change can not be handled by ANOVA. On the other hand, a health index which has a wide range of possible scores, can be used in this type of analysis. Obviously an index is not a continuous random variable, but if the range covers, for example 50 points, the violation of the normality assumption of this test is not so serious as to negate its use and indeed the robustness of this test compensates well for this violation. In addition, when differences are found by ANOVA one of the appropriate multiple comparison tests can be used.

EXAMPLES OF HEALTH INDICES

Two health indices have been developed at the Ohio State University. The first was constructed to be used with a

Streptococcus zooepidemicus model in the beagle dog and the second was for the same pathogenic model in the horse. Tables 40.1 and 40.2 describe the details of the index for the dog and horse respectively.

By comparing the individual components of the two indices, it is possible to observe the similarities and differences of the clinical manifestations in the two species. Moreover, the issue addressed earlier regarding "equally competent" clinicians is exemplified by the lameness and respiratory scoring in the horse. Each of these components requires a competent eye and ear respectively.

The health index for the dog model was used to evaluate the efficacy of a combination product of trimethoprim and sulphadiazine[3].

References
1. Powers, J.D. and Powers, T.E. (1977). A health index to quantitate disease states in animal models. Proceedings of the 10th International Congress of Chemotherapy.
2. Powers, J.D., Powers, T.E., Varma, K.J., Gabel, A.A. and Spurlock, S.L. (1984). A health index to clinically evaluate Strep disease model in the horse. J. Vet. Pharm. Ther. 7:213-217.
3. Powers, T.E., Powers, J.D. et al. (1980). Trimethoprim and sulfadiazine experimental infection of beagles. Am. J. Vet. Res. 41:1117-1122.

41
Pharmacology of carbadox in the pig

L. P. JAGER, E. J. VAN DER MOLEN, G. J. DE GRAAF,
T. H. J. SPIERENBURG, M. J. A. NABUURS AND A. J. BAARS

ABSTRACT

An evaluation has been made of the in vitro minimal
inhibitory concentrations (MIC) of carbadox against
various bacterial species in relation to the carbadox
levels obtained in the gastrointestinal tract and in the
blood after in-feed medication of carbadox. Although a
prophylactic efficacy against orally transmitted
enteropathogenic spirochaetes and anaerobic bacilli seems
warranted, no justification for the therapeutic
application of carbadox was found. In fact, therapeutic
dosages were found to induce hypoaldosteronism in young
pigs. A direct anabolic action of carbadox could not be
reproduced in healthy young pigs fed a standard commercial
feed. The widespread use of carbadox in pig husbandry
constitutes a selection pressure towards Escherichia coli
strains with MIC values above the carbadox levels in the
small intestines. Carbadox R-plasmids in E. coli strains
can be transmitted to other gram-negative bacilli but not
to Treponema hyodysenteriae. Prevention of swine
dysentery seems now to be the only indication for in-feed
administration of carbadox. A lower dosage and a shorter
treatment period than those currently advised might
provide a marginal safety factor while still being
effective.

INTRODUCTION

Most of the pigs raised each year in the Netherlands (1983 :17 million) receive carbadox in their feed, either as a feed additive, as in-feed medication or as feed contamination. Despite the widespread use of this drug, relatively little is known about the effects carbadox can induce in weaned pigs. As new data concerning its modes of action are emerging, further pharmacological evaluation of carbadox is required to reassess the desirability of its use in pig husbandry.

In this overview the pig, as a target animal, will serve as a focal point in a discussion of the pharmacology of carbadox. Subsequently the "desired" effects of carbadox, as deduced from the indications for its current use, and the side-effects, will be discussed and an attempt will be made to estimate the therapeutic margin of carbadox in pig husbandry.

PHARMACOLOGICAL CHARACTERISTICS

Antimicrobial activity

The antimicrobial activity of carbadox involves use as a prophylactic by in-feed medication of pigs at levels of 50-55 mg.kg^{-1} (ppm), whereas a therapeutic effect is sought with in-feed dosages of 100-150 mg.kg^{-1} (ppm). The available data concerning in vitro studies of its minimal inhibitory concentration (MIC) against several pathogens (Table 41.1) indicate that its antimicrobial activity under aerobic circumstances is poor. Under anaerobic circumstances much lower MIC values are reported especially for enteropathogenic bacilli and Treponema hyodysenteriae, supposedly the causative agent in swine dysentery (dysentery Doyle). In vitro MIC values of about 40 ng.ml^{-1} imply that carbadox might be an effective drug[6].

The pharmacokinetic characteristics of carbadox after oral administration however, do raise doubts about its probable efficacy[14]. As the infection is transmitted by the oral route, the amount of carbadox in the contents of

Table 41.1 In vitro susceptibility of bacteria for carbadox

Species	Minimal inhibitory concentration (MIC)*		References
	aerobic μg.ml⁻¹	anaerobic μg.ml⁻¹	

Species · Minimal inhibitory concentration (MIC)* aerobic μg.ml⁻¹ / anaerobic μg.ml⁻¹ · References

Species	aerobic $\mu g.ml^{-1}$	anaerobic $\mu g.ml^{-1}$	References
Escherichia coli	6	0.2	9
(chicken 1976)		0.31 ± 0.03	10
(cattle 1976)		0.31 ± 0.04	10
(swine 1976)		1.45 ± 0.17	10
(swine 1980)	131 ± 18	16.13 ± 2.57	10
	6-12		2
(swine 1978-80)	30 ± 2		2
	12-25	0.4-1.6	12,13
Klebsiella pneumoniae	25	0.8	10,13
Citrobacter freundii		0.4	10
Shigella flexneri		0.4	10
Shigella sonnei	25		13
Salmonella typhi		0.2	10
Salmonella typhimurium	12-50	0.8-1.6	12,13
Salmonella dublin		1.6	12
Salmonella chole-raesuis	1.6-25	1.6	12,13
Salmonella spp.	6-50	0.8-1.6	12,13
Lactobacillus spp.		8.0 ± 1.3	3
Staphylococcus aureus	25-50		2
Streptococcus faecalis	12-25		2
Treponema hyodysen-teriae		<0.01-0.04	12
		<0.01	6
		<0.05-0.08	16
		<0.02-0.04	17
		<0.01	18

* Average (m ± SEM), range or single value of the MICs
  reported.

the gastrointestinal tract proximal to the jejunum after in-feed medication with 50 ppm carbadox seems to be high enough to kill invading treponemes. Also, carbadox levels in the stomach and duodenum might be effective against invading bacilli, assuming anaerobic conditions. The MIC values reported under aerobic conditions are often well above the levels present after in-feed medication.

With regard to a therapeutic application of carbadox the prospects are less promising than for prophylaxis. In-feed medication of carbadox at therapeutic dosages (100 ppm) yields carbadox levels which, even in the distal half of the jejunum, are below the anaerobic MIC values. The pathogenic activity of T. hyodysenteriae includes penetration of mucosal cells of the colon, but even after in-feed medication with 100 or 150 ppm carbadox the level of carbadox in the contents of this part of the gastrointestinal tract can, by extrapolation, be assumed to be virtually zero. The blood levels of carbadox after in-feed medication might just attain the MIC values, but the concentration gradient across the colonic mucosa makes it unlikely that significant amounts of carbadox reach the infected mucosal cells. In outbreaks of dysentery (or diarrhoea) in-feed medication with carbadox (50 ppm) can be used to protect the animals not yet infected, but for the treatment of infected animals other drugs should be used.

With regard to the development of resistance of intestinal bacteria carbadox is notable. The widespread use of this drug as a feed additive constituted an enormous selection pressure in favour of intestinal bacilli with low sensitivities[2]. Ohmae et al.[10] reported that in 1980 more than 80% of the E. coli isolates from pigs had aerobic MIC values above 10 $\mu g.ml^{-1}$, and from the anaerobic MIC values 33% exceeded this value, while a few years earlier less than 1% of the isolated strains exceeded this value. It seems safe to assume that, on farms where carbadox is used as a standard feed additive, the aerobic sensitivity of all intestinal bacilli present is such that they will not be affected by the carbadox concentrations encountered in the gastrointestinal tract. With the increase of aerobic MIC values an increase of the anaerobic MIC values was observed, but the difference between these two values remained on the average 10-fold.

Not surprisingly with this selection for carbadox-insensitive strains, R-plasmids were found in E. coli isolates[9]. Their existence and the reported transfer to other gram-negative bacilli has consequences for an assessment of the usefulness of this drug. The already meagre prospects for prophylactic efficacy against enteropathogenic bacilli, because of the heavy reliance on anaerobic conditions in the gut, are now zero. Moreover, the possibility that multiple resistant gram-negative bacilli are selected might reduce the efficacy of other antimicrobial drugs. However, there is evidence indicating that carbadox actually reduces the incidence of multiple resistant strains of enteric bacteria and thus increases the efficacy of other antimicrobial agents[4]. The R-plasmid-eliminating activity of carbadox seems to be directly related to its inhibition of DNA-synthesis[4]. Also, the persistence of transposed carbadox resistance is short in the absence of selection pressure, therefore the introduction of a carbadox resistant gene might ultimately facilitate the disappearance of all resistant traits, encoded in the same plasmid as the carbadox resistance.

So far neither selection pressure nor R-plasmids have impaired the efficacy of carbadox against T. hyodysenteriae[1,10]. The difference between the highest reported MIC-value and the concentrations of carbadox in the stomach and duodenum after in-feed medication is 100-fold. In order to obtain a safety margin (see below) a lower dosage for carbadox as a preventive feed additive seems possible without attenuation of its efficacy.

Growth-promoting activity
The in-feed medication with carbadox up to 50 ppm has become popular in pig husbandry mainly because it is a

cheap growth promoter. As with other antimicrobial agents, growth-promoting activity was found to increase with infection pressure. Furthermore, a growth-promoting effect not attributable to the antimicrobial activity of carbadox or direct anabolic action of carbadox is claimed. Although there are reports indicating that with SPF pigs a significant growth-promoting effect was observed[5], in two different experiments we were unable to detect a growth-promoting activity in MD pigs. In field trials carbadox is reported to have a growth promoting effect of almost 25% in weight gain which can decrease to 18% in "clean uninfected university" pigs[13].

In our experiments we concluded that there was no basis for a growth-promoting effect of 10% or more by 50 ppm carbadox. The animals were fed ad libitum to enhance a growth-promoting effect. Frequent faecal samples indicated the absence of pathogens to ensure the detection of a direct anabolic action. The feed conversion of the control animals was ⩽ 2 during the treatment, which reduces the margin for growth promotion to the lower values reported[13]. The normal commercial pig feed used in these experiments, however, contained 11‰ lysine, well above the 8‰ lysine reported to be the upper limit for an improvement of the feed conversion by carbadox[5]. This might explain our negative findings, but also casts doubts about the justification for the use of carbadox as the ever-present growth promoter in pig feed.

From our observations of young pigs fed 0.25 or 50 ppm carbadox in their rations we concluded that carbadox at the 50 ppm dosage induced urine-drinking behaviour. It is tempting to speculate that this behaviour is brought about by salt-craving, an early symptom of hypoaldosteronism[7].

Toxic activity

The outstanding characteristic of the toxicology of carbadox is the seemingly highly selective and specific effect on the glomerular zone of the adrenal cortex after a few weeks of carbadox medication in feed at levels of

100 ppm and higher[8]. This histological observation was subsequently corroborated by the finding that even after a short period of carbadox administration aldosterone (released from the adrenal zona glomerulosa), sodium and potassium ion levels in blood are significantly altered[7]. It is doubtful whether the adrenal damage induced by carbadox is reversible. To date, we have not found an explanation for this specific and selective action of carbadox on the adrenals. Preliminary experiments did not confirm a supposed accumulation of carbadox in the adrenals. That the glomerular zone of the adrenals is a first site of action for carbadox is indirectly shown by our observation that within a week of the start of the administration of 100 ppm carbadox the aldosterone levels are reduced to 35% of the control values. The sodium and potassium levels in the blood only start to deviate from controls after 4 weeks.

Other, longer known aspects of the toxicological profile of carbadox are its mutagenicity in bacteria[15], and its genotoxic action in mammals[11]. It is possible that the toxic effects of carbadox are related to its antibacterial activity. The proposed mechanism of this action of carbadox is that it affects nucleic acid metabolism, and it was found to bind to DNA in bacteria. A similar interaction with mammalian DNA cannot be excluded. In this respect the difference between bacterial and mammalian cells might not be large for carbadox. At least in weaned pigs the factor between the prophylactic, growth-promoting dosage used and the lowest dosage studied with an undeniable toxic effect is only two.

CONCLUSION
The conclusion is reached that the current almost unrestricted use of carbadox as a feed additive for piglets is hardly justified. The prophylactic medication with 50 ppm only prevents orally invading T. hyodysenteriae, the protection against other

enteropathogens having become negligible. A direct
anabolic effect of carbadox seems doubtful with the high
lysine content of commercial Dutch pig feed. A reliable
protection against swine dysentery with a safety margin
might be provided by in-feed medication with 25 ppm
carbadox. The current therapeutic use of carbadox to
"cure" diarrhoea has a questionable efficacy because it
alters the aldosterone regulation of extracellular fluid
electrolyte concentration, extracellular fluid volume,
blood volume, arterial pressure and renal function; in
short it induces hypoaldosteronism.

References
1. Baumgartner, A., Meyer, J., Lebek, G. and Nicolet, J.
   (1985). Natur und Verbreitung der Carbadoxresistenz
   bei Escherichia coli, isoliert von Mastschwenen,
   -Kälbern und Geflügel. Schweiz. Arch. Tierheilk.
   127:339-347.
2. Das, N.K. (1984). In vitro susceptibility of Escherichia coli of swine origin to carbadox and other anti-
   microbials. Am. J. Vet. Res. 45:252-254.
3. Dutta, G.N. and Devriese, L.A. (1981). Sensitivity
   and resistance to growth promoting agents in animal
   lactobacilli. J. Appl. Bact. 51:283-288.
4. Gedek, B. (1979). Bewertung der Leistungsfähigkeit
   von Carbadox als Wachstumsförderer nach mikrobio-
   logischen Kriterien. Zbl. Vet. Med. B. 26:7-19.
5. Gropp, J. (1976). Der Einfluss von Fortigro bei
   Schweinen auf die Nährstoffverwertung. In : Wissen-
   schaftliche Vortragstagung über wirtschafliche
   Schweineproduktion :Fortigro R (carbadox) zwei Jahre
   im Einsatz, pp.67-94. Karlsruhe :Pfizer GmbH.
6. Kitai, K., Kashiwazaki, M., Adachi, Y., Kume, T. and
   Arakawa, A. (1979). In vitro activity of 39
   antimicrobial agents against Treponema hyodysenteriae.
   Antimicrob. Agents Chemother. 15:393-395.
7. Van der Molen, E.J., de Graaf, G.J. and Baars, A.J.
   (1985). Carbadox-induced changes in aldosterone and
   ion levels in the blood of weaned pigs. In : Van
   Miert, A.S.J.P.A.M., Bogaert, M.G. and Debackere, M.
   (eds). Comparative Veterinary Pharmacology, Toxicology and Therapy. Proc. 3rd EAVPT Congress, Part I,
   Abstracts, p.247. Utrecht: EAVPT.
8. Van der Molen, E.J., Nabuurs, M.J.A. and Jager, L.P.
   (1985). Clinical and pathological changes related to
   toxicity of carbadox in weaned pigs. Zbl. Vet. Med.
   B. 32: 540-550.
9. Ohmae, K., Yonezawa, S. and Terakado, N. (1981).
   R-Plasmid with carbadox resistance from Escherichia
   coli of porcine origin. Antimicrob. Agents Chemother. 19:86-90.

10. Ohmae, K., Yonezawa, S. and Terakado, N. (1983). Epi-
    zootiological studies on R Plasmid with Carbadox
    resistance. Jap. J. Vet. Sci. 45:165-170.
11. Oud, J.L., Reutlinger, A.H.J. and Branger, J. (1979).
    An investigation into the cytogenetic damage induced
    by the coccidiostatic agents amprolium, carbadox,
    dimetridazole and ronidazole. Mut. Res. 68:179-182.
12. Pfizer (1983). Mecadox (carbadox) vs. olaquindox.
    Technical information update, no. 8307. New York:
    Pfizer International Inc.
13. Pfizer (undated). Mecadox (carbadox) technische hand-
    leiding. Rotterdam: Pfizer BV.
14. Spierenburg, Th.J., De Graaf, G.J. and Jager, L.P.
    (1985). Levels of carbadox in porcine blood and
    gastrointestinal contents after in-feed administra-
    tion. In : Van Miert, A.S.J.P.A.M., Bogaert, M.G. and
    Debackere, M. (eds). Comparative and Veterinary
    Pharmacology, Toxicology and Therapy. Proc. 3rd EAVPT
    Congress , Part I, Abstracts, p.91. Utrecht :EAVPT.
15. Voogd, C.E., Van der Stel, J.J. and Jacobs, J.J.J.A.A.
    (1980). The mutagenic action of quindoxin, carbadox,
    olaquindox and some other N-oxides on bacteria and
    yeast. Mut. Res. 78:233-242.
16. Williams, B.J. and Babcock, W.E. (1976). In vitro
    susceptibility of Treponema hyodysenteriae to carba-
    dox, virginiamycin, and tylosin. Vet. Med. Small
    Anim. Clin. 71:957-959.
17. Williams, B.J. and Shively, J.E. (1978). In vitro
    antitreponemal activities of carbadox, virginiamycin,
    olaquindox and tylosin as indices of their
    effectiveness for preventing swine dysentery. Vet.
    Med. Small Anim. Clin. 73:349-351.
18. Williams, B.J. and Babcock, W.E. (1978). In vivo and
    in vitro susceptibility of Treponema hyodysenteriae to
    carbadox before and after repeated in vitro passage in
    sublethal concentrations of drug. Vet. Med. Small
    Anim. Clin. 73:432-436.

Opiates, Opioids
and
Neuropeptides

42
Opioid peptides and their receptors

R. A. LEFEBVRE

ABSTRACT

The endogenous opioid peptides belong to three groups : the endorphins, the enkephalins and the dynorphins. These three groups are clearly distinct chemical families deri- ved from three different precursor peptides : pro-opio- melanocortin, proenkephalin and prodynorphin. Endogenous opioid peptides are present as well in the brain as in the periphery and interact with opioid receptors. Three subtypes of opioid receptors are now generally accepted : mu, delta and kappa. Enkephalins are preferentially active at delta-receptors, beta-endorphin is very potent at both mu- and delta-receptors, while dynorphins show kappa-receptor preference.

INTRODUCTION

The effects of opiates have undoubtedly been known for many centuries. In the 1960s, it became clear that these effects are due to interaction with specific receptors, which were called "opiate receptors". In the early 1970s, evidence for the existence of endogenous ligands for the opiate receptor was obtained and in 1975 the structures of [Leu]enkephalin and [Met]enkephalin were elucidated. Since then, many other endogenous ligands acting on opiate receptors have been discovered.

The term "opioids" is now used to indicate directly acting compounds with effects that are stereospecifically antagonized by naloxone. The term "opiates" should be reserved for products derived from the opium poppy and related synthetic alkaloids. The endogenous ligands are mainly peptides; they should be called "endogenous opioid peptides"; as they are the physiological ligands for the opiate receptors, the latter should be called "opioid receptors".

CLASSES OF ENDOGENOUS OPIOID PEPTIDES

The endogenous opioid peptides belong to three major groups : the endorphins, the enkephalins and the dynorphins[2,3,5,6]. Some opioid peptides cannot be classified within these groups; these include the exorphins, which are present in body fluids (for example, beta-casomorphin in bovine milk).

The three main groups of endogenous opioid peptides are clearly distinct chemical families, each group being derived from another precursor peptide or prohormone. These prohormones contain from 256 to 265 amino acids and are genetically coded; after translation of the messenger RNA into the protein sequence of the prohormone, smaller fragments of the prohormone are cleaved out. In the prohormones, the peptides are surrounded by a pair of basic amino acid residues, which are presumed to be recognition sites for the cleavage by processing enzymes.

Endorphins

Endorphins are derived from pro-opiomelanocortin (POMC; Figure 42.1). POMC contains, at its C-terminal side, beta-lipotropin (a 91 amino acid sequence) : beta-endorphin, the main representative of the endorphin group, is the terminal 31 amino acid sequence of beta-lipotropin and has also been called C-fragment. Smaller fragments of beta-endorphin have also been extracted : beta-endorphin(1-16) or alpha-endorphin, beta-endorphin(1-17) or gamma-endorphin, beta-endorphin(1-26) and beta-endorphin(1-27), which is also known as delta-endorphin or C'-fragment. POMC further contains adrenocorticotrophic hormone (ACTH) and three copies (alpha, beta and gamma) of melanocyte-stimulating hormone (MSH).

High concentrations of endorphins are present in the pituitary. In the anterior lobe, a small number of cells produces beta-endorphin; in the intermediate lobe, which is not present in humans, all cells produce beta-endorphin-related peptides. In the brain, the distribution of endorphin-containing cell bodies is limited. A high concentration is found in the hypothalamus; from this area, fibres project to many areas of the brain. Endorphins have also been found in peripheral organs such as the pancreas.

Enkephalins
The enkephalins are derived from the prohormone proenkephalin (see Figure 42.1). Proenkephalin contains once the [Leu]enkephalin sequence and 4 times the [Met]enkephalin sequence. [Leu]enkephalin and [Met]enkephalin are both 5 amino acid peptides. From the brain, two extensions of [Met]enkephalin at its C-terminal end were extracted : [Met]enkephalinyl-Arg-Phe and [Met]enkephalinyl-Arg-Gly-Leu. Both of these peptides are present once in proenkephalin. Proenkephalin also contains three longer peptides, which were extracted from the adrenal medulla, that is, peptide F, peptide I and peptide B. These three peptides contain one or more of the smaller sequences, cited previously.

The enkephalins are much more widely distributed in the brain than the endorphins; the highest concentrations are found in the striatum and in the hypothalamus. High concentrations of enkephalins are also present in the brain stem, in the spinal cord, and in the periphery, mainly in the nervous plexus of the gastrointestinal tract and in the adrenal medulla.

PRO-OPIOMELANOCORTIN

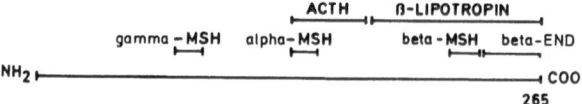

PROENKEPHALIN

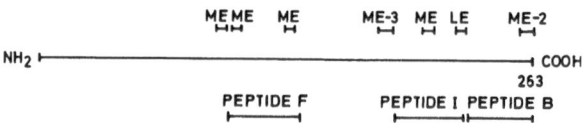

PRODYNORPHIN

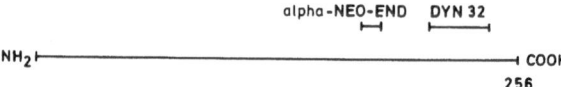

Figure 42.1 Schematic structure of pro-opiomelanocortin, proenkephalin and prodynorphin. The number of amino acids present in the prohormone is indicated. beta-END : beta-endorphin; ACTH : adrenocorticotrophic hormone; MSH : melanocyte stimulating hormone; LE : [Leu]enkephalin; ME : [Met]enkephalin; ME-2 : [Met]enkephalinyl-Arg-Phe; ME-3 : [Met]enkephalinyl-Arg-Gly-Leu ; alpha-NEO-END : alpha-neo-endorphin; DYN32 : dynorphin 32.

Dynorphins

Dynorphins all contain the [Leu]enkephalin sequence but are derived from a different precursor to proenkephalin, that is, prodynorphin (see Figure 42.1). Because of the similarity of this precursor peptide to proenkephalin, it is also known as proenkephalin B. Prodynorphin contains two opioid peptides : dynorphin 32 (32 amino acids) and alpha-neo-endorphin (10 amino acids). Smaller fragments of these peptides have also been isolated : dynorphin(1-8), dynorphin A and dynorphin B, which represent, respectively, sequences 1-8, 1-17 and 20-32 of dynorphin 32, and beta-neo-endorphin, which is alpha-neo-endorphin without the C-terminal lysyl group.

Dynorphins are widely distributed. High concentrations of peptides of the prodynorphin group are found in the posterior lobe of the pituitary, the hypothalamus, the spinal cord and the periphery, for example, in the nervous plexus of the gastrointestinal tract.

OPIOID RECEPTORS

The opioid receptor is the receptor with which opiates and opioids interact and which is blocked by naloxone. The existence of several subtypes of opioid receptor was first postulated in 1976 by Martin and his co-workers[8] on the basis of the pharmacological profile of opioids in neurophysiological and behavioural tests in the dog. Three types of opioid receptors were proposed : - mu, delta and sigma - for which the prototype agonists are morphine, ketocyclazocine and N-allylnormetazocine (SKF 10047), respectively.

On the basis of pharmacological assays on guinea-pig ileum and mouse vas deferens and binding assays in guinea-pig brain, Kosterlitz and his co-workers[7] suggested in 1977 that two types of opioid receptors are present both in brain and in peripheral organs : the mu-receptor and the delta-receptor, interacting preferentially with the enkephalins. The existence of other opioid receptor types has been proposed : epsilon-receptors - selective for beta-endorphin - in rat vas deferens[10] and brain[1]; iota-receptors in dog and rabbit ileum[9]; lambda-receptors - selective for 4,5-epoxymorphinans such as naloxone and morphine - in rat brain[4].

There is now firm evidence for the existence of three different opioid receptors, the delta-, kappa- and mu-subtypes. This conclusion is based mainly on the results of binding assays in brain homogenates but is parallelled by results obtained by in vitro assay systems, such as the guinea-pig ileum and the mouse and rabbit vas deferens.

The three main groups of opioid peptides seem to possess selectivity for these three types of opioid receptors. The enkephalins show preferential delta-receptor activity, beta-endorphin is equally potent at delta- and mu-receptors and the dynorphins interact pre-ferentially with kappa-receptors[2]. Further studies are needed to investigate whether there is a relationship between the anatomical distribution of the three families of opioid peptides and that of the three types of opioid receptors. In vitro results suggest that there is a relationship between the distribution of enkephalins and delta-receptors, and between the distribution of dynorphins and kappa-receptors.

ROLE OF ENDOGENOUS OPIOID PEPTIDES

The pharmacological properties of the endogenous opioid peptides resemble those of the opiates. They induce analgesia, respiratory depression, hypothermia, beha-vioural changes, alterations of endocrine secretions and gastrointestinal motility; tolerance and dependence occur with chronic administration. This variety of effects, the wide distribution and other experimental data suggest that endogenous opioid peptides could be involved in the regulation of functions such as nociception, cardiovascular and respiratory control, behaviour, temperature regulation, gastrointestinal motility, appetite and thirst, and several endocrine secretions.

Most work has been undertaken to determine a possible role of endogenous opioid peptides in pain regulation. Endogenous opioid peptides are probably involved in pain regulation at the level of the periaqueductal grey matter in the midbrain and of the dorsal horn of the spinal cord. It is thought that the endogenous opioid systems involved in pain control are relatively dormant under physiological conditions. In stressful situations, however, endogenous opioid peptides are released and they could then play a role in the regulation of pain sensation; opioid peptides released from the anterior pituitary and adrenal medulla could also be important.

References
1. Akil, H., Hewlett, W.A., Barchas, J.D. and Li, C.H. (1980). Binding of ^{3}H-ß-endorphin to rat brain membranes : characterization of opiate properties and interaction with ACTH. Eur. J. Pharmacol. 64:1-8.
2. Akil, H., Watson, S.J., Young, E., Lewis, M.E., Khachaturian, H. and Walker, J.M. (1984). Endogenous opioids : biology and function. Ann. Rev. Neurosci. 7:233-255.
3. Cox, B.M. (1982). Endogenous opioid peptides : a guide to structures and terminology. Life Sci. 31:1645-1658.
4. Grevel, J. and Sadée, W. (1983). An opiate binding site in the rat brain is highly selective for 4,5-epoxymorphinans. Science 221:1198-1201.
5. Hughes, J. (ed.). (1983). Opioid peptides. Br. Med. Bull. 39:1-100.
6. Kitchen, I. (1985). Endogenous opioid nomenclature : light at the end of the tunnel. Gen. Pharmacol. 16:79-84.
7. Lord, J.A.H., Waterfield, A.A., Hughes, J. and Kosterlitz, H.W. (1977). Endogenous opioid peptides : multiple agonists and receptors. Nature 267:495-499.
8. Martin, W.R., Eades, C.G., Thompson, J.A., Huppler, R.E. and Gilbert, P.E. (1976). The effects of morphine- and nalorphine-like drugs in the nondependent and morphine-dependent chronic spinal dog. J. Pharmacol. Exp. Ther. 197:517-532.
9. Oka, T. (1981). Enkephalin (opiate) receptors in the intestine. TIPS, December:328-340.
10. Schulz, R., Faase, E., Wüster, M. and Herz, A. (1979). Selective receptors for ß-endorphin on the rat vas deferens. Life Sci. 24:843-850.

43
Endorphin systems, pain and addiction

J. M. VAN REE

ABSTRACT

Several endogenous peptides with morphine-like properties (endorphins) are present in the pituitary, brain and various peripheral tissues. The presently known endorphins belong to three major families, arising from three distinct systems : pro-opiomelanocortin, proenkephalin and prodynorphin. There is some evidence that the opioid peptides belonging to a certain family can activate a specific subclass of opioid receptors. Endorphins may be concerned in motivational processes implicated in pain sensation, pain tolerance and the integrated response to pain and less in pain perception. Multiple endogenous analgesic systems are present in the body. Both neural and humoral pathways and both opioid and non-opioid substances play roles in the complex modulation of pain transmission. These various systems can be selectively activated by different environmental manipulations. Endorphins have inherent addictive properties and they have been implicated in reward mechanisms in the brain. It is postulated that they may facilitate "physiological" feelings of euphoria and lead to a state of ecstasy, which may be an important factor in addiction to various substances and habits.

INTRODUCTION

For many centuries it has been known that opium, derived from the poppy plant, causes pain relief and euphoria. This latter property is thought to be an important factor in the addictive properties of opium[13]. After the discovery of morphine as the most effective analgesic and addictive component of opium, morphine-related drugs have been developed in order to separate the desired analgesic and the undesirable addictive properties. Although these attempts were not very successful, the structure-activity relationship studies have revealed that specific opiate receptors are present in the body. The existence of such receptors was further supported by the finding showing specific binding of opiates to brain tissue[11]. Subsequently, the presence of endogenous substances that can interact with these receptor systems was postulated. This suggestion accords well with the idea that animals and humans have to a certain extent control over pain sensation. It was found in 1975 that brain tissue contains two pentapeptides, called enkephalins, that have morphine-like properties as assessed using isolated tissue preparations in vitro[6]. Since then several peptides with morphine-like action have been isolated from the brain and other tissues. These substances are called endorphins (endogenous morphine). Soon after their discovery these peptides were implicated in pain-related mechanisms, in chronic pain and various psychopathological disorders such as psychosis, depression, mania and addiction. The present survey will mainly focus on pain and addiction.

ENDORPHIN SYSTEMS

The several endorphins presently known belong to three major families, arising from three distinct systems, each containing a large precursor molecule of about 240 amino acids. Enzymatic processing of this molecule can generate peptide fragments with certain biological functions. These fragments are, however, also precursor molecules for smaller peptides with other biological activities. This

illustrates   the   neuropeptide   concept,   that   enzymatic
processing   of   peptide   molecules   can   evoke   specific
information enclosed in the molecule[4]. The three endorphin
systems   are   designated   as   pro-opiomelanocortin,
proenkephalin and prodynorphin (Table 43.1).

Pro-opiomelanocortin is located predominantly in the
pituitary, but it is also present in neuronal pathways in
the   brain[6].   From   the   basal   hypothalamus   (nucleus
arcuatus)   and the brain stem (nucleus tractus solitarius)
these pathways spread to several structures of the limbic
system   and   the   brain   stem.   In   addition,   pro-opiomelanocortin is present in the gut and in peripheral nerves.
Enzymatic processing can release from pro-opiomelanocortin
the hormones beta-lipotropin (beta-LPH) and adrenocortico-
tropin   (ACTH).   Beta-LPH   is   further   processed   to   the
opioid peptide beta-endorphin, which is the precursor
molecule for at least two other opioid peptides, alpha-
and gamma-endorphin. The structure of the N-terminal part
of   these   opioid   peptides   is   identical   to   that   of
(Met)-enkephalin, but this enkephalin is not derived from
these peptides.

Proenkephalin is located peripherally (for example, in
the adrenal medulla) and in widespread short neuronal
pathways in the brain[6]. Peptides belonging to this system
have been demonstrated, among other sites, in the basal
ganglia, hypothalamus, midbrain and spinal cord. Several
opioid peptides are derived from proenkephalin. These are
the   pentapeptides   (Met)-enkephalin   and   (Leu)-enkephalin,
but   also   larger   sequences   including   (Met)-enkephalin-
Arg-Phe and BAM-22P.

Prodynorphin is also synthesized throughout the brain
in a wide variety of neuronal systems[6]. Cell bodies
containing this molecule are present in several cerebral
cortical areas, basal ganglia, hippocampus, brain-stem
areas and certain hypothalamic nuclei, including those of
the   hypothalamic-hypophyseal   neuronal   pathway.   The
N-terminal part of the sequence of the opioid peptides
derived from prodynorphin, for example, dynorphin and

Table 43.1 Endorphins and opiate receptors

- Endorphins derived from Pro-opiomelanocortin (245 AA)
     Alpha-endorphin (16 AA)
     Gamma-endorphin (17 AA)
     Beta-endorphin (31 AA)
   Structure
     Tyr-Gly-Gly-Phe-Met ...
   Prototype
     Beta-endorphin
   Opiate receptor
     Mu (delta)
- Endorphins derived from Proenkephalin (239 AA)
     (Met)-enkephalin (5 AA)
     (Leu)-enkephalin (5 AA)
     Heptapeptide (7 AA)
     Octapeptide (8 AA)
   Structure
     Tyr-Gly-Gly-Phe-Met (or Leu) ...
   Prototype
     Met/Leu-enkephalin
   Opiate receptor
     Delta (mu)
- Endorphins derived from Prodynorphin (236 AA)
     Dynorphin (8 AA)
     Beta-neo-endorphin (9 AA)
     Alpha-neo-endorphin (10 AA)
     Dynorphin (17 AA)
     "New" big dynorphin (29 AA)
   Structure
     Tyr-Gly-Gly-Phe-Leu ...
   Prototype
     Dynorphin
   Opiate receptor
     Kappa

AA = Amino acids

alpha- and beta-neo-endorphin, is identical to that of (Leu)-enkephalin. In the brain the prodynorphin and proenkephalin systems are often anatomically contiguous, which may suggest that these peptides participate in a number of related brain functions.

Several subpopulations of opioid receptors have been proposed. Some information is available that the opioid peptides belonging to a certain family can activate a specific subclass (see Table 43.1) : beta-endorphin may activate the mu-receptor, but also the delta-receptor, enkephalins may activate the delta and to some extent the mu-receptor, while dynorphin may activate predominantly the kappa-receptor[19]. However, the exact relationship between these subclasses of opioid receptors and the physiological roles of the different opioid peptides have so far not clearly been elucidated.

When injected into body fluids, beta-endorphin is the most potent peptide in mimicking morphine-like actions. The other endorphins are also active, but more of these peptides is needed, presumably because of the more rapid degradation of the shorter endorphins. Accordingly, enkephalin analogues such as FK 33-824 which are less susceptible to enzymatic degradation than (Met)-enkephalin, are indeed more potent in eliciting morphine-like actions in vivo. Intracerebroventricularly injected beta-endorphin induces antinociception, hypothermia, hormonal changes, excessive grooming, and at higher dose levels profound immobilization and muscular rigidity[14]. Most, if not all, of these effects are mimicked by morphine and related drugs and are blocked by the specific opiate antagonists naloxone and naltrexone. Beta-endorphin also shows common actions with morphine-like drugs after repeated administration. Thus, tolerance develops to the effect of beta-endorphin on pain perception following repeated treatment[15]. Chronic administration of beta-endorphin induces physical dependence, characterized by opiate withdrawal symptoms[18]. Low doses of beta-endorphin causes self-injecting behaviour, indicating inherent addictive properties[16]. Most of these effects are, however, elicited by injecting rather high doses as compared to the amount of beta-endorphin available in the brain, and can therefore be considered as pharmacological rather than physiological actions.

ENDORPHINS AND PAIN

Opioid receptors and various endorphins are present at different levels of the spinal cord and in brain pathways, activated by painful stimuli and involved in pain detection, pain sensation, tolerance to pain and the response to pain. Different strategies have been followed to study the significance of endorphins for pain-related mechanisms, for example, antagonizing the opiate action of endorphins by opiate antagonists or by specific antisera which inactivate the physiologically available endorphins; the administration of endorphins or the release of endogenously available endorphins during pain; measurement of endorphin levels in body fluids in the presence and absence of pain.

The studies with the opiate antagonists in both animals and humans do not indicate a major role of endorphins in pain perception. In general, these substances failed to affect pain threshold of animals and humans without pain. However, when pain is present certain effects of naloxone have been described, which may suggest that pain may activate endorphin systems. The behavioural changes elicited by pain stimuli in animals and the pain sensation of humans are facilitated by naloxone[7]. The diurnal rhythm of the response to pain stimuli is absent after treatment with opiate antagonist. It has been suggested that endorphins are implicated in motivation and adaptive behaviour. Thus, the endorphins may be more concerned in motivational processes implicated in pain sensation, pain tolerance and the integrated response to pain than in pain perception.

As mentioned previously, endorphins, especially

beta-endorphin, produce long-lasting analgesia when injected into the cerebrospinal fluid. As with morphine, both the perception of pain and the response to pain are diminished. Several procedures have been applied to mobilize the endogenously available endorphins. These procedures include electrical stimulation of certain brain structures, stress-inducing stimuli (such as immobilization) and acupuncture and transcutaneous nerve stimulation. Electrical stimulation of structures in the brain-stem of animals and patients with chronic pain results in release of endorphins into the cerebrospinal fluid and in pain relief without sedation, which can partly be blocked by opiate antagonists[1]. Severe stress-inducing stimuli may be followed by a period of analgesia, which is abolished by removal of the pituitary and can partly be antagonized by opiate antagonists. There is evidence that acupuncture analgesia, induced by mechanical manipulation (classical) or electrical stimulation of the needles (electro-acupuncture), is accompanied by release of endorphins in body fluids and may be sensitive to treatment with opiate antagonists[5]. These data suggest a certain relation between the mobilization of endorphins in the body and pain relief.

Some patients suffering from chronic pain have a lower level of endorphin-like material in the cerebrospinal fluid as compared to healthy subjects[12]. This lower level was particularly apparent in patients with organic pain syndromes. Subnormal levels have been reported in patients with headache and with chronic pain. These findings, together with the increased endorphin levels after some procedures resulting in pain relief, suggest that a low level of endorphins may be related to some pain syndromes. However, the available data do not allow definite conclusions to be drawn in this respect.

Several procedures exist to treat clinical pain. Most of them were developed before information about endogenous systems involved in pain control became available. Evidence has been presented for multiple endogenous analgesia systems[17]. Both neural and hormonal pathways and both opioid and non-opioid substances play roles in the complex modulation of pain transmission. These various systems can be selectively activated by different environmental manipulations. For example, the neural-opioid system may be activated by morphine treatment and the hormonal-opioid system by stress, classical acupuncture and variants of acupuncture, such as the twitch procedure in horses, which calms down the animals and activates pain-decreasing mechanisms[9]. Electrical brain stimulation may activate both neural-opioid and neural-non-opioid systems, while transcutaneous nerve stimulation may enhance activity in opioid or non-opioid systems, depending on the type of stimulation.

ENDORPHINS AND ADDICTION

Repeated administration of psychoactive drugs may lead to a state of drug dependence characterized by the drug user exhibiting erratic behaviour leading specifically to further administration of the drug. Severe degrees of dependence are commonly labelled as addiction, particularly in clinical practice. Extensive studies in animals have revealed that the self-administration technique, in which drug administration is contingent on the occurrence of a prior response, is a useful method to predict the abuse potential of drugs. It establishes the reinforcing (rewarding) efficacy of drugs and is reliably applicable to evaluate the variables that interfere with drug-taking behaviour[13]. Morphine and related drugs are abused, self-administered and interfere with brain reward mechanisms. The presence of endorphins in the pituitary and brain led to the postulate that these peptides may be involved in the functioning of physiological systems that are implicated in reward and which are susceptible to narcotic drugs. Thus, the endorphins may have intrinsic reinforcing efficacy and may mediate or modulate brain reward, which can be studied by intracranial electrical self-stimulation.

Beta-endorphin has been found to support self-administration when administered intracerebroventricularly[16].
The same has been reported for synthetic enkephalin
analogues that are resistant to enzymatic breakdown.
Thus, beta-endorphin and enkephalin analogues can serve as
positive reinforcers. Other data suggest that these
peptides also possess discriminative internal stimulus
properties similar to those of narcotic drugs. Both the
positive reinforcing and the discriminative stimulus
properties of beta-endorphin indicate that this peptide
may exert powerful control over behaviour. This action of
beta-endorphin may be mimicked by narcotic drugs, and in
this way organisms may become dependent on these drugs.

The involvement of endorphins in reward is suggested by
the decreasing influence of opiate antagonists or brain
electrical self-stimulation. This may suggest that
endorphins are also implicated in dependence with other
than narcotic drugs and in reward mechanisms in general.
It has been shown that blockade of opioid receptor systems
with opiate antagonists decreases the reinforcing effects
of ethanol. In alcoholics, the concentration of
beta-endorphin in the cerebrospinal fluid was markedly
decreased as compared to that of normal individuals. In
addition, other brain endorphins, such as enkephalins,
have been implicated in drug addiction especially with
ethanol consumption in experimental animals[2]. Naloxone
has been reported to reduce the amount of cigarettes
smoked by chronic smokers. Nicotine has been shown to
increase the plasma level of beta-endorphin[10]. Thus,
endorphins may be a common factor in drug dependence.

The involvement of endorphins in brain reward and drug
dependence permits questions to be raised as to whether
these entities are involved in the functioning of
physiological systems involved in euphoria, a feeling of
wellbeing. Certainly, euphoria can be induced or
facilitated by many addictive drugs, even resulting in a
state of ecstasy or trance, but feelings of wellbeing

(physiological euphoria) are also present after a good performance, delicious meals, sexual behaviour and enjoyable social contacts among others. There is some evidence that endorphins are indeed implicated in food, sexual and social behaviour; for example, beta-endorphin facilitates social contact behaviour of animals. However, whether this and other endorphins mediate the euphoria of these behaviours is not yet known.

CONCLUSION

Endorphin systems are implicated in several mechanisms controlling pain, which are present in the brain as well as in the spinal cord. The endorphin systems can be activated by procedures such as stress, electrical stimulation and acupuncture, resulting in relief of pain. Different endorphin systems and various types of opioid receptors are present in the brain, but their distinct role in processes involved in pain is still under debate. Developing substances or procedures that can selectively activate one of the endorphin systems or one of the non-opioid analgesic systems may lead to a more goal-directed treatment of the symptom pain, a frequently occurring symptom and sometimes markedly resistant to treatment.

Endorphins may also be concerned in dependence not only for morphine-related drugs but also for other addictive drugs. In particular, they may be implicated in brain reward mechanisms and "physiological" feelings of euphoria. Excess of endorphins may lead to a state of ecstasy or trance, which may be an important factor in addiction to various substances and habits. In view of the properties of morphine-related drugs, analgesia and addiction, which can hardly be separated, it may be proposed that a balanced system is operative in the body, characterized by the continuum affection(anhedonia)-dysphoria(pain)-euphoria-ecstasy, in which endorphins may play a profound role. Morphine and endorphins may move the continuum to the right, and when this happens frequently addictive behaviour may occur. This could suggest that addiction to endogenously available endorphins would be possible (for example, gambling) and that (mental or physical) pain and dysphoria-inducing situations would facilitate the release of endorphins in order to restore the balance. Chronic exposure to these latter situations may result in abundant release of endorphins and addictive-like behaviour may be elicited. An example of such a process may be the development of stereotyped behaviour of tethered sows, induced by the housing conditions in present use[3]. This stereotyped behaviour can be markedly decreased by treatment with naloxone.

References
1. Basbaum, A.I. and Fields, H.L. (1984). Endogenous pain control systems : brainstem spinal pathways and endorphin circuitry. Ann. Rev. Neurosci. 7:309-338.
2. Blum, K. (1984). Psychogenetics of drug seeking behaviour. In : Müller, E.E. and Genazzani, A.R. (eds). Central and Peripheral Endorphins : Basic and Clinical Aspects, pp.339-356. New York : Raven Press.
3. Cronin, G.M., Wiepkema, P.R. and Van Ree, J.M. (1985). Endogenous opioids are involved in abnormal stereotyped behaviours of tethered sows. Neuropeptides 6:527-530.
4. De Wied, D. (1977). Peptides and behavior. Life Sci. 20:195-204.
5. Han, J.S. and Terenius, L. (1982). Neurochemical basis of acupuncture analgesia. Ann. Rev. Pharmacol. Toxicol. 22:193-220.
6. Hughes, J., Smith, T.W., Kosterlitz, H.W., Fothergill, L.A., Morgan, B.A. and Morris, H.R. (1975). Identification of two related pentapeptides from the brain with potent opiate agonist activity. Nature 258:577-579.
7. Jacob, J.J.C. and Ramabadran, K. (1981). Role of opiate receptors and endogenous ligands in nociception. Pharmacol. Ther. 14:177-196.
8. Khachaturian, H., Lewis, M.E., Schäfer, M.K.-H. and Watson, S.J. (1985). Anatomy of the CNS opioid systems. TINS March:111-119.
9. Lagerweij, E., Nelis, P.C., Wiegant, V.M. and Van Ree, J.M. (1984). The twitch in horses : a variant of acupuncture. Science 225:1172-1174.
10. Pomerleau, O.F. and Pomerleau, C.S. (1984). Neuro-regulators and the reinforcement of smoking : towards a biobehavioral explanation. Neurosci. Biobehav. Rev. 8:503-513.
11. Terenius, L. (1973). Characteristics of the "recep-

tor" for narcotic analgesics in synaptic plasma membrane fraction from rat brain. Acta Pharmacol. Toxicol. 33:377-384.

12. Terenius. L. (1978). The implication of endorphins in pathological states. In : Van Ree. J.M. and Terenius. L. (eds). Characteristics and Function of Opioids. pp.143-158. Amsterdam : Elsevier/North Holland Biomedical Press.

13. Van Ree. J.M. (1979). Reinforcing stimulus properties of drugs. Neuropharmacology 18:963-969.

14. Van Ree. J.M. and De Wied. D. (1983). Behavioral effects of endorphins : modulation of opiate reward by neuropeptides related to pro-opiocortin and neurohypophyseal hormones. In : Smith, J.E. and Lane. J.D. (eds). The Neurobiology of Opiate Reward Processes. pp.109-145. Amsterdam: Elsevier Biomedical Press.

15. Van Ree. J.M., De Wied. D., Bradbury, A.F., Hulme, E.C., Smyth. D.G. and Snell, C.R. (1976). Induction of tolerance to the analgesic action of lipotropin C-fragment. Nature 264:792-794.

16. Van Ree. J.M., Smyth. D.G. and Colpaert, F. (1979). Dependence creating properties of lipotropin C-fragment (ß-endorphin) : evidence for its internal control of behavior. Life Sci. 24:495-502.

17. Watkins. L.R. and Mayer. D.J. (1982). Organization of endogenous opiate and nonopiate pain control systems. Science 216:1185-1192.

18. Wei. E. and Loh. H. (1976). Physical dependence on opiate-like peptides. Science 193:1262-1263.

19. Wood. P.L. (1982). Multiple opiate receptors : support for unique mu. delta and kappa sites. Neuropharmacology 21:487-497.

44
Opioid effects on gastrointestinal motor and secretory functions

Y. RUCKEBUSCH AND G. SOLDANI

ABSTRACT

The term "opioid" refers to morphine, similar synthetic drugs (opiates) and exogenous or endogenous opioid peptides (EOP), and it corresponds to substances which share, in common, modulation of nociceptive processes and regulation of gastrointestinal (GI) functions. Opioids strongly affect gastric and colonic motility in non-ruminant species, resulting in a delayed gastric emptying and constipation. The main site of action is peripheral and involves cholinergic and non-cholinergic enteric neurones rather than the muscle cells.

Opioids can stimulate gastric secretion via the release of histamine or gastrin and by increasing mucosal blood flow rather than by a primary action on the parietal cells. However, there is also a strong inhibition of acid secretion by delta and mu opioid agonists which is mainly centrally mediated via a reduction in the vagal tone. The anti-secretory effects of opioids on pancreaticobiliary and intestinal secretions are also centrally mediated, possibly through decreased vagal activity and increased sympathetic activity on the proximal part of the small intestine.

INTRODUCTION

Any coherent picture of the imposing amount of data on gastrointestinal motility and secretions as affected by opioids must take into account considerable species differences. These have long been known in the effect of morphine and similar drugs on the central nervous system (CNS), for example, excitation and mydriasis in horse, cattle and cats versus sedation and myosis in dogs and rodents as described in 1898 by Guinard[8]. The use of inbred strains of mice has confirmed the genetic influence on the density of opiate receptors and their subtypes[13]. The mode of action of opioids on gastrointestinal motility patterns in carnivores and rodents has been recently reviewed. The effects range from inhibition of propulsive activity via the release of acetylcholine and substance P from enteric neurones in the guinea-pig ileum to a spasmogenic action via increased release of acetylcholine and/or serotonin (5-hydroxytryptamine, 5-HT) in the ileum of most species. The abolition of naloxone-induced withdrawal diarrhoea by indomethacin and 5-HT suggests that 5-HT and prostaglandins (PG) are involved in the antidiarrhoeal activity of EOP[2]. On the other hand, suppression of the EOP antisecretory activity by adrenergic agonist pretreatment indicates participation of the sympathetic nervous system[4], either locally or at the spinal cord level[17].

In this chapter, special attention will be given to the opioid effects on digestive functions of herbivores as compared to carnivores, the former group including species with enlargement for plant fibre fermentation of the foregut (ruminants) or the hindgut (rabbit, horse). These will be contrasted with the effects in rats, the species in which the majority of studies on secretory functions have been carried out.

MOTOR FUNCTIONS

Oesophagus

The oesophagus smooth muscle is richly supplied with

adrenergic, cholinergic and peptidergic (vasoactive intestinal polypeptide, VIP)-containing nerves. In cattle subjected to rumen insufflation, naloxone and methyl-naloxone increase the volume of gas expelled without changes in ruminal motility, and these drugs alleviate gas accumulation resulting from the inhibition of reticulo-ruminal cycles by morphine and loperamide. Furthermore, the alpha₂-adrenoceptor blocker, tolazoline, reduced the bloating effect in cattle, but not in sheep, of morphine or loperamide when given systemically, a finding in agreement with the recent claim of involvement of adrenoceptors in the effect of morphine[25].

Stomach

Reduction of antral spike electrical activity and, at higher doses, gastric relaxation, is a common effect of morphine and fentanyl in dogs. The effects are blocked by naloxone. Fentanyl, unlike morphine, does not elicit vomiting in dogs, but like morphine, induces regular spiking activity (RSA)-like events on the proximal duodenum followed by a period of quiescence.

Pylorus

Duodenal acidification induces pyloric closure associated with duodenal contractions which are blocked by naloxone and atropine, respectively[14]. In sheep, both tonic and phasic contractions of the pylorus are likewise associated with duodenal activity elicited by an opioid peptide agonist, dermorphin, or following an enkephalinase inhibitor, thiorphan.

Forestomach

The inhibition of reticulorumen cyclical contractions by mu opiate agonists given systemically is similar to the effect of alpha₂-adrenoceptor agonists in that it does not affect the secondary ruminal contractions which depend on the enteric nervous system (ENS)[11], thus it indicates a centrally mediated effect. Evidence for a central opioid inhibitory system involved in the reticular contractions associated to a regurgitation and subserved by mu and delta receptor subtypes has been documented[19]. The classical competitive antagonism between morphine and nalorphine of respiratory movements in rabbits has also been found between fentanyl-ethylketazocine concerning the frequency of reticular contractions in sheep.

Small intestine

The major effect of several opiate agonists like fentanyl or D-Ala[2]-D-Leu[5]-enkephalin (DADLE) administered centrally is an inhibition of motility corresponding to a supraspinal inhibition of the intestinal motor functions[20]. The motor effects of intraluminal opioids (loperamide) on the small intestine or the release of endorphin (END) into the systemic circulation consist of an increased motor activity with for beta-endorphin in dogs, a regional specificity of enzymatic processing[7]. These effects are blocked by atropine or tetrodotoxin pretreatment in dogs, but not in ruminants, in which, because of the length of the bowel and the large amount of contents, minimal changes in the motility index are accompanied (in sheep) by dramatic changes in the net flow of digesta.

Large intestine

The existence of differential affinity of the proximal versus distal colon for mu, kappa or delta opiate agonists with considerable species differences is becoming more apparent[1,12]. As shown in Figure 44.1, the distal portion of the rabbit colon exhibits an opposite response, compared to the proximal colon, to the EOP dynorphin. This stimulatory effect of a kappa agonist on the distal colon is lacking in the dog where mu opiate agonists have stimulatory effects instead. In the horse, opioids, after a shortlived stimulation of the replicated colon have a dose-related inhibitory effect which resembles that obtained in other species[16].

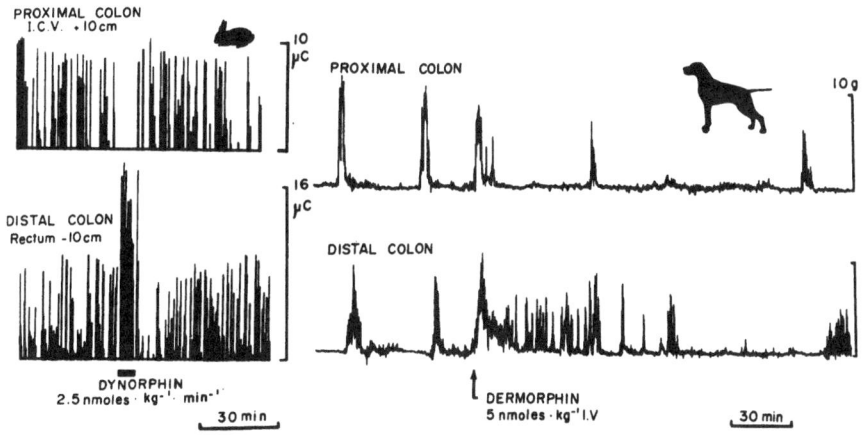

Figure 44.1   Stimulation of rabbit distal colonic electrical activity (integrated record) by dynorphin and of
canine distal colon (mechanical activity) by dermorphin.

SECRETORY FUNCTIONS
Gastric secretion

Although Riegel[15] described an excitatory effect of
morphine on gastric acid secretion as early as 1900,
opiates are usually considered inhibitors of gastric
secretion. Using the mu opioid agonists dermorphin and
morphine, we have found a significant increase in acid
secretion in dogs[24]. These stimulatory effects were
prevented by naloxone and also by peripheral opioid
antagonists. However, dermorphin did not modify acid
output stimulated by 2-deoxy-D-glucose (2DG) from gastric
fistulae, while morphine significantly inhibited it
(Figure 44.2). These results may thus be explained, as for
clonidine [23], on the basis of simultaneous yet opposite
effects of opioids on interdependent regulatory pathways
in the stomach. This involves inhibition related to impairment of the vagal tone and excitation related to a direct stimulation of peripheral opioid receptors. This, in
turn, increases mucosal blood flow, induces the release of
histamine and gastrin, and inhibits somatostatin release.

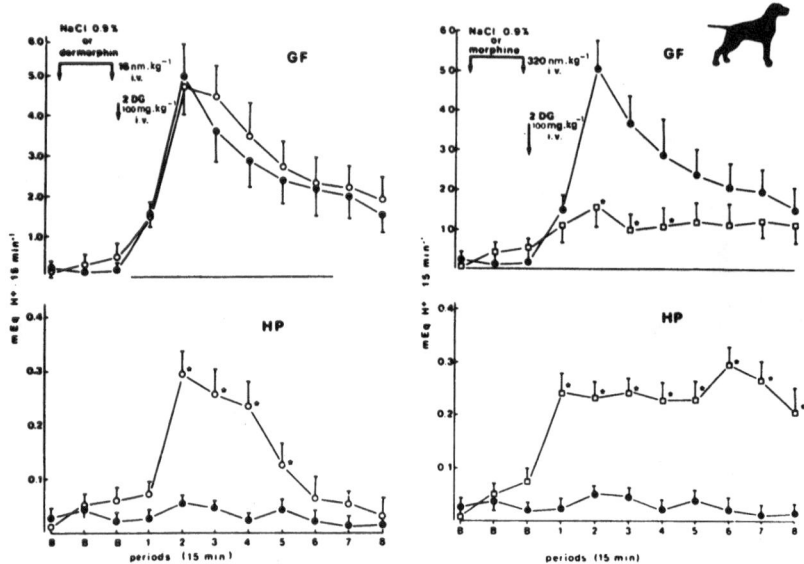

Figure 44.2 Effects of dermorphin or morphine on 2DG-sti-
mulated gastric acid secretion from gastric fistulae (GF)
and Heidenhain pouch (HP) dogs. Note that morphine
possesses two simultaneous yet opposite effects (inhibitory and excitatory) on vagally stimulated secretion
(*P < 0.01).

Pancreatic secretion

Opiates generally have direct inhibitory effects on both
bicarbonate and enzyme secretion. For example, methadone
inhibits both bicarbonate and protein output induced by
vagal stimulation, whereas the effects of direct
cholinergic stimulation remain unchanged[18]. Since the
intracerebroventricular administration of doses of
D-Ala[2]-D-Met[5]-enkephalin (DAMA) which are inactive by the
systemic route strongly inhibits both basal and
2DG-stimulated secretion[3], and this effect is not blocked
by methylnaloxone, it seems that the inhibitory effects on
pancreatic secretion resemble those on gastric secretion
and likewise involve a vagal pathway at the central
level[5].

Intestinal secretion

Morphine inhibits PG-induced and VIP-induced secretion by the rat jejunum in vivo[10]. Similarly, loperamide increases absorption and inhibits secretion provoked by prostaglandins and Escherichia coli enterotoxin in isolated rabbit ileal mucosa[9]. Such an antisecretory effect has been also observed for morphine in E. coli enterotoxin-exposed pig jejunum[27]. The fact that the effects of morphine on short-circuit current are increased by the presence of low Ca^{2+} bathing solution on the serosal surface indicates that the opiates alter intestinal transport by Ca^{2+} or calmodulin-dependent mechanisms. Accordingly, loperamide and diphenoxylate possess a high affinity for calmodulin binding sites, the potency in binding calmodulin being correlated to their antidiarrhoeal activity[26].

DISCUSSION AND CONCLUSIONS

Concepts of an EOP system in the gastrointestinal tract are closely linked to the roles of neuropeptides : ENK-like peptides located in the ENS and END-like peptides in the CNS and adrenals. Whether different receptors subserve different functions in the gastrointestinal tract remains to be determined, except that the occupation of opiate receptor sites within the villus core and intestinal glands leads to profound effects on the handling of fluid and electrolytes[6], and the occupation of receptors within the ENS leads to changes in the motility patterns. Since the potency of intracerebroventricular morphine in inhibiting gastrointestinal transit is about 50 times that when given intravenously, and this effect can be blocked by vagotomy, it has been concluded that morphine produces most of its motor effects by acting supraspinally via the vagal nerves. The fact that the synthetic opiate agonists diphenoxylate and loperamide, given intraluminally, are selective for peripheral gastrointestinal opiate receptors suggests that peripheral effects are also important. The use of opiate receptor antagonists which do not cross the blood-brain barrier to a large extent[21],[24], in conjunction with agonists acting on the CNS, represent interesting means of dissociating the centrally mediated effects from those corresponding to local effects via the ENS. Recently, the synthetic enkephalin analogue (Hoe 825), a mixed mu-delta opiate agonist, was shown to cause, in dogs, the appearance of a premature myoelectric migrating complex. These stimulating effects were of peripheral origin since this opioid peptide does not penetrate into the CNS. They were prevented in part (70%) by atropine and fully suppressed by naloxone[3]. Thus the EOP can stimulate small intestinal motility by enhancing acetylcholine release and by a direct action on muscle, and these stimulating effects might be of therapeutic benefit for treating humans under conditions where gastrointestinal motility is diminished or absent.

Prevention of the influx of Ca^{2+} in epithelial cells by opioid agonists such as loperamide results in an inhibition of the propulsion of fluid through the gut[22], hence the possibility of the existence of a peripheral mechanism in the inhibition of secretory functions by EOP. However, the intestinal[4] and pancreatic[5] antisecretory activity of opiates administered into the CNS is also relevant, and furthermore, its adrenergic mediation via the spinal cord is likely. It is thus tempting to speculate that the motor functions of the gastrointestinal tract are modulated by the opiates peripherally and via a parasympathetic pathway at the supraspinal level, while the modulation of secretory functions by opiates also involves peripheral receptors but works at the spinal level via a sympathetic pathway. This indicates that the EOP can work both centrally and peripherally and that the major site of action would depend on species-specific differences in the location and types of receptors, and in the autonomic nervous system as well.

References
1. Bardon, T. and Ruckebusch, Y. (1985). Comparative effects of opiate agonists on proximal and distal colonic motility in dogs. Eur. J. Pharmacol. 110:329-334.
2. Beubler, E., Bukhave, K. and Rask-Madsen, J. (1984). Colonic secretion mediated by prostaglandin E_2 and 5-hydroxytryptamine may contribute to diarrhea due to morphine withdrawal in the rat. Gastroenterology 87:1042-1048.
3. Bickel, M. and Belz, U. (1985). Initiation of the interdigestive motor complex by a synthetic enkephalin analogue in the dog. IRCS Med. Sci. 13:525-526.
4. Brown, D.R. and Miller, R.J. (1984). Adrenergic mediation of the intestinal antisecretory action of opiates administered into the central nervous system. J. Pharmacol. Exp. Ther. 231:114-119.
5. Chicau-Chovet, M., Chariot, J. and Rozé, C. (1985). Central inhibition of exocrine pancreatic secretion by D-Ala²-Metenkephalinamide in rats. Gastroenterol. Clin. Biol. 9:220-222.
6. Dashwood, M.R., Debnam, E.S., Bagnall, J. and Thompson, C.S. (1985). Autoradiographic localisation of opiate receptors in the rat small intestine. Eur. J. Pharmacol. 107:267-269.
7. Davis, T.P., Culling, A.J., Schoemaker, H. and Galligan, J.J. (1983). Beta-endorphin and its metabolites stimulate motility of the dog small intestine. J. Pharmacol. Exp. Ther. 227:499-507.
8. Guinard, L. (1898). Etude expérimentale de la pharmacodynamie comparée sur la morphine et l'apomorphine. Thèse Doct. Méd. Lyon, 728.
9. Huges, S., Higgs, N.B. and Turnberg, L.A. (1982). Antidiarrhoeal activity of loperamide : studies of its influence on ion transport across rabbit ileal mucosa in vitro. Gut 23:974-979.
10. Lee, M.K. and Coupar, I.M. (1980). Opiate receptor-mediated inhibition of rat jejunal fluid secretion. Life Sci. 27:2319-2325.
11. Maas, C.C. (1982). Opiate antagonists stimulate ruminal motility of conscious goats. Eur. J. Pharmacol. 77:71-74.
12. Pairet, M. and Ruckebusch, Y. (1984). Opioid receptor agonists in the rabbit colon : comparison of in vivo and in vitro studies. Life Sci. 35:1653-1658.
13. Przewlocki, R. (1984). Some aspects of physiology and pharmacology of endogenous opioid peptides. Pol. J. Pharmacol. Pharm. 36:137-158.
14. Reynolds, J.C., Ouyang, A. and Cohen, S. (1984). Evidence for an opiate-mediated pyloric sphincter reflex. Am. J. Physiol. 246:G130-G136.
15. Riegel, F. (1900). Ueber den Einflusse der Morphins auf die Magensaftsecretion. Z. Klin. Med. 40:347-350.
16. Roger, T., Bardon, T. and Ruckebusch, Y. (1984). Colonic motor responses in the pony : relevance of colonic stimulation by opiate antagonists. Am. J.

Vet. Res. 46:31-35.

17. Romagnano, M.A. and Hamill, R.W. (1984). Spinal sympathetic pathway : an enkephalin ladder. Science 225:737-739.

18. Rozé, C., Chariot, J., De La Tour, J., Souchard, M., Vaille, C. and Debray, C. (1978). Methadone blockade of 2-deoxyglucose-induced pancreatic secretion in the rat. Gastroenterology 74:215-220.

19. Ruckebusch, Y., Bardon, T. and Pairet, M. (1985). Opioid control of the ruminant stomach motility : functional importance of mu, kappa and delta receptors. Life Sci. 35:1731-1738.

20. Ruckebusch, Y., Ferré, J.P. and Du, C. (1984). In vivo modulation of intestinal motility and sites of opioid effects in the rat. Regul. Peptides 9:109-117.

21. Russell, J., Bass, P., Goldberg, L.I., Schuster, C.R. and Merz, H. (1982). Antagonism of gut, but not central effects of morphine with quaternary narcotic antagonists. Eur. J. Pharmacol. 78:255-261.

22. Schiller, L.R., Santa Ana, C.A., Morawski, S.G. and Fordtran, J.S. (1984). Mechanism of antidiarrheal effect of loperamide. Gastroenterology 86:1475-1480.

23. Soldani, G., Del Tacca, M., Bernardini, C., Martinotti, E. and Impicciatore, M. (1984). Evidence for two opposite effects of clonidine on gastric acid secretion in the dog. Naunyn-Schmiedeberg's Arch. Pharmacol. 327:139-142.

24. Soldani, G., Del Tacca, M., Mengozzi, G., Bernardini, C. and Bartolini, D. (1985). Central and peripheral involvement of mu receptors in gastric secretory effects of opioids in the dog. Eur. J. Pharmacol. 117:295-301.

25. Wong, C.L. (1984). Involvement of adrenoceptors in the intestinal effect of morphine in mice. Clin. Exp. Pharm. Physiol. 11:605-611.

26. Zavecz, J.K., Jackson, T.E., Limp, G.L. and Yellin, T.O. (1982). Relationship between antidiarrheal activity and binding to calmodulin. Eur. J. Pharmacol. 78:375-377.

27. Zhu, B. and Ahrens, F. (1983). Antisecretory effects of berberine with morphine, clonidine, L-phenylephrine, yohimbine or neostigmine in pig jejunum. Eur. J. Pharmacol. 96:11-19.

45
Central nervous system control of feeding behaviour by some neuropeptides in sheep

L. BUÉNO, C. HONDÉ, A. DURANTON AND J. FIORAMONTI

ABSTRACT

The hypothalamus is a major site responsible for the control of food intake. Many peptides are able to modify feeding behaviour when centrally administered in sheep. They may be classified into two categories : (1) CCK8, CRF and calcitonin which reduce food intake by affecting the rate of eating (CCK8), the frequency and the duration of meals (CRF, calcitonin), while the gastrin group of peptides promotes rumination; (2) GRF and CGRP which increase food intake by delaying satiety.

INTRODUCTION

The hypothalamus is a major site responsible for the integration of information in the regulation of energy balance. From the pioneering work of Della-Fera and Baile[6], showing that centrally administered cholecystokinin-octapeptide (CCK8) exerted anorectic effects in sheep, much information has been accumulated concerning the involvement of neuropeptides in the control of food intake in sheep[13] : the CCK family of peptides initiates satiety and opioid peptides (enkephalins, beta-endorphin and dynorphin) increase feeding. However, separation into these two classes is not wholly satisfactory in view of recent findings. For example, naloxone, an opioid mu and delta receptor antagonist, does not reduce food intake as expected but, in contrast, can block the anorectic effects of centrally administered CCK8 and it antagonizes the inhibitory effect of CCK8 on postprandial ruminoreticular motility in sheep[3].

We report herein the results of experiments performed to determine the nature of behaviour disturbances responsible for short-term anorexia produced by some peptides administered centrally to hay-fed animals.

CCK8 AND GASTRIN GROUP PEPTIDES
Mammalian brain extracts contain peptides which cross-react in gastrin radioimmunoassay, the majority of this immunoreactivity being due to the presence in such brain extracts of a peptide mainly corresponding to the C-terminal octapeptide of cholecystokinin.

However, using a sequence-specific radioimmunoassay, the presence of a smaller molecular form probably corresponding to the C-terminal tetrapeptide common to gastrin and CCK has been identified in brain extracts of rats[12].

The comparative influence of these peptides administered centrally was analysed in Lacaune ewes (50-60 kg) equipped with a stainless steel cannula 29 mm in length and 1-2 mm in diameter inserted into one of the cerebral ventricles[3].

Figure 45.1 summarizes the influence of these treatments on feeding behaviour and permits the conclusion that gastrin group peptides (tetragastrin, pentagastrin and gastrin 17), but not CCK8, administered intracerebroventricularly reduced food intake from 0 to 120 min after their administration by promoting an early rumination. This finding suggests that the C-terminal tetrapeptide or a smaller form is the probable fragment of gastrin 17 responsible for this action.

In contrast, CCK8 affected food intake by reducing the rate of ingestion over 3 h of feeding without affecting rumination[3]. The lack of an immediate anorectic effect of CCK4, compared to CCK8, reinforces previous results

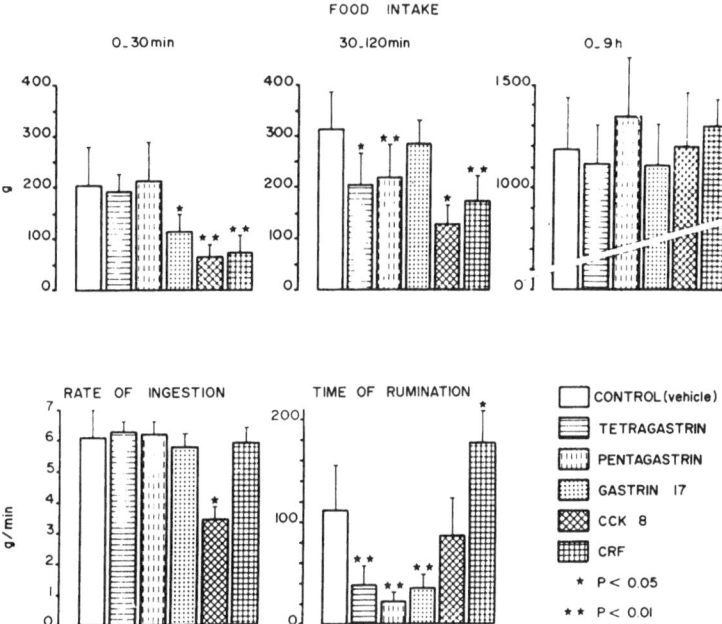

Figure 45.1 Comparative effects of intracerebroventricular (ICV) administration of tetragastrin, pentagastrin,
gastrin 17, CCK8 and CRF on feeding behaviour in hay-fed
ewes (mean ± SD; experiments in duplicate in six ewes).
Note that gastrin group peptides induced premature rumination, while CCK8 and CRF affect food intake by reducing
the rate of ingestion and the time spent eating respectively.

showing that the satiety properties of CCK8 are associated
with the presence of a sulphydryl bond and that CCK4 in
the brain is more representative of the gastrin peptides
than the cholecystokinin residue.

CORTICOTROPIN-RELEASING FACTOR AND CORTISOL
A peak of plasma corticoids has been found just prior to
feeding[18], and treatment with glucocorticoids results in
an increased appetite[7]. These observations suggest that
plasma glucocorticoids interact with feeding behaviour,
but the specific nature of the site and mode of action,

whether peripheral or central, remain unknown[15].

Recently we have shown[5] in sheep as previously found in rats[16] that CRF administered intracerebroventricularly induces rapid anorexia by limiting the time spent eating (Figure 45.1).

Using a similar methodology to that for comparing the effects of CCK8 and gastrin group peptides, we have tested the effects of intracerebroventricular versus intravenous administration of cortisol injected at 9.00 or 12.00 h. Furthermore, we have evaluated the nature of the action of cortisol by measuring the effects of its administration on CRF-induced anorexia and plasma cortisol levels.

Cortisol administered intracerebroventricularly at a dose of 40 ng/kg at 9.00 h prior to feeding did not affect the first hour food intake but increased ($P < 0.01$) by 29.4% the 3 h (morning) food intake without affecting the daily consumption or the rate of ingestion. A similar increase (31.9%) in afternoon food intake was observed when cortisol was injected intracerebroventricularly at noon and this also resulted in an increase in daily food intake. Cortisol (40 ng/kg) administered intracerebroventricularly 5-10 min before CRF (100 ng/kg) partially reduced the first 30 min period of anorexia induced by CRF, abolished the 2 h effects and restored to normal rumination altered by CRF.

These results are in agreement with the observation that corticoids interact permissively with noradrenaline injected into paraventricular nuclei (PVN) to elicit feeding[15], while CRF suppressed feeding induced by noradrenaline[16]. The existence of steroid-sensitive single neurones in the hypothalamus and midbrain has been demonstrated[17] and corticoid-induced behavioural effects are observed independently of the feedback effect of plasma hormonal level on the hypothalamo-pituitary adrenocorticoid (HPA) system[2] or spontaneous variations[6]. The present results indicate that cortisol interacts in the brain at a site involved in the control of food intake in sheep independently of its feedback action on the HPA system.

CALCITONIN AND CALCITONIN GENE-RELATED PEPTIDE (CGRP)

Calcitonin is considered to be one of the major factors concerned in satiety[9-11]. Calcitonin gene-related peptide (CGRP), a product of alternative processing of RNA transcripts, to form the calcitonin gene, has been found in the brain[1] and mRNA encoding CGRP is found in several brain nuclei important in ingestive behaviour. Centrally administered CGRP inhibits both spontaneous and starvation-induced food intake in rats[14] but only with a 1000 times higher dose rate than calcitonin, and with a low ratio (1:2) between intracerebroventricular and intravenous administration.

In sheep, intracerebroventricular calcitonin at a dose level of 2-200 mU/kg, reduced, in a dose-related manner, the immediate (0-60 min) food intake. The daily food intake was also significantly (P < 0.05) decreased with doses up to 20 mU/kg. In contrast, CGRP given intracerebroventricularly did not affect the first 3 h period of food intake, while a significant increase (27.8%) in daily food intake was observed at a dose of 20 ng/kg. Furthermore, CGRP given intracerebroventricularly (100 ng/kg) did not antagonize the immediate anorectic effects of calcitonin (200 mU/kg), although it delayed commencement of rumination and partially restored the daily food intake (Figure 45.2).

The fact that CGRP increases food intake in sheep, at doses as low as 20 ng/kg intracerebroventricularly, contrasts with the anorectic action observed in rats for intracerebroventricular doses of 1-10 µg by Krahn et al.[14] emphasizing the species differences in action. The hypothesis that these two peptides affect food intake by acting selectively on two parts of the hypothalamus is not in agreement with our observations that CGRP failed to antagonize the early (0-180 min) anorectic effect of calcitonin and produced a slight immediate (0-60 min) inhibition of food intake at the highest intracerebroventricular dose (100 ng/kg).

Finally, it is tempting to speculate from our results

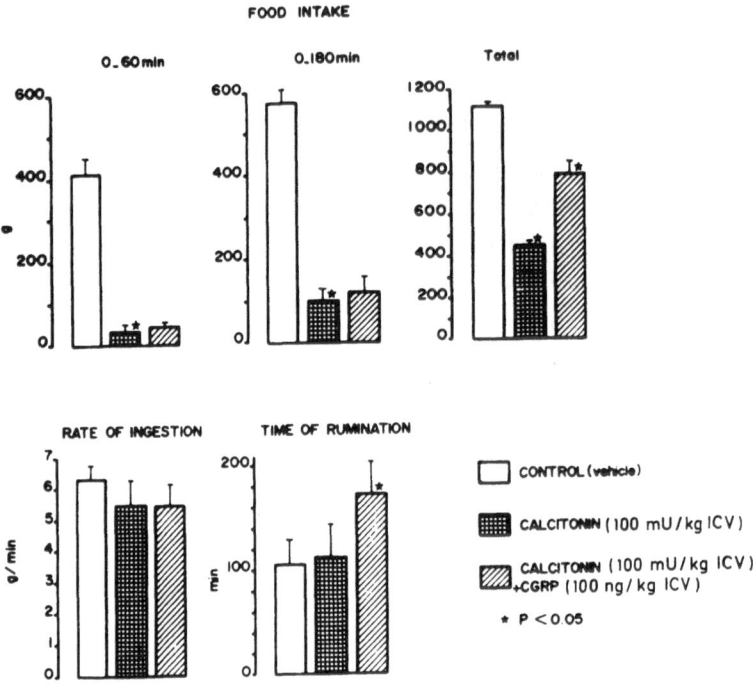

Figure 45.2 Influence of intracerebroventricular administration of calcitonin with or without previous intracerebroventricular injections of CGRP on feeding behaviour
in sheep (means ± SD, n = 6).

that CGRP increases food intake when centrally administered at relative low doses by (1) inhibiting the release or
the synthesis of calcitonin and/or its precursors by the
thyroidal "C" cells; or (2) affecting the structure of
hypothalamic receptors for calcitonin.

GROWTH HORMONE RELEASING FACTOR AND DOPAMINE
GRF immunoreactivity has been found in rat hypothalamus,
being localized in neurones bordering the ventromedial
hypothalamic nucleus[19]. It has recently been shown in rats
that intracerebroventricular administration of hpGRF and
rhGRF stimulates food intake in rats[20]. The increased
milk production observed in cows injected with GRF has
prompted us to investigate the effects of GRF on short—

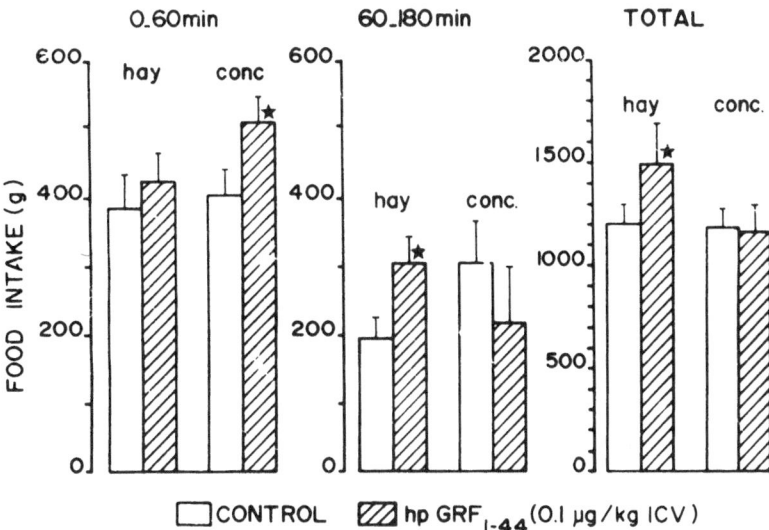

Figure 45.3 Effect of central intracerebroventricular administration of hGRF₁₋₄₄ on food intake level and profile
in hay and concentrates-fed ewes (mean ± SD, n = 4).

term satiety in sheep submitted to two different feeding
regimens : hay and concentrates. In hay-fed sheep, GRF
administered intracerebroventricularly at a dose of 0.1
µg/kg did not affect (0-60 min) food intake significantly
(P > 0.05) while a 25.5% increase was noticed over the 3 h
post-treatment. This effect mainly corresponded to an
increased number and duration of meals without affecting
the rate of ingestion or the occurrence of rumination. In
concentrate-fed animals only the early (0-60 min) food intake was increased while no effect was observed on the total daily consumption (Figure 45.3). As previously observed for the gastrointestinal motor effects[4], the orectic
action of GRF on hay-fed animals was abolished when administered after intravenous administration of metoclorami-
de suggesting a mediation through dopaminergic receptors.

CONCLUSIONS
It is clear that several brain peptides play important
roles within the CNS in the control of feeding behaviour

in sheep. These peptides may be divided into two main groups :

(1) CCK8, CRF and calcitonin seem to act as short-term satiety factors, acting respectively on the rate of eating (CCK8), number and duration of meals (CRF, calcitonin), while gastrin group peptides modulate rumination.

(2) CGRP and GRF delay satiety without affecting either immediate feeding behaviour or appetite.

Feed intake is an important component in the regulation of energy balance and peptides are likely to be involved at the interface between the energy balance regulator and controller of feed intake. The use of new behavioural and anatomical approaches may lead to a better understanding of peptidergic influences in long-term regulation and to the development of new ways of increasing the efficiency of production in ruminants.

References
1. Amara, S.G., Jones, V., Rosenfeld, M.C., Ong, E.S. and Evans, R.M. (1982). Alternative RNA processing in calcitonin gene expression generates mRNAs encoding different polypeptide products. Nature 298:240-244.
2. Buckingham, J.C. (1982). Corticotrophin releasing factor. Pharmacol. Rev. 31:253-275.
3. Buéno, L., Duranton, A. and Ruckebusch, Y. (1983). Antagonistic effects of naloxone on CCK-octapeptide induced satiety and ruminoreticular hypomotility in sheep. Life Sci. 32:855-863.
4. Buéno, L., Fioramonti, J. and Primi, M.P. (1985). Central effects of growth hormone-releasing factor (GRF) on intestinal motility in dogs : involvements of dopaminergic receptors. Peptides 6:403-407.
5. Buéno, L., Hondé, C., Duranton, A. and Fioramonti, J. (1985). CNS control of feeding behavior by some neuropeptides (gastrin, CCK8 and CRF) in sheep. Rep. Nutr. Dev. 2:456-457.
6. Chestworth, J.M. and Easdon, M.P. (1983). Effect of diet and season on steroid hormones in the ruminant. J. Steroid Biochem. 19:715-723.
7. Dallman, M.F. (1984). Viewing the ventromedial hypo-thalamus from the adrenal gland. Am. J. Physiol. 246:R1-R12.
8. Della-Fera, M.A. and Baile, C.A. (1979). Cholecysto-kinin octapeptide continuous picomolar injections into

the cerebral ventricles suppress feeding. Science 206:471-473.

9. Fargeas, M.J., Fioramonti, J. and Buéno, L. (1984). Prostaglandins E2 : a neuromodulator in the central control of gastrointestinal motility and feeding behavior by calcitonin. Science 225:1050-1052.

10. Fischer, J.A., Henke, H., Petermann, J. and Ischopp, F.C. (1984). Calcitonin gene related peptide (CGRP) and calcitonin (CT) and their binding sites in the central nervous system. In : Pecile, A. (ed.). International Symposium on Calcitonin. Abstract n°66.

11. Freed, W.J., Perlow, M.J. and Wyatt, R.J. (1979). Calcitonin : inhibitory effect on eating in rats. Science 206:850-852.

12. Halmy, L., Nyakas, C. and Walter, J. (1982). The C-terminal tetrapeptide of cholecystokinin decreases hunger in rats. Experientia 38:873-874.

13. Hondé, C. and Buéno, L. (1984). Evidence for central neuropeptidergic control of rumination in sheep. Peptides 5:81-83.

14. Krahn, D.D., Gosnell, A., Levine, A.S. and Morley, J.E. (1984). Effects of calcitonin gene-related peptide on food intake. Peptides 5:861-864.

15. Leibowitz, S.F., Roland, D.R., Hor, L. and Squillary, V. (1984). Noradrenergic feeding elicited via the paraventricular nucleus is dependent upon circulating corticosterone. Physiol. Behav. 32:857-864.

16. Levine, A.S., Rogers, B., Kneip, J., Grace, M. and Morley, J.E. (1983). Effects of centrally administered corticotropin releasing factor (CRF) on multiple feeding paradigms. Neuropharmacology 22:337-339.

17. Mandelbrod, I., Feldman, S. and Werman, R. (1974). Inhibition of firing is the primary effect of micro-electrophoresis of cortisol to units in the rat tuberal hypothalamus. Brain Res. 80:303-315.

18. Moberg, G.P., Bellinger, L.L. and Mendel, V.E. (1975). Effect of meal feeding on daily rhythms of plasma corticosterone and growth hormone in the rat. Neuroendocrinology 19:160-169.

19. Smith, R.M., Howe, P.R.C., Oliver, J.C. and Willoughby, J.O. (1976). Growth hormone releasing factor immunoreactivity in rat hypothalamus. Neuropeptides 4:109- 115.

20. Vaccarino, F.J., Bloom, F.E., Rivier, J., Vale, W. and Koob, G.F. (1985). Stimulation of food intake in rats by centrally administered hypothalamic growth hormone-releasing factor. Nature 314:167-168.

Drug Use and Regulation

46
The use in animals of drugs licensed for human use only

A. S. J. P. A. M. VAN MIERT

ABSTRACT

In relation to the use in animals of drugs licensed for human use only, extrapolation of dosages based on body weight is open to objections. Conversion based on the two-thirds or three-quarters power of the body weight is regarded as preferable. Some examples are given of conversion of dosages for one species of animal (including man) into those suitable for other mammals (including dogs and cats).

INTRODUCTION

When faced with a patient who needs treatment, the veterinarian must make a choice among a variety of possible drugs and devise a dosage regimen that is likely to produce maximal benefit and minimal toxicity. The choice of a drug not only depends upon the effect desired, but is also influenced by the species of animal undergoing therapy. For instance, lincomycin is contraindicated for hamsters, guinea-pigs and rabbits. Low doses in these species cause severe enterocolitis, anorexia, diarrhoea, and death within 2 days[9]. On the other hand, the mechanism of action of a drug is often the same in humans and other mammalian species, whereas the intensity and duration of the effects produced can vary widely. This implies that in most cases, species variations in response produced by a fixed dose of drug can be attributed to differences in pharmacokinetic processes.

Patients may differ in the rate of absorption of a drug[22], in distributing it through body compartments[2,3], in metabolizing it[2], or in clearing the drug from the body[3]. Any of these pharmacokinetic differences may alter the concentration of drug that reaches relevant receptors and thus alter the clinical response. Repeated measurements of drug concentrations in blood during the course of treatment are often helpful in dealing with the variability of clinical response caused by pharmacokinetic differences due to pathophysiological processes. These pharmacokinetic differences can be used to guide quantitative decisions regarding an initial dosing regimen. For example, the kinetics of chloramphenicol in veal calves experimentally infected with Salmonella dublin, showed that the plasma elimination half-life of the drug rose from a value of 7.5 ± 0.8 h (mean $\pm$ SD) in healthy calves to 13.6 ± 1.5 h in infected animals[8]. On the basis of a MIC value of 3 $\mu g.ml^{-1}$, Groothuis[8] therefore advises an initial intravenous dose of 40 $mg.kg^{-1}$ followed by an oral maintenance dose every 24 h of about 35 $mg.kg^{-1}$.

Because the patient is never an idealized system, the veterinarian will not have precise information about the physicochemical nature of the receptors involved, the number of receptors, or their affinity for drugs. Nonetheless, in order to make rational therapeutic decisions, the veterinarian must understand how drug-receptor interactions underlie the relations between dose and response in non-ideal patients, the nature and causes of variation in pharmacological responsiveness, and the clinical implications of selectivity of drug action. Experimental studies have documented changes in drug responsiveness caused by increases or decreases in the number of receptor sites or by alterations in the efficiency of coupling of receptors to distal effector mechanisms. These differences account for much of the individual variability in response to some drugs, particularly those that act at receptors for hormones, biogenic amines, and neurotransmitters. In some cases, the change in receptor number is caused by bacterial fragments: for example, Haemophilus influenzae endotoxin can affect negatively the functioning of the beta-adrenergic system on cells involved in anaphylactic mediator release and respiratory smooth muscle. Secondarily, the cholinergic bronchoconstrictive impulses are elevated by this bacterial product[18].

In small animal medicine, a rather high number of drugs licensed for human use only are used, but may be often misused because of the lack of specific data in these species of animal. There are several possible ways to tackle this problem. Very often, pharmaceutical firms do have information about the pharmacokinetics and side-effects of their products in small animal species. For example, the beagle is often used in pharmacokinetic and toxicity studies, whereas the cat is a well-known experimental animal in research projects concerning the development of new non-steroidal anti-inflammatory agents (NSAIDS).

THE INFLUENCE OF THE SIZE OF AN ANIMAL
There can only be a question of a real difference in responsiveness for a drug or poison between man and other mammals if in one way or another the difference in body size is taken into account. Taking full account of the body size is also essential if calculating doses of drugs based on data obtained from other animal species, and for instance for extrapolation of toxic doses or no-effect dosages from laboratory animals to man. Within one single species the dosage based on body weight can as a rule be a usable starting point provided that the very special position of very young animals is taken into account. However, as soon as extrapolation from man to cat is necessary, a dosage calculated on body weight, which can

be correct for an adult human patient, can be ineffective in a cat.

When one realizes that processes in the pharmacokinetic phase of the action of drugs which influence the concentration in the blood are related to the functions of the liver and the kidneys, it will be clear that special attention should be paid to the relationship of these functions with the size of the body. It can be taken for granted that the capacity of the liver and kidneys are adapted to the requirements resulting from normal food intake and digestion, which means with normal metabolism. For example, excretion of a drug and its metabolites is promoted by larger kidneys. In rats, the ratio between the weight of the kidneys and body weight is 0.7%. In man, goats (40 kg), and dogs (15 kg), these values are 0.35, 0.46 and 0.61% respectively[13,15].

It is known that basic metabolism of warm-blooded animals is a function of surface of the body rather than that of the body weight. Smaller animals have greater body surface area when related to body weight (Table 46.1). To maintain a steady body temperature, a higher heat production is required, which is achieved by a higher level of metabolism. Many investigators have studied the relationships between doses, body surface area, plasma levels and elimination half-life values to responses in various species[13,23]. They have found that the difficulty in relating results from one species to another (including man) may be partly overcome if the dosage is adjusted in relation to body surface area.

Table 46.1 represents a proposal taken from Mellet[13] and Spector[19], to use the Km factor for the modification of mg.kg^{-1} dosage into mg.m^2 dosage. By dividing one Km factor by another, we can find the mg.kg^{-1} dose ratio between two species (mg.kg^{-1} equivalents). This extrapolation is, of course, not sufficient for calculating a safe drug dose for cat and dog from data obtained from other animal species (including man). The area under the serum curve for the various doses tested

Table 46.1 Representative body surface area to body weight ratios for various species (after Mellett[13] and Spector[19], modified)

Species	Body weight (kg)	Surface area (m²)	Km factor*	Dose equivalent (kg⁻¹)+
Man adult	60	1.6	37.5	1
Man child	20	0.8	25	1.5
Mouse	0.02	0.0066	3	12.5
Rat	0.15	0.025	6	6.3
Cat	3	0.24	12.5	3
Dog	16	0.65	24.5	1.5
Sheep/goat	50	1.1	45.5	0.8
Pig	75	1.5	50	0.75
Cow	150	2.4	62.5	0.6
Cow	500	5.0	100	0.4
Pony	280	4.4	63.5	0.6
Horse	350	4.0	87.5	0.4
Horse	650	5.9	110	0.3

* To express a $mg \cdot kg^{-1}$ dose in any given species as an equivalent $mg \cdot m^2$ dose, multiply the dose by the appropriate Km factor. In the cat, $10 \ mg \cdot kg^{-1}$ is equivalent to $10 \ mg \cdot kg^{-1} \times 12.5 = 125 \ mg \cdot m^2$.

+ Setting the dose equivalent for man (adult, 60 kg) as 1, we may obtain the dose equivalent kg^{-1} (in relation to man) by dividing the Km factor for humans through the Km factor for any species given in the table.

should bear a linear relationship to the dose in $mg \cdot m^2$. If this relationship holds for various other species, it is likely to hold for the cat and the dog. If one observes great variations in the response of various species that bear no relationship to the size of the animals, then it is unlikely that any prediction can be made for the dog and the cat[13].

Other authors have found that the metabolic activity on the whole range from mouse to cow can be placed on one line in a double logarithmic diagram and that it is approximately proportional to the weight of the body to the three-quarter power (the computed regression line corresponds to an exponent 0.756).

In his computation over a large range of warm-blooded animals, Brody[5] found the regressions indicated in Table 46.2, in which some additional values for the number of nephrons and the hippurate clearance[1] are included. Based on these data, it is to be expected that it will be possible to approximate the dosage in relation to the size of the body by the three-quarters power of body weight. Extrapolation of dosages using this formula is not a simple matter; therefore, some ratios are given in Table 46.3 (taken from Van Genderen[21]).

CORRELATION BETWEEN DOSE, BASIC METABOLISM AND RESPONSE

It is the quantitative rate of drug disposition that is of practical importance in determining optimal dosage schedules. Therefore, some examples were selected based on the availability of quantitative data in various species after various doses of drugs. In rabbits procaine penicillin G (40,000 IU.kg^{-1} intramuscularly for 5 days) is often the antibiotic of choice to treat pasteurellosis[9]. In vitro, Pasteurella multocida is sensitive to penicillin G, although sensitivity varies from isolate to isolate (MIC values : 0.27-5 IU.ml^{-1}). Furthermore, there are penicillin G-resistant strains. The calculated doses based on metabolic weight (G.$^{0.75}$) for dogs, cattle, swine and piglets from rabbit data for procaine penicillin G are remarkably close to the doses advised by pharmaceutical firms : dogs 30,000 IU.kg^{-1}, cats 40,000 IU.kg^{-1}, piglets 25,000 IU.kg^{-1}, swine 20,000 IU.kg^{-1} and cows 15,000 IU.kg^{-1}[4,16].

The efficacy of this drug can be expected to be related to levels of penicillin G in the plasma. Penicillin G concentrations in dog serum after parenteral

Table 46.2 Body weight (G) in relation to various factors
(taken from Van Genderen[21])

Basic metabolism (cal)	70.5 $\times G^{0.73}$
Weight of liver (adult) kg	$0.0333 \times G^{0.87}$
Weight of kidneys (adult) kg	$0.0073 \times G^{0.85}$
Number of nephrons (adult)	2600 $\times G^{0.62}$
Hippurate (PAH) clearance	5.4 $\times G^{0.80}$
Blood (kg)	$0.0507 \times G^{0.99}$

---

administration (thoracic wall) of 30,000 IU.kg^{-1} were more
than 0.5 IU.ml^{-1} at 12 h, whereas at 24 h this was still
the case in nine out of 11 animals[10]. In pigs (30–68 kg)
the mean concentrations of penicillin G in serum after an
intramuscular injection of 21,000 IU.kg^{-1} (calculated dose
range 19,000–25,000 IU.kg^{-1}) were 0.25 and 0.05 IU.ml^{-1} at
the 12th and 24th h after treatment, respectively[14].
Similar results were obtained in cows after an
intramuscular dose of 13,000 IU.kg^{-1}[17], whereas in serum
samples from steers (182–314 kg) given a massive dose of
33,000 IU.kg^{-1}, concentrations were 0.25 and 0.05 IU.ml^{-1}
at the 24th and 36th h after treatment[20]. In these
species, comparison of serum concentrations in relation to
the doses used is somewhat complicated by the fact that
the injection sites were not systematically reported. When
drug suspensions are used, the absorption rate depends on
the injection site, being superior for the cervical area
in comparison with other regions such as the gluteal
muscles[12]. In the study with steers the injection site
was in the gluteal region. Nevertheless, the published
data do suggest a reasonable correlation between dose,
basic metabolism and serum profile.
    A second example are the liver-fluke anthelmintics
bromophenophos (Acedist[R]) and nitroclofene (Distoject[R]).
In rats bromophenophos is highly active (95–100%) at an
oral dosage of 60 mg.kg^{-1}[11]. When this value is used
for computing highly effective doses for cattle and sheep

Table 46.3 Proportion scheme of dosages on basis of body weight : $G.^{0.75}$ (taken from Van Genderen[21])

Body weight	Dosage given to man (60 kg) = (A)mg.kg^{-1}	Dosage given to rat (0.2 kg) = (B)mg.kg^{-1}
corresponds		
0.2 kg (rat) to	4.2(A) mg.kg^{-1} or to	1.0(B)mg.kg^{-1}
1 kg to	2.8 mg.kg^{-1}	0.67 mg.kg^{-1}
10 kg to	1.5 mg.kg^{-1}	0.37 mg.kg^{-1}
60 kg (man) to	1.0 mg.kg^{-1}	0.24 mg.kg^{-1}
100 kg to	0.89 mg.kg^{-1}	0.22 mg.kg^{-1}
500 kg to	0.58 mg.kg^{-1}	0.14 mg.kg^{-1}

(see Table 46.3), the following results will be obtained : sheep 14.4 mg.kg^{-1} and cattle 8.4-10 mg.kg^{-1}. Efficacy studies have proved that an oral dose of 10 mg.kg^{-1} is highly effective in cattle; in sheep this is 15 mg.kg^{-1}[11]. For practical reasons the advised doses to be administered to cattle and sheep are 12 and 16 mg.kg^{-1}, respectively. In the mouse and rat nitroclofene is highly active against 12-week-old Fasciola hepatica after an intramuscular injection of 40 and 10 mg.kg^{-1} respectively[11].

The calculated doses based on metabolic weight (Tables 46.1 and 46.3) for cattle and sheep from these data are : 1.6 mg.kg^{-1} and 2.5 mg.kg^{-1}, respectively. These values are remarkably close to the effective doses against 16-week-old F. hepatica infections in cattle (ED$_9$$_8$: 2.6 mg.kg^{-1}) and sheep (ED$_9$$_8$: 2.1 mg.kg^{-1}). From clinical efficacy studies based on the permanent reduction of the excretion of fluke ova as well as on the eradication of liver flukes, Ladage[11] concluded that 3 mg.kg^{-1} intramuscularly is the dose that may be used for treatment of cattle suffering from chronic fascioliasis; for sheep a dosage of 4 mg.kg^{-1} intramuscularly is recommended. The elimination half-life values in goats, sheep and cattle for nitroclofene are : 22.5 ± 5.3, 46 ± 4.6 and 62.1 ± 1.1 h, respectively[11].

Another example is proligestone, which is used to suppress or to postpone oestrus in the bitch and the female cat[24]. In rats proligestone delayed the onset of pregnancy for 4-5 weeks after subcutaneous injection of 50-55 mg.kg^{-1}. The efficacy of proligestone can be expected to be related to levels of active compound in the plasma. This is essentially the difference between the amount released from the subcutaneous injection depot and that inactivated mainly by biotransformation in the liver. Therefore Van Os[24] compared the effectiveness of the advised doses with doses based on metabolic weight $(G.^{0.75})$.

With the advised doses smaller animals were somewhat overdosed and larger animals underdosed. A significant trend ($p < 0.01$) was found for advised dosages towards a higher efficacy for smaller dogs, and a lower efficacy for larger animals. In cats the efficacy was 96% (500 injections). Furthermore, a lower efficacy for correct doses was found for some breeds only : Siamese and Angora cats, Alsatians and Great Danes. Van Os concluded that his results seem to confirm the correctness of dosing according to metabolic weight calculated according to the formula $G.^{0.756}$[24].

LACK OF CORRELATION BETWEEN DOSE, BASIC METABOLISM AND RESPONSE

The examples just discussed were intended to call attention to the fact that important quantitative differences in rates of drug excretion and metabolism are to be expected in various species and in the same species when the subjects differ greatly in size. In general, excretion and metabolism of drugs does occur more rapidly in small animal species than in large ones. There are, of course, exceptions to this generalization. For example phenylbutazone is more rapidly metabolized in laboratory species than in cattle[6,7]; however, the horse[4] also metabolized this drug at about the rate of the smaller animal species (phenylbutazone half-life values in hours in the rabbit, rat, horse, cow and man are : 3, 6, 3.5-8.6, 31-82 and 72, respectively). Another example are the aminoglycosides, which have a limited distribution volume, are not metabolized and are excreted by passive glomerular filtration. Therefore, it is not surprising that the advised dosages in mg.kg^{-1} in various species are rather uniform for these drugs.

There are a number of other phenomena which may cause complications : (a) the plasma level of a drug may exceed protein-binding capacity; (b) distribution may increase at higher blood levels; (c) an enzyme system metabolizing a drug may become saturated at higher blood levels; (d) a drug's metabolism may be stimulated by the drug itself; or (e) a drug's metabolism may be stimulated or inhibited by another agent. Nevertheless, for many drugs there exists a valid relationship between dose, plasma levels, body size and response. However, if one sees great variations in response of some animal species that bear no relationship to the size of the animals, then it is unlikely that any prediction can be made for other animal species. The approaches suggested in the foregoing discussion to the solution of the problem may help to expand the extrapolation of drug dosages in laboratory animals, man or large animal species to those effective in dogs and cats.

References
1. Adolph, E.F. (1949). Quantitative relations in the physiological constitution of mammals. Science 109:579.
2. Anika, S.M., Nouws, J.F.M., Van Duin, C.T.M., Nieuwenhuijs, J. and Van Miert, A.S.J.P.A.M. (1986). Tick-borne fever : efficacy and effects on pharmacokinetics of some chemotherapeutic agents in the goat. In: Van Miert, A.S.J.P.A.M., Bogaert, M.G. and Debackere, M. (eds). Comparative Veterinary Pharmacology, Toxicology and Therapy. Proc. 3rd EAVPT Congress, Part II. Invited lectures. Lancaster : MTP Press.
3. Baggot, J.D. (1977). Principles of Drug Disposition

in Domestic Animals. Philadelphia: W.B. Saunders.

4. Bogan, J.A., Lees, P. and Yoxall, A.T. (1983). Pharmacological Basis of Large Animal Medicine. Oxford: Blackwell Scientific.

5. Brody, S. (1968). Bioenergetics and Growth. New York: Hafner Publishing Company.

6. De Backer, P., Braeckman, R., Belpaire, F. and Debackere, M. (1980). Bioavailability and pharmacokinetics of phenylbutazone in the cow. J. Vet. Pharmacol. Ther. 3:29-33.

7. Eberhardson, B., Olsson, G., Appelgren, L. and Jacobsson, S. (1979). Pharmacokinetic studies of phenylbutazone in cattle. J. Vet. Pharmacol. Ther. 2:31-37.

8. Groothuis, D.G. (1983). Pharmacokinetics of some antimicrobial drugs in veal calves and their activity in relation to Salmonella dublin infections. Utrecht: Ph.D thesis.

9. Harkness, J.E. and Wagner, J.E. (1983). The Biology and Medicine of Rabbits and Rodents, 2nd ed. Philadelphia: Lea and Febiger.

10. Hartman, E.G. (1985). Influence of the injection site on the depot-effect of procaine-penicillin G in dogs. In: Van Miert, A.S.J.P.A.M., Bogaert, M.G. and Debackere, M. (eds). Comparative Veterinary Pharmacology, Toxicology and Therapy. Proc. 3rd EAVPT Congress, Part I, Abstracts, p.52. Utrecht: EAVPT.

11. Ladage, C.A. (1979). The development of a new injectable anti-liver fluke compound. Utrecht: PhD thesis.

12. MacDiarmid, S.C. (1983). The adsorption of drugs from subcutaneous and intramuscular injection sites. Vet. Bull. 53:9-23.

13. Mellett, L.B. (1969). Comparative drug metabolism. In: Jucker, E. (ed.). Progress in Drug Research 13, pp.136-169. Basel: Birkhäuser Verlag.

14. Mercer, H.D., Righter, H.F. and Carter, G.G. (1971). Serum concentrations of penicillin and dihydrostreptomycin after their parenteral administration in swine. J. Am. Vet. Med. Assoc. 159:61-65.

15. Neff-Davis, C., Davis, L.E. and Powers, T.E. (1975). Comparative body compositions of the dog and goat. Am. J. Vet. Res. 36:309-311.

16. Rossoff, I.S. (1974). Handbook of Veterinary Drugs. New York: Springer.

17. Schipper, I.A., Filipors, D., Ebeltoft, H. and Schermeister, L.J. (1970). Blood serum concentrations of various benzyl penicillins after their intramuscular administration to cattle. J. Am. Vet. Med. Assoc. 158:494-500.

18. Schreurs, A.J.M. and Nijkamp, F.P. (1984). Haemophilus influenzae and the ß-adrenergic system : a review. Vet. Res. Commun. 8:1-14.

19. Spector, W.S. (1961). Handbook of Biological Data. Philadelphia: W.B. Saunders.

20. Teske, R.H., Rollins, L.D. and Carter, G.G. (1972). Penicillin and dihydrostreptomycin serum concentrations after administration in single and

repeated doses to feeder   steers.   J.   Am.   Vet.   Med.
Assoc. 160:873-878.
21. Van Genderen, H. (1975).   Combined use of drugs and
    variations   in   action   in various animals.   Tijdschr.
    Diergeneesk. 100:25-36.
22. Van Gogh, H., Van Deurzen, E.J.M., Van Duin, C.T.M.
    and   Van   Miert,   A.S.J.P.A.M.   (1984).   Effect   of
    staphylococcal   enterotoxin B-induced diarrhoea on the
    pharmacokinetics of sulphadimidine in   the   goat.   J.
    Vet. Pharmacol. Ther. 7:303-305.
23. Van Noordwijk, J. (1964).   Communication between the
    experimental   animal   and   the   pharmacologist.
    Statistica Neerlandica 18:403.
24. Van Os, J.L. (1982).   Oestrus control in the bitch
    with proligestone.   Utrecht: PhD thesis.

47
The use in small animal medicine of drugs licensed for human purposes

A. R. M. KIDD

ABSTRACT

Products licensed for human medical purposes in the United Kingdom may also be legally obtained and used under UK medicines legislation by qualified veterinarians. Many of the disease conditions encountered by veterinary surgeons in small animal medicine require treatment with products for which there is usually a very limited veterinary market. As a result it is often necessary to employ products which have been designed for use in man. This chapter describes some of the disease conditions encountered in small animal medicine which can be treated with products licensed for human use in the United Kingdom.

Under United Kingdom legislation drug substances are classified for distribution purposes into one of three categories. Most of the products considered in the paper are classified as prescription-only medicines. The possibility of misuse is considered in relation to the disciplinary procedures applied by the veterinary profession to its members and the legal strictures which apply in the United Kingdom where the veterinary profession has the freedom to prescribe licensed human products.

This chapter also emphasizes the importance of

reporting adverse reactions and of applying principles of clinical pharmacology in pioneering new developments in veterinary medicine.

INTRODUCTION

The licensing of veterinary medicines in the United Kingdom is controlled by legislation enacted in 1968 under the Medicines Act. This Act requires that for any veterinary product which is sold or supplied, parameters of safety, quality and efficacy must be fully taken into account and the product recommended for licensing by an independent Committee of Experts, the Veterinary Products Committee. The licensing authority responsible for issuing the licence is the Ministry of Agriculture, Fisheries and Food (MAFF).

The same piece of legislation and the same criteria of safety, quality and efficacy apply in the case of products intended for use in man. Applications for product licenses are also considered by an independent expert committee known as the Committee of Safety of Medicines and product licenses or clinical trials certificates are issued by the licensing authority which in the case of human medicines is the Department of Health and Social Security.

Licensed veterinary products must also satisfy the requirements of the Veterinary Medicines Directives (EC 82/851 and EC 82/852) and equally those licensed for use in man are licensed in accordance with the requirements of the parallel human directives.

Products which have been fully licensed for medical purposes in the United Kingdom may normally be legally obtained or administered by qualified veterinarians for the treatment or prevention of disease or for other veterinary purposes (such as anaesthesia) in animals under their care.

Certain disease conditions, especially some encountered by veterinarians involved in small animal species, are not necessarily very common and the volume demand for products to treat these conditions may not be high. As a result there is no great incentive for a commercial company to develop specific veterinary products for a very limited market. The veterinarian is therefore often obliged to seek and use alternative products and turns to those designed primarily for use in man.

For discussion at this congress the question "which drugs are essential in small animal medicine" (that is, human drugs) has been posed. The following examples of drugs and the uses to which they are put will hopefully serve to illustrate that, although not always essential, a considerable number of substances are used on occasion. In this era of fast-moving advances in our knowledge of small animal medicine there is clearly a need for such drugs to improve the welfare of the animals with which we as veterinarians have to deal.

DISEASES SUITABLE FOR TREATMENT WITH LICENSED MEDICAL PRODUCTS

For the purpose of this paper examples have been selected of various types of condition which seem particularly suitable for treatment with approved and licensed medical products. Some of the diseases involved are often unrewarding to treat, irrespective of the drugs available and the prognosis may frequently be poor.

Skin diseases

Skin diseases of the dog and cat associated with autoimmune phenomena have been well described in recent papers. Wilkinson[7] for example refers to three major types and indicates drugs which may be valuable for treatment. The feline pemphigus group and feline ulcerative pododermatitis may be resistant to conventional immunosuppressive doses of prednisolone but may respond to aurothiomalate or aurothioglucose. For systemic lupus erythematosus Wilkinson suggests immunosuppressive drugs such as melphalan with monitoring for myelosuppression. Bennett[2] in a review in 1984 alludes to the use of cytotoxic drugs to treat pemphigus vulgaris particularly in cases which do not respond to steroids. He specifically mentions cyclophosphamide and azathioprine. Chlorambucil has also been recommended. Combinations of steroids and cytotoxic drugs are suggested where the main advantage lies in being able to employ lower doses of each.

Cushing's syndrome

Cushing's syndrome is a condition associated with hyperadrenocortism caused by excessive glucocorticoid production usually because of increased adrenocortico-tropin hormone secretion; it is characterized by polyuria, polydypsia, and polyphagia. There are no products licensed for use in the United Kingdom for the treatment of the condition but mitotane (United States Pharmacopoeia - USP) has been recommended.

Addison's disease

Addison's disease is a condition of hypoadrenocortism associated with vomiting, diarrhoea, muscular weakness, dehydration, polyuria, polydypsia, trembling and weight loss. Some human preparations not licensed for veterinary use have been used in the United Kingdom. These include mineralocorticoids such as deoxycortisone pivalate, and fludrocortisone acetate.

Lymphosarcoma

Lymphosarcoma is seen in both cats and dogs and it has been treated with a variety of immunosuppressive substances such as azathioprine, chlorambucil, vincristine sulphate as well as L-asparaginase. Close collaboration between veterinary and human oncologists is clearly very desirable since tumours exist where the histological appearance in dogs and cats resembles that seen in man.

In addition to those drugs already mentioned, methotrexate, cytosine arabinoside, and doxorubicin have been used. Combination therapy using vincristine, cytosine arabinoside, cyclophosphamide and prednisolone give median survival times of 6 months in canine lymphosarcoma.

Diabetes

Diabetes mellitus is a condition which is not uncommon in dogs, and as no insulin preparations are licensed for use in animals, licensed human products have been used in the United Kingdom for many years. It is generally thought desirable to use depot insulin for stabilization and maintenance. It is also worth mentioning that as yet there is no evidence to suggest that any of the oral hypoglycaemics have been used with success.

Diarrhoeal conditions

It has been said that colitis and proctitis account for half of all cases of chronic diarrhoea in the dog. Similarities with Crohn's disease have been postulated, especially in the case of histiocytic ulcerative colitis in boxers and regional enterocolitis in the cocker spaniel. These are conditions where recourse to human products has been associated with iatrogenic problems. Wilson[6] has reported the successful use of a 5 day regimen of sulphasalazine and Isogel in cases which were a sequel to chronic rectal impaction. Sulphasalazine has been particularly useful in older dogs, where due to other disease conditions the use of steroids has been contraindicated. Because of differences in the metabolism of sulphonamides in man and the dog the possibility exists of unusual side-effects. Sansom et al.[5] reported 13 cases of iatrogenic and bilateral keratoconjunctivitis sicca following the use of sulphasalazine for the treatment of colitis in dogs. The lacrimotoxic effect of sulphasalazine was permanent in all except one case. Other drugs used for colitis include metronidazole and diphenoxylate.

HUMAN PRODUCTS AND CONDITIONS IN SMALL ANIMALS

Reports and recommendations exist for the use of human products against a variety of other conditions seen in small animals. Licensed veterinary preparations are available which can be used for treatment but alternative human drugs and products exist which veterinarians choose to use on an occasional basis. For convenience of presentation these conditions can be divided into five categories : eye conditions, central nervous system and skeletal conditions, intestinal conditions, cardiac and respiratory conditions, and a range of miscellaneous conditions.

Eye conditions

In the case of eye conditions, they include anterior uveitis, conjunctivitis, corneal oedema, glaucoma, keratitis, and keratoconjunctivitis sicca. Some of the drugs used for treatment are atropine, pilocarpine, proxymetacaine, acetazolamide, demecarium bromide, dichlorphenamide, idoxuridine and N-acetylcysteine, the latter in cases of keratoconjunctivitis sicca.

Central nervous system and skeletal conditions

Central nervous and skeletal conditions are clearly varied in character and severity of symptoms, but nervous problems such as narcolepsy, Scottie cramp or convulsions may benefit from treatment with substances such as amphetamines, imipramine, methylphenidate, phenytoin and diazepam. Skeletal or arthritic conditions may respond to treatment with sodium aurothiomalate, aspirin, pethidine or ibuprofen, bearing in mind that toxicity to some of these substances in the dog and cat is well recognized.

Intestinal tract disorders

A vast range and diversity of substances is used to treat disorders of the intestinal tract many of them antimicrobial and designed to deal with specific infections. Cimetidine, however, may have a place in treating gastritis especially where a reduction in acidity is likely to be beneficial. Medium-chain triglycerides are useful in malabsorption syndromes; also of value in dealing with persistent vomiting and diarrhoea are drugs such as metoclopramide, prochlorperazine, loperamide and diphenoxylate, the latter in combination with atropine. Spironolactone is one substance which is marketed under a number of different trade names in the United Kingdom and is considered to be of value in the treatment of chronic liver disease, or for idiopathic oedema.

Cardiac and respiratory diseases

As with intestinal disease, many drugs in suitable veterinary formulations are available to treat cardiac and respiratory diseases. For congestive heart failure and feline cardiomyopathy, digoxin and digitalis remain high in popularity. Non-specific cough, not associated with known specific disease agents may on occasion be treated with codeine, acetylcysteine or carbocisteine.

Miscellaneous conditions

A number of miscellaneous conditions are not readily classified into any of the above groups. Cat leprosy associated with infection with Mycobacterium lepramurium has been treated with dapsone, and cryptococcosis with amphotericin. Chlorpropamide has been used in cases of diabetes insipidus, chlorpheniramine in urticarial conditions and allopurinol to treat urolithiasis.

IDENTIFYING AND CLASSIFYING SUBSTANCES

Altogether, without attempting to be comprehensive, it has been possible to identify some 50 different compounds available in human medicine which are used to treat or alleviate up to 40 different disease conditions in dogs and cats. It is important to recognize, however, that limitations exist. In a recent review on canine glaucoma, Bedford[1] emphasizes differences in approach between man and animals. The use of miotics has little place in the dog, and suppression of aqueous humour is much more effectively carried out with carbonic anhydrase inhibitors. Sympathomimetic agents and beta-blockers are therefore not much used.

Under United Kingdom legislation drug substances used in human medicine are classified for distribution purposes into three categories. Some substances such as aspirin are classified as suitable for general sale (GSL) but the vast majority of those mentioned in this paper come within the prescription-only (POM) category. The distribution of some of these is restricted to hospitals only. Those substances which are not listed in either of these categories are sold only under the direction of a pharmacist (category P). The same categories also exist for veterinary medicines, but an additional category exists for certain substances considered suitable for sale from agricultural merchant's premises (category PML). Examples include sheep dips, as well as many of the anthelmintics used for treating agricultural livestock. Substances used in small animal medicine are not normally considered suitable for this category.

MISUSE OF DRUGS

The misuse of drugs is a matter raised for discussion within the framework of this congress. The sale and supply of licensed products is controlled under the terms of the Medicines Act and the sale or supply of unlicensed products is therefore an offence subject to prosecution. The practising veterinary surgeon is free to prescribe licensed products, whether human or veterinary. If he advocates a product's use in accordance with the data sheet recommendations (and these reflect the terms of the licence) responsibility for the product lies with the product licence holder. While the veterinary surgeon is free to use the product outside the terms of the data sheet, he then does so on his own responsibility. The governing body of the veterinary profession in the United Kingdom, the Royal College of Veterinary Surgeons, also exercises control over the profession in general as well as providing guidance to it on a wide range of issues including the use of drugs.

ADVERSE REACTIONS TO DRUGS

Licensed products are regarded as safe when used in accordance with experimentally determined dosage, but the Medicines Act requires the reporting and collection of suspected adverse reactions. When a veterinarian administers to animals products recommended only for use in man, he should be aware of increased chances of adverse drug reactions occurring. A recent example has been the reporting of keratoconjunctivitis sicca in dogs treated for colitis with sulphasalazine.

Another recent review by Taylor[6] dealing with the use of analgesics in small animal medicine lists a number of preparations for which no veterinary licensed product is available as well as referring to some of the older opiates now no longer so readily obtainable. Non-steroidal anti-inflammatory drugs (NSAIDS) such as indomethacin and ibuprofen are becoming more commonly used, but problems of gastric irritation with vomiting and diarrhoea as well as occasional blood dyscrasias indicate the potential for adverse reactions.

A review article by Keen and Livingston[3] on adverse reactions to drugs published in 1983 referred to several preparations not licensed in the United Kingdom for use in the dog, but which though effective gave rise to unacceptable side-effects. One example quoted was the prostaglandin dinoprost used in the treatment of pyometra, which may give rise to bronchoconstriction and gastrointestinal side-effects. Another drug sometimes used to treat gastrointestinal disorders is clioquinol and when used in dogs it can cause a fatal encephalitis. Keen also emphasized that cats are only poorly able to metabolize phenolic derivatives and are therefore susceptible to toxic side-effects from such compounds. In the case of salicylates, cats should therefore receive a lower dose than the dog. Lees et al.[4] drew attention to the need for great care in prescribing aspirin in the cat and suggested it should not be used at all in either very young and very old cats. Keen observed that paracetamol is also toxic to the cat, and recent reports of incidents of paracetamol poisoning include one where cats were able to obtain access to tablets and then exhibited symptoms of vomiting, diarrhoea, cyanosis, ataxia, and hypothermia.

It therefore seems desirable to ensure that the use of human drugs in animals, especially in small animals, is accompanied by a system of reporting and investigating adverse reactions so that more information can be made available on the pharmacological effects of such products in these species.

CONCLUSIONS

This paper has attempted to take account of many types of situation under which products licensed for human use are employed in small animal medicine in the United Kingdom. It is necessary, however, to bear in mind that human health and safety problems might arise if human products are used to treat animals destined for human consumption, and the question of residues is especially important. The majority of products licensed for human use are not, however, of suitable pack size to be widely used in agricultural situations. Thought has nevertheless been given in the United Kingdom to cater for situations where human or veterinary products are administered despite no residue data having been generated. In such circumstances a standard withdrawal period of 28 days for meat and meat products, and 7 days for milk has been proposed. As mentioned earlier there is little incentive for companies to generate data such as no effect levels and acceptable daily intakes for products which are old or have a limited market. In the case of products possessing antimicrobial properties the possibility, however remote, that residues may give rise to plasmid-mediated resistance also needs to be considered, and resolved.

References
1. Bedford, T.G.C. (1985). The treatment of glaucoma in the dog. Vet. Annual 25:352-357.
2. Bennett, D. (1984). Skin diseases of the dog and cat associated with autoimmunity. Vet. Annual 24:198-207.
3. Keen, P. and Livingston, A. (1983). Adverse reactions to drugs. Practice 5:174-180.
4. Lees, P., Higgins, A.J. and Sedgwick, E.D. (1985). Aspirin in cats. Vet. Rec. 116:479.
5. Sansom, J., Barnett, K.C. and Long, R.D. (1985). Keratoconjunctivitis sicca in the dog associated with the administration of salicylazosulphapyridine (sulphasalazine). Vet. Rec. 116:391-393.
6. Taylor, P. (1985). Analgesia in the dog and cat. Practice 7:5-13.
7. Wilkinson, G.T. (1985). Autoimmune skin disease in the cat. Vet. Annual 25:248-253.
8. Wilson, N.D. (1985). Proctocolitis in the dog. Vet. Rec. 116:503.

48
The use in animals of drugs licensed for human use: the situation in Sweden

K. BINGEFORS

ABSTRACT

Use of human drugs in the treatment of animals was studied by means of a cross-sectional prescription survey. Human drugs were primarily prescribed to small animals. Dogs in particular received a great variety of human drugs. The most frequent prescribing of human drugs occurred in the chemotherapeutics group, but drugs from all pharmacological groups were used in animal treatment. Some human drugs are more often prescribed for animals than for people. Availability of substances, more suitable formulations and strengths and manufacturer preference were considered important factors in choosing human drugs in the treatment of animals.

INTRODUCTION

In Sweden all drugs, veterinary and human, are distributed only via the National Corporation of Swedish Pharmacies (NCSP). The only exception to this monopoly is the distribution of antibiotic feed additives. As from 1 January 1986, growth promoting antibiotics will not be allowed on the market while therapeutic antibiotics will fall under the same legislation as licensed pharmaceutical specialities. In contrast to many other countries, veterinarians may only dispense drugs to a limited extent

513

as part of a consultation within their clinic or in acute situations in the field.

Veterinarians are qualified to prescribe practically all drugs on the market as long as they can be shown to be justified in the treatment of animals. Drugs registered for veterinary use are licensed for use in one or more specified species. They may, of course, be prescribed for use in other species but in this case, as is also true for human drugs, the responsibility lies with the prescribing veterinary practitioner. In Sweden very comprehensive drug utilization statistics are published yearly, mainly based on wholesale statistics. It is not possible, however, to study the use of human drugs in veterinary practice via the official drug utilization data. Human drugs sold for use in animals are recorded as if they were used in humans. Also, there are no possibilities for studying the use of drugs in different species.

MATERIALS AND METHODS

The monopolized drug distribution system in Sweden has made possible a study of the use in animals of drugs registered for human use. This study was designed as a cross-sectional prescription survey[1]. All veterinary prescriptions completed throughout the whole country during 2 weeks in the autumn of 1981 were collected and analysed. The study also included drug requisitions from surgeries and animal hospitals. For each prescription item the type of drug, quantity dispensed and species were recorded. A computerized analysis was performed with the help of central drug registers at the NCSP.

Naturally, there are some limitations in using the prescription survey method. The main objection is that the study tends to be purely descriptive and very few valid analytical studies can be made on the material collected. However, further studies of a more explanatory nature can be made with a descriptive study as a basis. Another objection is that over-the-counter drugs are poorly represented even though they are included in the

pharmacy   monopoly.   There are few incentives to actually
prescribe   over-the-counter   drugs   since   there   are   no
economic   benefits   in   buying   them   with a prescription.
Rather a large proportion of the drugs   are   delivered   to
veterinary surgeries and hospitals.   It is not possible to
determine the species for which these drugs are   intended.
In   spite of these limitations, the results of the present
study ought   to   be   representative   of   the   prescription
pattern for human drugs in veterinary therapy.

    In   contrast   to the situation in many other countries,
all   pharmaceutical   specialities   have   to   be   sold   in
unbroken   manufacturer's   packages.   In   the absence of a
better measure of the volume prescribed, we decided to use
the number of packages dispensed as our unit of measure in
this study.   Furthermore, this is the   unit   used   in   all
available   sales   statistics.   Thus   we were able to make
direct comparisons with this.

RESULTS

In 1981 there were about 2500 pharmaceutical   specialities
on the market in Sweden.   Our survey showed the use of 900
separate entities in animals, two-thirds   of   these   being
drugs   licensed for human use only.   By volume, 20% of the
45,798 packages dispensed during the period of study   were
human   drugs.   Human   drugs   from   all   19 officially
classified   pharmacological   groups   were   prescribed   for
animal   treatment.   Since drug use in other than the major
species (such as dogs, cats, horses, cattle and swine)   is
negligible,   only   drug   use   in   major   species   and   in
veterinary clinics will be considered.

    As expected, most human drugs were prescribed for small
animals   and for use in veterinary surgeries (Table 48.1).
More than half of all human drugs prescribed were intended
for   use in dogs, and in this species the most varied drug
prescribing also occurred.   Almost a third   of   all   drugs
prescribed   for   dogs were human drugs (Figure 48.1) while
other species received smaller proportions of their   total
drug   use   as   human   drugs.   A great variety of different

Table 48.1 Human drugs, distribution on major species, n = 9023

Dogs	57.7%
Cats	9.5%
Horses	4.8%
Cattle	1.6%
Swine	1.5%
Veterinary practice	24.9%

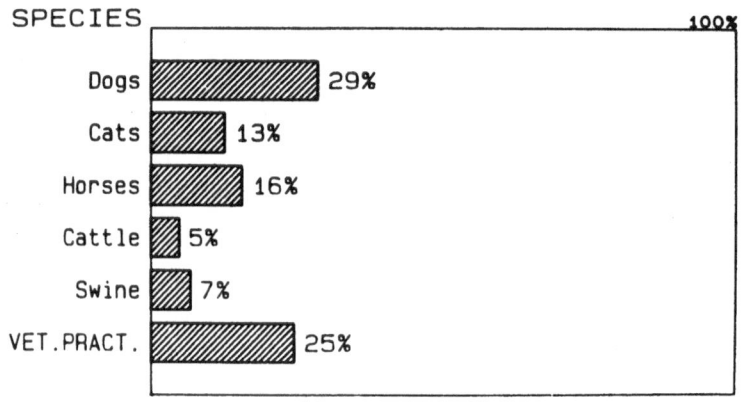

Figure 48.1 Human drugs as a proportion of the total prescribing for each species and for use in veterinary clinics.

drugs were prescribed for dogs even if most of them were not frequently used. On the other hand, use of human drugs in food-producing animals can be considered as relatively low. For this chapter we have selected some of the more interesting pharmacological groups for a closer study.

By far the largest prescribing of human drugs occurs in the chemotherapeutic drug group. This was almost totally restricted to use in cats and dogs, more than a third of the total chemotherapeutics used for these species being human drugs (Figure 48.2). A large part of the pre-

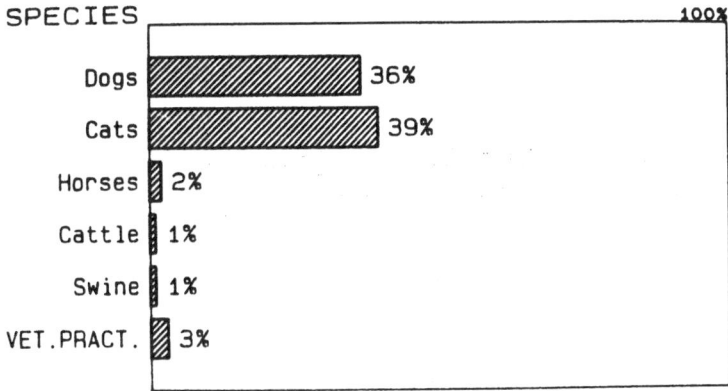

Figure 48.2 Chemotherapeutic agents : human   drugs   as   a
proportion   of   the   total prescribing of chemotherapeutic
agents for each species and for use in veterinary clinics.

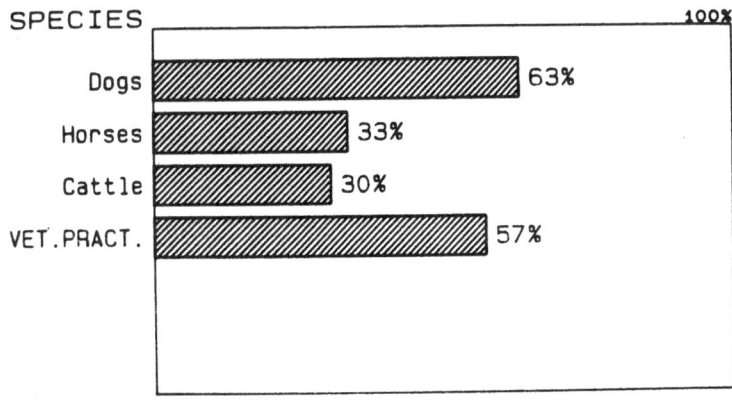

Figure 48.3 Analgesics : human drugs as a   proportion   of
the   total   prescribing of analgesics for each species and
for use in veterinary clinics.

scribing in this   group consisted of synonymous preparations of penicillins and tetracyclines. Sulphonamides,
erythromycin,   trimethoprim-sulphamethoxazole,   nitrofurantoin and chloramphenicol were commonly used in small
animals.   In fact, the relatively high sales   figures   for
chloramphenicol tablets (licensed for human use) have been

discussed, but according to our data 80% of sales are actually consumed by dogs. In cats there was a frequent use of demeclocycline paediatric drops, a drug which is apparently hardly ever used for children, an amount corresponding to the total sales of this drug being prescribed for cats. The proportion of human drugs used in the analgesics/anaesthetics group was also high in some species (Figure 48.3). Most of this drug use is phenylbutazone tablets where veterinarians seem to prefer the synonyms licensed for human use. Phenylbutazone is not licensed at all for use in cattle, due to problems with residues[3], and yet it was used in cattle to some extent. The use of drugs from this group in veterinary clinics was dominated by the use of human anaesthetics.

Dermatological agents had a widespread use in animals. All species received between a third and a half of their use in this group as human specialities (Figure 48.4). Commonly used preparations were corticosteroids in different combinations.

Respiratory drugs (Figure 48.5) only licensed for humans, mainly bronchodilators, were used to some extent in dogs and in horses. Dogs were also treated with different kinds of cough mixtures.

CONCLUSIONS
The market for animal drugs in Sweden is very small. Consequently, it is not economically feasible for drug companies to keep a large variety of drugs licensed for veterinary use only. Registration and marketing of veterinary drugs entail fees and costs for maintaining information that in many cases would exceed the earnings. Thus there is a definite need to use human drugs, particularly in small animal practice. Many drugs used are substances with a fairly good documentation in veterinary medicine but many "new" drugs are also used, particularly in species for which the documentation of effects and kinetics is still not reliable. This is especially true in drug treatment of dogs.

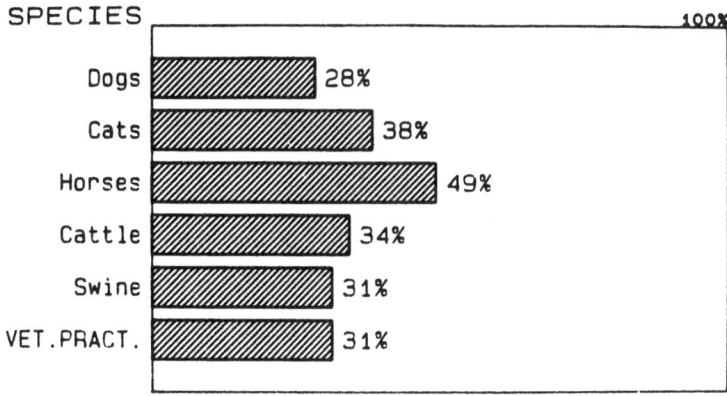

Figure 48.4   Dermatological agents : human drugs as a proportion of   the total prescribing of dermatological drugs
for each species and for use in veterinary clinics.

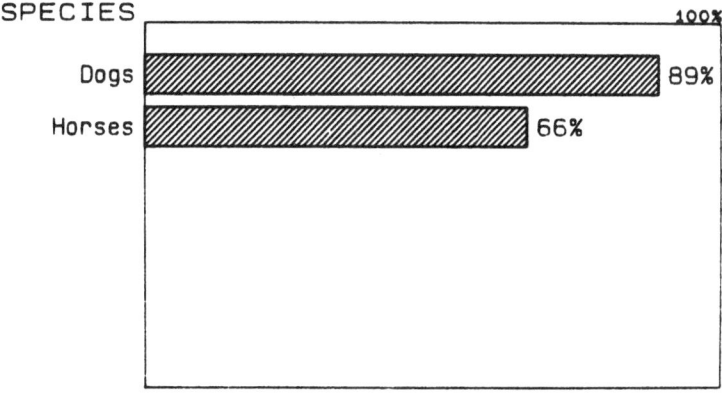

Figure 48.5   Respiratory drugs : human drugs as a proportion of the total prescribing of respiratory drugs for
each species and for use in veterinary clinics.

    In some cases, notably penicillins and phenylbutazone,
veterinarians prefer to prescribe human synonyms rather
than their veterinary equivalents. This phenomenon seems
to be partly the result of manufacturer preference; for
example, a manufacturer with a good reputation in the
veterinary market also gets a certain amount of their

human drugs used in animal therapy in spite of the fact
that unlicensed promoting is prohibited. Apart from the
above-mentioned reasons, the most important factors in
choosing human drugs seem to be the more suitable
formulations and strengths for use in small animal
medicine.

In conclusion, there is a widespread use of human drugs
in veterinary practice today. A wide variety of human
drugs are tried in therapy and quite a few are also widely
used.

The results of this study have been used as a guidance
for analysis of residues in meats and in malfunctioning
fermentation processes[2]. They may also be used by
manufacturers and licensing boards in determining which
drugs should be licensed for use in animals or, in some
cases, regulated due to their use in food-producing
animals.

References
1. Bingefors, K., Isacson, D. and Hamring, A. (1982).
   Veterinär läkemedelsförskrivning- en receptstudie.
   Copenhagen : Proc. of the 14th Nordic Veterinary
   Congress.
2. Hagelberg, M., Mathiesen, B., Sandkvist, A. and Söder-
   lind, I.-L. (1984). Effekt på biogasprocesser av vete-
   rinärmedicinska preparat. Stockholm : Royal Institute
   of Technology Report Trita-Vat-3843.
3. Martin, K., Andersson, L., Stridsberg, M., Wiese, B.
   and Appelgren, L.-E. (1984). Plasma concentration,
   mammary excretion and side-effects of phenylbutazone
   after repeated oral administration in healthy cows. J.
   Vet. Pharmacol. Ther. 7:131-138.

49
Regulation of drug usage in veterinary medicine: the situation in Germany

J. FINK

ABSTRACT

The legislative basis of drug usage in veterinary medicine is discussed following the outline of the German Medical Act. Different drug formulations and their regulations are mentioned including the procedure of drug registrations.

The historical right of veterinarians to dispense drugs and to have their own supplies, as well as the legal possibility to use drugs from human medicine in veterinary therapeutics include a high responsibility for the individual practitioner. Usage of homeopathic formulations and administration of "home made" formulations need a clear legal definition, especially when these formulations are administered to food producing animals.

The development of drug legislation is determined by increasing awareness of the risks in drug usage and the fear of undesirable effect and hazards. This is of special concern in the regulation of veterinary drug usage. Considering the specific term "drug", German drug legislation covers all subjects of both human and veterinary medicine under one Medical Act.

THE MEDICAL ACT

The "II. Medical Act" consists of different sections which should be interpreted from a veterinary point of view.

Definition of "drug"

In the first section (Table 49.1) the term "drug" is defined as a compound which is used for the treatment of diseases and disorders including substitutive and sympto-matic administration, prophylactic therapy and use for diagnostic purposes. For a precise explanation of margi-nal "therapeutic" areas, a clear demarcation with other administrative and legal fields is often used. There is interaction with other areas of German legislation for cosmetics, disinfectants and mineral water which are covered under food regulations, as well as for food additives that are regulated with the foodstuff law.

Quality and declaration of drugs

The second section of the Medical Act gives detailed information about the quality and declaration of drugs including prohibited compounds. This part also contains an obligation not to supply drugs which are sterilized by gamma-radiation. Where there is no alternative method this is only possible with special additional permission of the Ministry of Internal Affairs.

Commercial production

The third section defines commercial production. Accor-ding to this section a veterinarian or physician has to prove his participation in special pharmaceutical courses, which are not included in the regular studies. Thus, prac-tically only pharmacists have the right to supervise com-mercial drug manufacturing.

Veterinarians may only produce special formulations for their clients; quality of these formulations is defined by the regulations of the national pharmacopoeia and quantity by the needs (cfr. number of clients) of the veterinarian. Physicians are almost totally excluded from the field of

Table 49.1 Legislative definition

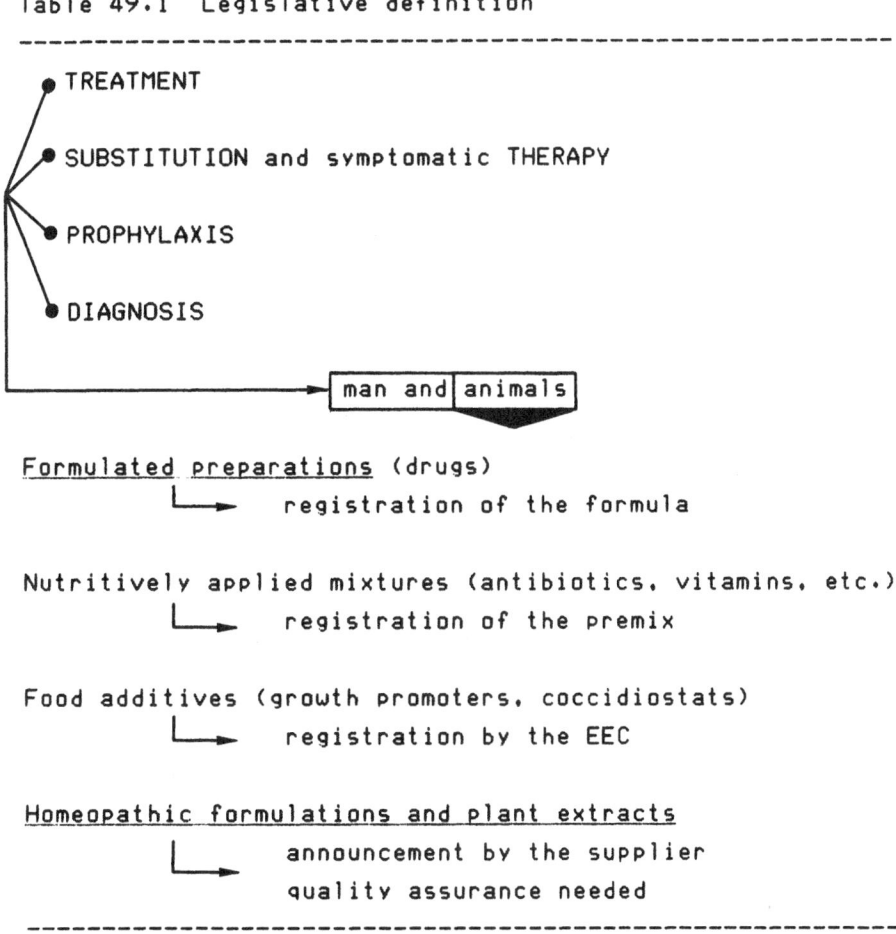

Formulated preparations (drugs)
        └──► registration of the formula

Nutritively applied mixtures (antibiotics, vitamins, etc.)
        └──► registration of the premix

Food additives (growth promoters, coccidiostats)
        └──► registration by the EEC

Homeopathic formulations and plant extracts
        └──► announcement by the supplier
             quality assurance needed

---

drug production.

Registration

The fourth section of the Medical Act deals with registration requirements. Registration of a veterinary drug
involves four dossiers : (a) the analytical dossier; (b)
the results of pharmacological and toxicological trials;
(c) efficacy and clinical data including species-specific
tolerances and interactions with other drugs; and (d)
pharmacokinetic data, residue levels in edible tissues and
the proposal of a withdrawal time based on the no-effect
level.

PROVIDING DATA FOR THE AUTHORITIES

To provide these data for the authorities, a company can include its own original investigation or provide general documentation with data available in the scientific literature, if these are reviewed by an independent expert.

In the daily practice of registration, discussions with the authorities commonly arise about questions of experience at the time of introduction of a new compound. Another crucial point is the definition of safety, including primary and secondary toxicity considerations. The determination of specific side-effects such as neurotoxicity, endocrinological effects and alterations in the immunological status are still the subject of discussion because of the need for basic research in order to understand and interpret biochemical mechanisms.

Secondary toxicity summarizes possible hazards for the consumer in correlation with the incidence and toxicity of drug residues. The FDA proposed the use of score-factors according to the frequency of drug administration, but this concept is not generally accepted. Therefore, the threshold limit is based on a no-effect level established by experiments in at least two different laboratory animal species.

PRACTICAL USE OF VETERINARIAN DRUGS

Apart from general scientific questions surrounding legislation, there is still the problem of supervising the practical usage of veterinary drugs.

For the latter, the company has to provide a precise description of a simple and reproducible analytical procedure. The task is to monitor actual drug residue levels as "routinely carried out food control" by governmental health institutes throughout the country. As this prediction is part of the latest modification of the Medical Act for public interest, only little experience is currently available on its success, but the financial burden, for laboratory equipment and staff to monitor experiments, is enormous.

HOMEOPATHIC FORMULATIONS

Official registration is also necessary for homeopathic formulations, but at a different level. Formulations have to be manufactured according to the generally accepted principles of homeopathy, laid down in a special national pharmacopoeia. Substance specific data including toxicity and safety evaluations are not generally required, which seems illogical considering the fact that, for example, food additives are administered in "homeopathic" dosages.

DELIVERY OF DRUGS

A special section of the Medical Act refers to the delivery of drugs. Distribution of drugs as "pharmacologically active compounds" is controlled by pharmacists for human drugs; but veterinarians still have the right to dispense and prescribe drugs for their clients - that is, all species of animal. They also have the right to use their own supplies, with the sole restriction of only distributing drugs for specific clients. To sell drugs to a third person is only allowed for companies granted special permission. A directive to the Medical Act gives detailed information about the practical circumstances of an individual practitioner's dispensary (Table 49.2).

PRESCRIBING DRUGS FOR ANIMALS

Within the general right to dispense and prescribe drugs, a veterinarian can also use human medicines. However, the Medical Act prohibits the use of compounds for food-producing animals; if they are not registered definitively for this species, administration of such a compound is limited to emergency cases. This is at the practitioner's own risk, the question of legal responsibility not being completely clarified. The same legal situation exists for the practitioner's own formulations prepared in his laboratory. Although he has the legal right to use his own formulations, the administration is at his own risk. This

Table 49.2 Usage of human drugs in veterinary medicine

Prescription for an individual animal
At the risk of the veterinarian
For pet animals only ???
    Withdrawal time ? 5 days

Table 49.3 Experiences and problems

"Black market" - price limits
Important quality of living animals and food
Epidemic diseases and vaccinations
Natural products and endogenous compounds
----

situation is still unsatisfying especially when one con-
siders the fact that about 15% of practitioners increasingly use their right to dispense, due to the trend
towards alternative methods in veterinary medicine.

"BLACK MARKET" DRUG USE
The tasks of the latest revision of the Medical Act
were to consider the problems of the "black-market" use of
drugs and the increasing pressures and criticisms from the
public on the question of safe and residue-free foodstuffs
of animal origin (Table 49.3). Strict limitation of drug
distribution and increasing efforts in safety regulations
were the consequence.   For a practitioner working, perhaps, in poultry production the pathway to legal drug
usage is extremely narrow, thus producing criticism about
overregulation and suppression of new developments in
animal production.

50
Do residues of antimicrobial drugs constitute a microbiological risk for the consumer?

B. VAN KLINGEREN

ABSTRACT

In relation to the veterinary use of antibiotics the question has arisen whether ingestion of residues of these agents in food of animal origin might result in a build up of resistance in the human intestinal flora.

Since direct evidence is lacking the (im)probability of this presumed effect can be estimated from the intrinsic activity of a compound and its kinetics, that is its measured or calculated concentration in the lower intestinal tract.

The relevant data are reviewed for those antimicrobial drugs that are extensively used in human and veterinary medicine. They include the penicillins, tetracyclines, sulphonamides, trimethoprim, macrolides, aminoglycosides and chloramphenicol. It is argued that the microbiological risk of residues of these drugs is negligible as compared to the risk of resistance development as a consequence of their (sub)therapeutic and prophylactic use.

INTRODUCTION

Since it is obvious that resistance to antimicrobial drugs is a real threat to human health, every use of these drugs that can induce a rise in the level or incidence of resistance has to be considered thoroughly.

527

There has been and there is still much debate going on about the main causes of resistance development. There is a broad consensus now that resistance in human pathogens is in the first place caused by the therapeutic and prophylactic use of antibiotics in humans, and resistance in animal pathogens by the veterinary use, not only in therapeutic and prophylactic dosages but also by subtherapeutic low level feeding for growth promotion[11,18].

It is widely known that, in particular, the selection of R-plasmids in Enterobacteriaceae constitutes a major hazard, although the importance of a veterinary build up of an R-plasmid reservoir for human health is far from clear.

Within the framework of our subject we have to confine ourselves to the question : "Do residues of antimicrobial drugs in food of animal origin constitute a microbiological risk for the consumer ?".

Recently this topic has also been discussed during a joint FAO/WHO Expert Consultation on residues of veterinary drugs in foods (Rome, 1984). Quoting from the report of that meeting[12] :

"The principal question is whether the ingestion of residues of antimicrobial agents via food of animal origin poses a danger to human health either
(a) by exerting a selective pressure on the intestinal
    flora and thus favouring the growth of microorganisms
    with natural or acquired resistance; or
(b) by giving rise, directly or indirectly, to the deve-
    lopment of acquired resistance in pathogenic enteric
    bacteria.
The Consultation was not aware of any relevant studies which have been performed with food which contained residues of antimicrobial agents, hence no direct answer can be given to either question".

Because of this lack of direct information one has to

approach the matter indirectly and find arguments to convince the community that the presumed risk does or does not exist.

WHERE AND HOW COULD RESIDUES ACT UPON BACTERIA

A basic principle must be that in order to exert a selective pressure a residue should have at least some bacterial growth inhibiting effect.

It is obvious that the only candidate for antimicrobial attack by residues is the human gut flora. Theoretically one could argue that also the bacterial microflora of the oral cavity will come in contact with residues but the short time of exposure makes any selective pressure highly improbable if not impossible.

Subsequently we have to define how residues of antimicrobials could possibly influence the intestinal flora in human beings in a negative way. The following possibilities can be distinguished :

(1) selective pressure on Enterobacteriaceae, in particu-
    lar E. coli;
(2) impairment of the colonization resistance;
(3) promotion of R-plasmid transfer.

IN VITRO ACTIVITY OF RESIDUES

A well-known parameter for quantifying antibacterial activity is the MIC, defined as the lowest concentration at which no growth at all is visible in liquid or on agar media after appropriate incubation. It is widely recognized, however, that bacterial growth is already influenced (retarded) by sub-MIC concentrations. For instance Greenwood[5] showed that the growth rate of E. coli under the influence of chloramphenicol gradually decreases at increasing subinhibitory concentrations; with gentamicin a sub-MIC concentration-dependent delay of growth was observed. The lowest concentration at which any effect could be observed in vitro amounted to 1/16 of the MIC. Approximately the same value can be found in the proceedings of a symposium on the effects of subinhibitory concentrations of antibiotics on bacteria during the 10th International Congress of Chemotherapy in 1977[3]. Another parameter is the so called MAC (minimum antibacterial concentration) introduced by Lorian[10] who studied subinhibitory effects in great detail. The MAC is the lowest concentration of an antibacterial agent that will affect bacterial structure, the growth rate or both.

For beta-lactam antibiotics and aminoglycosides MIC/MAC ratios were usually found to be between 10 and 20, in other words concentrations of 1/10 to 1/20 of the MIC can be expected to exert a selective pressure in vitro. This has been confirmed more directly by Lebek and Egger[9]. These authors followed the growth of a tetracycline-susceptible E. coli strain and a clone of the same strain harbouring a tetracycline-resistant plasmid in a continuously growing mixed culture in a chemostat in the presence of varying subinhibitory concentrations of tetracycline. They found that concentrations as low as 1/10 of the MIC exerted a selective pressure on the susceptible strain resulting in overgrowth of the resistant clone. Therefore they suggested replacement of zero tolerances in food to levels equal to half of the minimal selection concentrations (MSC).

IN VIVO ACTIVITY OF RESIDUES

The question, of course, is whether this MSC-approach is relevant in the in vivo situation. It might be an oversimplification leading to tolerances that, although more realistic than zero tolerances, are lower than necessary. In the first place food of animal origin will be diluted within the total mass of food and water ingested. In total diet studies carried out in the Netherlands the mean daily food and water intake was found to be approximately 2.5 kg (losing 80% at drying). Assuming that the daily amount of meat and meat products is approximately 250 g it follows that residues will be diluted 10-fold in vivo. Moreover, many antimicrobial drugs will undergo chemical or bioinactivation or will be absorbed during their passage through the intestinal tract. So presumably the concentration of residues in the large intestine, where the influence (if any) on the microflora will take place, will be substantially lower than the residual level in the food of animal origin.

Other factors decreasing the risk of selective pressure of antibiotic residues in vivo are the interaction between the different organisms within the gut's ecosystem resulting in lower growth rates than under optimal in vitro circumstances, and the fact that exposure to residues will be pulsed so that a selective pressure, if any, will be significantly lower than under continuous in vitro exposure.

Nevertheless, it is quite understandable that attempts have been made to study the selective potential of food containing low levels of antibiotics under in vivo circumstances. In 1961, Goldberg et al.[4] studied the influence of long-term feeding of oxytetracycline in human volunteers. Daily dosages of 10 mg were given calculated to result in 5-10 ppm of their total diet. In half of the individuals an increase of oxytetracycline-resistant coliforms was observed. However, the discriminative power of studies in men is rather poor due to great natural fluctuations in the human gut flora. Studies by Rollins et al.[13] with beagle dogs showed a selective pressure of food containing 10 ppm oxytetracycline but not with food containing 2 ppm. The latter concentration is approximately the MIC for susceptible E. coli.

Recently, Corpet[2] has proposed an animal model using germ-free mice inoculated with a donor intestinal microflora, for instance human gut flora. As shown by Hazenberg et al.[7] this microflora will be stable for weeks in mice. In this model the selective pressure on Enterobacteriaceae, in particular E. coli, can be studied in mice drinking water ad libitum containing antibiotics in varying concentrations. In this model, water with 20 ppm of chlortetracycline was found to promote the prevalence of tetracycline-resistant E. coli. However, the question is whether this model is representative for the human in vivo situation. For instance, metabolism in mice differs from metabolism in men and the exposure via drinking water is closer to continuous exposure than to intermittent exposure.

To quote Corpet : "Due to species differences other than the flora, i.e. drug absorption or the enterohepatic cycle, direct extrapolation to animals or humans should not be considered".

Earlier the possibility of impairment of colonization resistance (CR), that is by interfering with the anaerobic intestinal bacteria which outnumber the coliform organisms by a factor of 100-1000, was mentioned. From studies carried out by van der Waay and others[16] it follows that for such an effect high therapeutic dosages of particular antibiotics are needed. It is evident that the local antibiotic concentrations in the lower gut that will induce CR impairment will never be obtained through ingestion of residues in food.

A third possibility of negative interference of antimicrobial residues in the lower intestinal tract might be the promotion of R-plasmid transfer. The author is not aware of published evidence for this. On the contrary, as early as 1965 Guinée[6] concluded from experiments with mice inoculated with multiresistant Salmonellae and fed on a diet containing tetracycline, streptomycin or chloram-phenicol: "There is no evidence that the frequency of resistance transfer itself is influenced by administration of antibiotics".

ANTIMICROBIAL DRUGS : RESIDUES AND TOLERANCES
It can be argued that primarily, or only, those antibiotics in veterinary practice that are also widely used in the treatment or prophylaxis of infectious diseases in humans will be of importance. However, one has to face the possibility that other agents might select for R-plasmids, encoding for combined resistance to

unrelated compounds.

The main compounds in veterinary and human use are penicillins, tetracyclines, sulphonamides, trimethoprim, macrolides, aminoglycosides and chloramphenicol. As recommended by the World Health Organization[17], low level feeding of virtually all of these compounds is prohibited in many European countries. Residue tolerances for most of the antibiotics have been established by several countries. Some relevant Dutch and American FDA values are shown in Table 50.1 together with the usual MIC values for E. coli.

Penicillins

The tolerance for penicillins is very low on immunological grounds (allergy). The MICs for Enterobacteriaceae are at least 50 times higher. Moreover, significant inactivation or absorption will take place before residual amounts reach the lower intestine. It is therefore very unlikely that these levels will do any microbiological harm.

Chloramphenicol

For chloramphenicol a zero tolerance has been established in many countries since even low doses may induce aplastic anaemia in susceptible individuals. One might expect that real tolerances of this drug will be fixed at ppb levels and thus will be well below antimicrobial concentrations.

Macrolides

Among the macrolides, tylosin is used extensively in veterinary practice, either therapeutically or as a growth promoter. It is not used in human therapy. Macrolides are not active against Enterobacteriaceae and most other gram-negative bacteria. Subinhibitory concentrations were found not to induce resistance in staphylococci and streptococci. Hence, it is very unlikely and there is no evidence that the use of tylosin will compromise human therapy[8,14]. The same argument is valid for the related antibiotic virginiamycin, which is only used as a feed

Table 50.1 Tolerances of antibiotics in muscle tissue
(μg/g)

Substance	Dutch Public Health Council	FDA	MIC (μg/ml) for E. coli
Penicillins	0.005	zero-0.05	2-R
Tetracyclines	zero	1	0.5-4
Chloramphenicol	zero	?	2-8
Neomycin	0.25 M	0.25	1-2
Erythromycin	0.03 M	0.1	R
Tylosin	0.03 M	0.2	R
Sulphonamides	1 M	0.1 (2?)	4-16
Trimethoprim	0.025 M	?	0.5-2

M = microbiological motives
R = resistant : > 64

additive.

Aminoglycosides

Aminoglycosides such as neomycin, kanamycin and gentamicin
are not, or only poorly, absorbed when given by the oral
route. Parenteral use in food-producing animals should be
restricted on toxicological and immunological grounds.
The present tolerance for neomycin (0.25 μg/g) is
approximately one-quarter of the MIC for E. coli.

So the discussion about a microbiological risk of
antimicrobial residues can mainly be reduced to an
evaluation of the risk involved with the use of a very
limited number of drugs widely used in animals as well as
in humans. They are the tetracyclines, the sulphonamides
and trimethoprim.

Tetracyclines

The present tolerance of tetracyclines in several European
countries is zero. In the United States a level of 1 ppm

is accepted. It follows from the literature that the probability of exposure to a residue of tetracyclines greater than 1 µg/g in meat is very low. In a USDA monitoring programme among 5300 animal tissue samples only 23 were found with tetracycline residues between 0.01 and 1 µg/g and only five with levels more than 1 µg/g[15]. Moreover, one has to realize that tetracyclines are unstable to the temperatures usually obtained in preparing food. Nevertheless, incidental exposure to food containing 1 or 2 µg/g tetracycline (only obtainable with therapeutic dosages) might occur. As discussed earlier, it is very unlikely that this will lead to any selective pressure in the lower gut.

Sulphonamides

The present FDA tolerance of 0.1 ppm is 10-fold lower than the level permitted in the Netherlands. However, in 1978 the American Food Safety and Inspection Service found more than 10% of pigs being slaughtered for human consumption with higher residue levels[1]. From current toxicological studies it is anticipated that the tolerance may be increased to 2 µg/g. The question is whether regular ingestion of food with 1 or 2 ppm sulphonamides will exert a selective pressure upon the intestinal flora. One should realize that this level is approximately the lower level of the MIC-range of susceptible E. coli. If present in the lower intestinal tract this concentration could possibly promote the growth of less susceptible bacteria. However, sulphonamides are absorbed in the upper intestinal tract; this makes, together with the dilution factor, a build-up of antimicrobial concentrations in the colon unlikely.

Trimethoprim

Trimethoprim (TMP) is usually given in combination with a sulphonamide, although monotherapy in humans is becoming more popular, in particular for the prophylaxis and treatment of lower urinary tract infections. Information on residues of TMP is lacking, but from the kinetics of this compound one can expect that immediately after treatment muscle tissue levels will not exceed 1 µg/g. This level is approximately the MIC for E. coli. However, in the presence of 1 µg/ml of a sulphonamide only 0.05 µg/ml TMP is sufficient to inhibit E. coli in vitro. For this reason a relatively low tolerance (0.025 µg/g) has been established by the Dutch Public Health Council. The most popular TMP/sulphonamide combination in human therapy is co-trimoxazole (TMP + sulphamethoxazole). It is frequently used for selective decontamination of immuno-compromised patients. High therapeutic dosages do not impair the colonization resistance[16].

CONCLUSION

From an assessment of the available information, the conclusion seems to be justified that the microbiological risk of eating food containing low levels of residues of antimicrobial substances is negligible as compared to the risk of resistance development as a consequence of the (sub)therapeutic and prophylactic use of these drugs.

There is indeed in vitro evidence that concentrations as low as 1/10 or 1/20 of the MIC might elicit some selective pressure but the extrapolation to tolerances of the same level is an unjustified simplification. The proposed animal model of Corpet[2] to study the influence of residues in germ-free mice inoculated with human gut flora is an interesting one from an academic point of view, but the results are, as with the in vitro information, hard to extrapolate to the conditions of real life.

As a consequence, establishing tolerances on microbiological grounds is a rather arbitrary exercise. One might choose a quarter or even 1/20 of the usual MIC for E. coli, but there is no evidence that even the daily ingestion of meat and meat products containing anti-microbials at MIC level will do any harm from a microbio-logical point of view.

With this in mind, and provided there are no

toxicological objections, it should be possible to establish realistic and safe tolerances that can be measured reliably and cheaply in routine control laboratories.

References
1. Bevill, R.F. (1984). Sulfonamides. In: CRC Handbook Series in Zoonoses, Section D: Antibiotics, Sulfon-amides, and Public Health, Vol. 1, pp.355-365. Boca Raton, Florida: CRC Press, Inc.
2. Corpet, D.E. (1984). The effect of bambermycin, car-badox, chlortetracycline and olaquindox on antibiotic resistance in intestinal coliforms : a new animal model. Ann. Microbiol. (Inst. Pasteur) 135A:329-339.
3. Effects of subinhibitory concentrations of antibiotics on bacteria (1978). In: Current Chemotherapy, pp. 72-78. Proc. of the 10th Intern. Congr. Chemother., Zurich, 1977.
4. Goldberg, H.S., Goodman, R.N., Logue, J.T. and Hand-ler, F.P. (1961). Long-term, low-level antibiotics and the emergence of antibiotic-resistant bacteria in human volunteers. Antimicrob. Agents Chemother.: 80-87.
5. Greenwood, D. (1981). In vitro veritas ? Antimicro-bial susceptibility tests and their clinical rele-vance. J. Inf. Dis. 144:380-385.
6. Guinée, P.A.M. (1965). Transfer of multiple drug resistance from Escherichia coli to Salmonella typhimurium in the mouse intestine. Antonie van Leeuwenhoek 31:314-322.
7. Hazenberg, M.P., Bakker, M. and Verschoor-Burggraaf, A. (1981). Effects of the human intestinal flora on germ-free mice. J. Appl. Bacteriol. 50:95.
8. Knothe, H. (1977). Medical implications of macrolides resistance and its relationship to the use of tylosin in animal feeds. Infection 5:137-139.
9. Lebek, G. and Egger, R. (1983). R-selection of sub-bacteriostatic tetracycline concentrations. Zbl. Bakt. Hyg. I. Abt. Orig. A. 255:340-345.
10. Lorian, V. (1985). Low concentrations of antibiotics. J. Antimicrob. Chemother. 15, Suppl. A:15-16.
11. National Academy of Sciences (1980). The effects on human health of sub-therapeutic use of antimicrobials in animal feeds. Washington DC: Report of the National Research Council.
12. Residues of veterinary drugs in food (1984). Report of a joint FAO/WHO Expert Consultation, Rome 29 October to 5 November 1984.
13. Rollins, R.D., Gaines, S.A., Pocurull, D.W. and Mer-cer, H.D. (1975). Animal model for determining the no-effect level of an antimicrobial drug on drug resistance in the lactose fermenting enteric flora. Antimicrob. Agents Chemother. 7:661-665.
14. Ten years on from Swann (1981). Proceedings of a sym-

posium organized by the Association of Veterinarians in Industry: London.

15. Timoney, J.F. The tetracyclines. In: CRC Handbook Series in Zoonoses, Section D: Antibiotics, Sulfonamides, and Public Health, Vol. 1, pp.267-279. Boca Raton, Florida: CRC Press, Inc.

16. Van der Waay, D. and Verhoef, J. (ed. 1979). New criteria for antimicrobial therapy: maintenance of digestive tract colonization resistance. Amsterdam, Oxford: Excerpta Medica.

17. World Health Organization (1974). The public health aspects of antibiotics in foodstuffs. Report of a Working Group, Bremen, 1-5 October 1973. Copenhagen: WHO Regional Office for Europe.

18. World Health Organization (1981). Antimicrobial resistance. Report of a Scientific Working Group, Geneva, 23-27 November 1981.

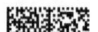